Basic Histopathology

This book is dedicated to the memory of

Paul Richard Wheater

Born 28th December 1951
Died 7th September 1989

A lost friend

Basic Histopathology

A COLOUR ATLAS AND TEXT

The late Paul Wheater
BA Hons (York), B Med Sci Hons (Nott), BM BS (Nott)

George Burkitt
BDSc Hons (Queensland), MB BChir (Cantab), MMed Sci (Nott), FRACDS

Medical Author, General Medical Practitioner, Newcastle, New South Wales, Australia

Alan Stevens
MB BS (Lon) FRCPath

Senior Lecturer in Pathology, University of Nottingham Medical School
Honorary Consultant Pathologist, Trent Regional Health Authority (T), UK

James Lowe
B Med Sci Hons (Nott), BM BS (Nott), MRCPath

Senior Lecturer in Neuropathology, University of Nottingham Medical School
Honorary Consultant Pathologist, Trent Regional Health Authority (T), UK

SECOND EDITION

CHURCHILL LIVINGSTONE
EDINBURGH LONDON MADRID MELBOURNE NEW YORK AND TOKYO 1991

CHURCHILL LIVINGSTONE
Medical Division of Longman Group UK Limited

Distributed in the United States of America by Churchill
Livingstone Inc., 650 Avenue of the Americas, New York, 10011
and by associated companies, branches and representatives
throughout the world.

First edition 1985
Second edition 1991
   Reprinted 1992

ISBN 0-443-04237-3

British Library Cataloguing in Publication Data
A catalogue record for this book is available from the British
Library.

Library of Congress Cataloging in Publication Data
Basic histopathology: a colour atlas and text / Paul Wheater
. . . [et al.]. – 2nd ed.
      p. cm.
   Includes index.
   1. Histology, Pathological – Atlases. I. Wheater, Paul R.
   [DNLM: 1. Histology – atlases.
   2. Pathology – atlases. QZ 17
B311]
RB33.B26 1991
611'.018 – dc20
DNLM/DLC
for Library of Congress

Publisher	Timothy Horne
Project Editor	Jim Killgore
Production	I Macaulay Hunter
Designer	Design Resources Unit
Sales Promotion Executive	Hilary Brown

Produced by Longman Group (FE) Ltd
Printed in Hong Kong

The
publisher's
policy is to use
**paper manufactured
from sustainable forests**

Preface to the second edition

In preparing this second edition we invited the comments of medical students and teachers of pathology who were familiar with the first edition. As a result of their helpful suggestions we have maintained the original format, with instructional text being largely in the form of expanded captions to colour photomicrographs, but have also attempted to improve the presentation of unavoidable blocks of text by the incorporation of lists, flow diagrams and simple line diagrams where relevant. We have also rearranged the introductory text in each chapter so that it is closely followed by appropriate illustrations. By using the new technology of 'desk-top publishing' it has been possible to fine-tune the text and layout while increasing the size of both running text and captions which we hope will make the book less of a strain to read.

We have, of course, up-dated the text, particularly the chapters on amyloid and disorders of the lymphoreticular, male reproductive and nervous systems, but have resisted the temptation to convert this into a comprehensive textbook of pathology.

We have taken the opportunity to add a number of new micrographs and to improve upon a number of others which failed our expectations once committed to the printed page. At the same time we have tried to keep the price within the bounds of the limited budget of the majority of medical students.

The preparation of the second edition was clouded by the tragic illness and death of one of the authorship team, Paul Wheater, at the early age of 37. His skills as a photomicrographer, and his humour and enthusiasm will be sadly missed.

Nottingham UK and Newcastle Australia, 1990

P.R.W.
H.G.B.
A.S.
J.L.

Preface to the first edition

Histopathology is an essential component of pathology teaching in all medical and dental courses, nevertheless the scope, content and emphasis on microscopy vary considerably between different centres. Adding to this diversity are the different stages in the preclinical and/or clinical years when the subject matter is presented. This book has been designed to meet as closely as possible the requirements of these many differing courses. We believe that practical microscopy is an important part of pathology teaching, and therefore we have chosen to centre our discussion around appropriate colour photomicrographs as might be done in the lecture room or microscope laboratory. The text has been designed as a series of amplified captions explaining not only the features visible in the labelled colour plates, but also providing some background text in order to relate the subject matter to the theoretical and clinical implications of the pathological processes. Consequently this book should not be regarded as a copiously illustrated introductory textbook of pathology, but rather it is intended as a histopathology companion to any of the many excellent standard pathology textbooks; the text, though more than normally found in an atlas, is thus by no means comprehensive.

The subject matter has been divided into two sections, the first covering basic pathological processes and the second encompassing the common diseases encountered in systems pathology. In general, our material has been taken from both surgical and necropsy specimens of common clinical conditions. Uncommon conditions have been included only where they illustrate important pathological principles. The haematoxylin and eosin staining method has mainly been employed as is standard practice in pathology laboratories, but special staining methods have been occasionally used where appropriate. Rather than specifying numerical magnification factors, each micrograph has been designated as low power, medium power or high power by the abbreviations LP, MP and HP respectively as this is probably more relevant to student needs.

It is our hope that this book will be useful both as a guide in formal practical classes, as well as assisting the student in private study. Although the book is primarily aimed at preclinical and clinical medical and dental students, it would also prove useful for other groups such as veterinary science students, medical laboratory scientists specialising in histopathology, and candidates for post-graduate examinations in surgery and pathology.

Nottingham, 1985

P.R.W.
H.G.B.
A.S.
J.L.

Acknowledgements

In a book such as this, the illustrations which finally appear represent only a minute fragment of the photographs taken and of the vast number of microscope slides which have been prepared for review and selection prior to photography. Our biggest debt of gratitude, therefore, is owed to Janet Palmer and Anne and Ian Wilson who, between them, skilfully sectioned an enormous number of paraffin blocks, often at many levels, staining the sections with a number of different haematoxylin and eosin schedules, to meet our frequently inordinate demands. Their skill, industry and patience have played an important part in the successful outcome of this enterprise. Mr. Stan Terras developed and printed the electron micrographs, and Jane Watson prepared the resin sections of bone.

We are most grateful to our many colleagues who helped us by providing suitable material from their own collections: in particular Professors Ian Dawson and D. R. Turner, Dr Peter James, Dr Alasdair Mackay, Dr Peter Smith, University Hospital, Nottingham; Dr David Howell of Derby Royal Infirmary; Dr Roy Reeve, Dr Jane Johnson, Professor Roger Cotton, Professor Stephen Jones of the City Hospital, Nottingham; Dr George Hall kindly gave us access to a personal index file of outstanding material and to the paraffin block stores at the General Hospital, Nottingham.

The text (with its many revisions) was originally typed by Christine Stevens and Isabella Streeter, to whom we would like to express our thanks. The second edition and its revisions was transcribed onto an Apple Macintosh by Linda Dewdney to whom we are especially grateful. All the colour illustrations were photographed by the authors using a Leitz vario-orthomat photomicroscope.

The text and layout for this book were performed by the authors using Apple Macintosh computers and QuarkXpress®. We would like to thank the staff at Churchill Livingstone who considerably rearranged production methods to allow us to create the second edition in this way.

P.R.W.
H.G.B.
A.S.
J.L.

Contents

PART 1

BASIC PATHOLOGICAL PROCESSES

1. Cellular responses to injury

Introduction

The constantly changing cellular environment demands a considerable degree of cellular adaptability. Most of these adaptations are at a biochemical level and represent fine regulation of metabolic function, however many adaptations are also accompanied by structural changes visible microscopically. Many such structural changes fall within the normal pattern of growth of a tissue; for example the thyroid gland enlarges in pregnancy due to the stimulus of thyroid stimulating hormone on thyroid epithelial cells. This is an example of *physiological cellular adaptation,* the stimulus for such a cellular change being part of the accepted normal physiological range. In contrast, certain environmental changes lie outside an acceptable range of normality and may then be termed *pathological stimuli*. Cells may respond to such pathological stimuli by extending their normal physiological adaptive processes. These broadly fall into three categories: *increased cellular activity*, *decreased cellular activity* or *alteration of cell morphology*.

The names given to describe the processes of cellular adaptive response are summarised in Figure 1.1 with examples overleaf. These are discussed in further detail in Chapter 5. The key feature of these cellular adaptive mechanisms is that cells and tissues become modified such that their function is suited to new demands placed upon them. Inability to adapt successfully to environmental change, and the structural consequences of such a failure, are the central themes of this chapter.

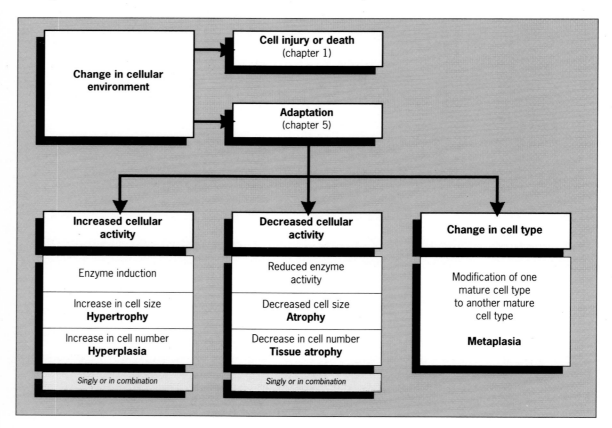

Fig. 1.1   Cellular adaptation

Examples of cellular adaptation to tolerable environmental change (see Chapter 5)

- In an athlete, skeletal muscle fibres increase in size in response to exercise and increased metabolic demands (*physiological hypertrophy*).

- When the aortic valve outlet is narrowed due to disease, cardiac muscle fibres increase in size in response to increased demands (*pathological hypertrophy*).

- Under the influence of endocrine stimulation in pregnancy, breast epithelial cells increase in size and number (*physiological hyperplasia*).

- Under the influence of abnormal endocrine stimulation from an oestrogen-secreting ovarian tumour, endometrial epithelial cells increase in number (*pathological hyperplasia*).

- With reduced activity of old age, skeletal muscle fibres decrease in size (*physiological atrophy*).

- After trauma to a supplying nerve root, skeletal muscle fibres are markedly reduced in size following loss of innervation (*pathological atrophy*).

- In the ageing parathyroid gland, hormone-secreting cells diminish in number with replacement by fat cells, the gland retaining its normal size (*functional organ atrophy*).

- In response to cigarette smoking, respiratory epithelium differentiates into stratified squamous epithelium in the bronchi (*metaplasia*).

Failure of cellular adaptation

Cells which are intrinsically unable to adapt, or which are approaching the limits of adaptability (Fig. 1.2), exhibit a variety of characteristic morphological changes at first seen ultrastructurally (Fig. 1.3) and later as easily visible light microscopic abnormalities.

Cells which have failed to adapt to metabolic stress, e.g. hypoxia, cease to produce structural proteins and begin to have difficulties supplying energy to preserve electrolyte gradients and sustain other membrane functions. Light microscopical examination of such failing cells typically shows fluid accumulation in cells which makes them pale-staining or vacuolated, giving rise to the widely used descriptive terms *cloudy swelling* or *hydropic degeneration* (Fig. 1.4). In special conditions, certain cell types respond to metabolic stress by failing to metabolise fatty acids, and thus accumulate lipid within cytoplasmic vacuoles, giving rise to the descriptive term *fatty change* (Fig. 1.5). Such early structural manifestations of cell failure are potentially reversible if the causative metabolic stress is removed or abates.

If a cell recovers from a metabolic stress then damaged proteins and organelles are removed through autophagy via the lysosomal system, new structural components being synthesised. In contrast, if the injury is irreversible there is progressive failure of key structural and metabolic components of the cell leading to death of the cell. This is termed *necrosis* and has several characteristic morphological features (Figs. 1.6 & 1.7). If a metabolic stress is severe, then there is not the progressive deterioration in function as described above but rather there is rapid cell death with the development of immediate structural features of necrosis.

In addition to the forms of cellular damage discussed above, certain harmful stimuli modify cellular responses to factors which control rate of growth and maturation. Such cells may grow in an uncoordinated manner and fail to reach a fully mature state, a phenomenon termed *dysplasia*. Other stimuli may cause irreversible changes to genetic material causing uncontrolled cell proliferation; this process is termed *neoplasia,* resulting in the formation of benign or malignant tumours. These changes in the patterns of cell growth are considered in detail in Chapters 5 and 6.

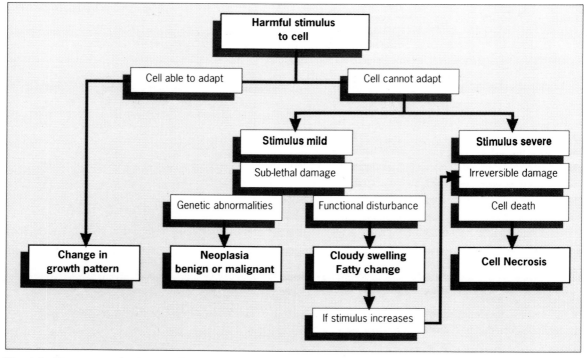

Fig. 1.2   Response of cells to injury

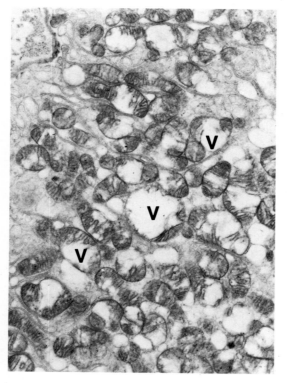

Fig. 1.3   Early cellular responses to injury (EM)

The first ultrastructural evidence of sub-lethal cell damage is swelling of membrane-bound organelles, particularly endoplasmic reticulum and mitochondria.

In this electron micrograph of a renal tubular epithelial cell damaged by hypoxia, most of the mitochondria are swollen. Instead of regular stacks of cristae (inner mitochondrial membrane) several of the mitochondria now contain spaces or vacuoles **V** pushing the cristae apart. This is probably due to accumulation of electrolytes and water due to early damage to the enzymes of the membrane sodium pump. This change is potentially reversible if the noxious stimulus is insufficient to cause cell death. Further insult leads to destruction of the cristae and more severe swelling of the mitochondria. At this stage the changes are probably not reversible and cell death occurs when ATP production is insufficient to maintain other cellular functions.

Another manifestation of early cell injury is loss of ribosomes, particularly those attached to the rough endoplasmic reticulum (not illustrated here). Lethal injury is marked by progressive disintegration of other organelles, particularly lysosomes which release hydrolytic enzymes causing auto-digestion of the cell (*autolysis*).

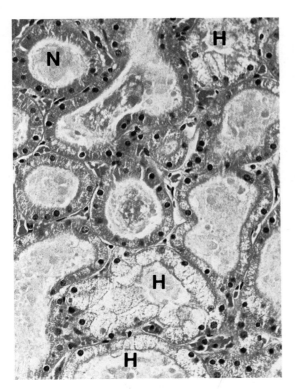

Fig. 1.4 Hydropic degeneration: kidney (HP)

The earliest light microscopic evidence of cellular injury is loss of normal staining intensity of the cytoplasm due to swelling of membrane-bound organelles. The normal cytoplasm stained with haematoxylin and eosin is light pink with a faint tint of blue; the blue tint (basophilia) is mainly due to the presence of ribosomal RNA. With sub-lethal cellular damage, ribosomes are reduced in number and the normal blue cytoplasmic tint is lost. Swelling of endoplasmic reticulum and mitochondria contribute to further cytoplasmic pallor. This is described as *cloudy swelling*. With further swelling of organelles, the cell becomes waterlogged and true vacuoles appear in the cytoplasm, which now stains faintly with total loss of basophilia. At this stage, cells are said to exhibit *hydropic degeneration*.

This micrograph shows a section of kidney deprived of blood flow due to severe hypotension. Undamaged tubules are seen lined by normal staining epithelial cells **N**. Some of the tubules are damaged, the cells being pale and vacuolated and exhibiting hydropic degeneration **H**. Such damage to the renal tubules may lead to acute renal failure.

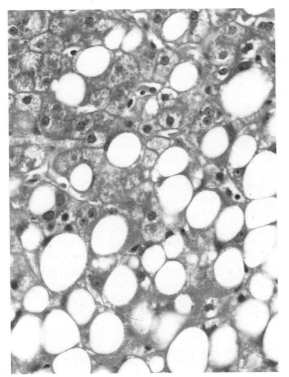

Fig. 1.5 Fatty change: liver (HP)

Fatty change is a manifestation of sub-lethal metabolic derangement seen in certain cell types with high energy demand. It is usually seen in liver, as in this example, but also occurs in the myocardium and the kidney. The common causes of fatty change are toxins (particularly alcohol and halogenated hydrocarbons such as chloroform), chronic hypoxia and diabetes mellitus. Impaired metabolism of fatty acids leads to accumulation of triglycerides (fat) which form vacuoles in cells.

This example of liver from an alcoholic shows large vacuoles in the hepatocytes. In conventionally processed tissue, organic solvents used in preparation dissolve out the fat to leave an empty, non-staining hole. Specialised frozen sections can however be prepared to preserve the fat which can then be specifically stained.

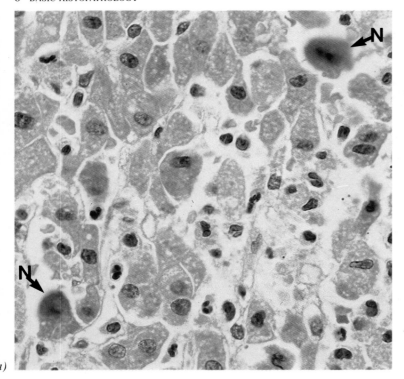

(a)

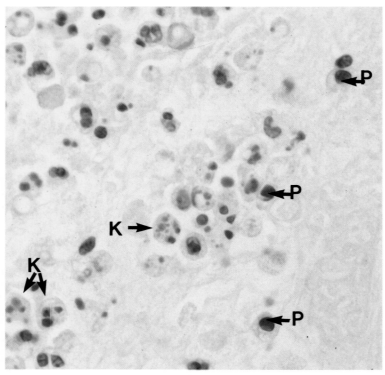

(b)

Fig. 1.6 Cell necrosis
(a) liver (HP)
(b) renal cortex (HP)

When a cell has sustained irreversible damage, a succession of histological changes occur which are grouped under the term *necrosis*.

Micrograph (a) is a section of liver from a person poisoned by paracetamol, an hepatic toxin. Many of the hepatocytes are pale stained and a few exhibit early vacuolation indicative of sub-lethal injury. Several cells also show histological features of necrosis **N**. The dead cells stain brightly pink (eosinophilic) and stand out from the other cells, due to the degeneration of structural proteins which form a compact homogeneous mass. Compared to living cells, the nucleus of each necrotic cell is smaller, condensed, and intensely stained with haematoxylin (basophilic). This condensed nuclear appearance is termed *pyknosis* and is the end result of changes which cause the chromatin to become progressively clumped, possibly due to reduced pH resulting from terminal anaerobic metabolism.

Further changes in the appearance of the nucleus of dead cells are seen in micrograph (b), which is a portion of necrotic kidney. Pyknotic nuclei **P** stand out as intensely basophilic (purple), round bodies.

With further degeneration, the pyknotic nuclei become fragmented into several minute particles which represent pieces of degenerate nuclear material, a change termed *karyorrhexis*. In the micrograph, several karyorrhectic nuclei **K** can be identified.

Complete breakdown of nuclear material then takes place by release of cellular hydrolytic enzymes, leading to loss of the groups which bind haematoxylin, a process termed *karyolysis*. When karyolysis is complete, the dead cell is seen as an anucleate and eosinophilic homogeneous mass.

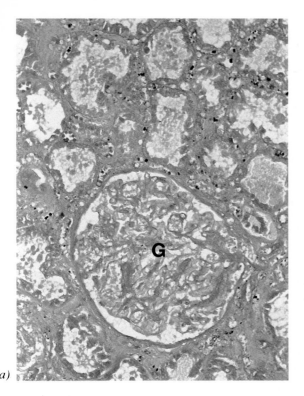

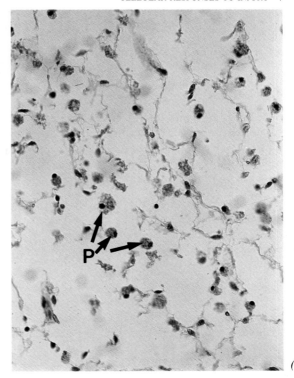

(a)   (b)

Fig. 1.7 Patterns of tissue necrosis
(a) coagulative necrosis: kidney (MP)   **(b) colliquative necrosis: brain** (HP)

Traditionally, three main patterns of tissue necrosis are described: coagulative, colliquative and caseous. Each term attempts to portray the macroscopic appearance of necrotic tissue. In coagulative necrosis, tissue appears firm as if cooked; in colliquative necrosis, the dead tissue appears semi-liquid; while in caseous necrosis, the dead tissue has a soft consistency reminiscent of cream-cheese. These gross patterns correlate closely with histological appearances.

In areas of coagulative necrosis, much of the cellular outline and tissue architecture can be discerned histologically even though the tissue components are dead. The commonest cause of such a pattern of necrosis is ischaemia due to occlusion of the arterial supply to a tissue.

In areas of caseous necrosis, cells die and form an amorphous proteinaceous mass in which no semblance of original architecture can be discerned. Such a pattern is invariably associated with tuberculosis.

The term colliquative necrosis was originally used to describe the macroscopic appearance of necrosis in the brain as a result of arterial occlusion (cerebral infarction), at a stage when the dead area was replaced by semi-liquid material. This appearance, however, is not a specific form of necrosis but results from dissolution of tissue after an initial phase of coagulative-like necrosis. Increased

knowledge of the changes occurring in dead tissues indicates that a coagulative-like phase of necrosis exists in all tissues, cell organisation and outline being initially preserved following cell death. The liquefaction of dead tissue is a function of both tissue composition and aetiology of the necrosis. In brain, the relative lack of extracellular structural proteins (reticulin and collagen) leads to rapid loss of tissue architecture as autolysis occurs, resulting in the early formation of a semi-liquid mass of dead cells. Otherwise, liquefaction of dead tissues is virtually confined to cases of necrosis associated with pyogenic bacteria such as in an abscess (Fig. 2.13).

Micrograph (a) is an example of coagulative necrosis in an area of kidney subject to infarction. Note that the architecture of a glomerulus **G** and surrounding tubules is still recognisable despite the fact that there is virtually no nuclear staining except for a few pyknotic and karyorrhectic remnants.

Micrograph (b) illustrates the phase of liquefaction in a cerebral infarct; the earlier phase of coagulative necrosis in brain can be seen in Figure 22.5 (a). No residual tissue architecture is preserved. The necrotic brain is now largely replaced by wisps of pink-staining cellular debris, with phagocytic cells **P** engulfing degenerate material.

Examples of caseous necrosis can be seen in tuberculous lesions in Chapter 3 (Figs. 3.6-3.17).

2. Acute inflammation, healing and repair

Introduction

When cells are damaged by any harmful stimulus, a sequence of responses is triggered in the surrounding tissue termed *acute inflammation*. This is a relatively non-specific but almost universal initial response which attempts to neutralise the damaging agent and restore injured tissue to useful function. The injured area becomes flooded with fluid, plasma proteins and neutrophil leucocytes emanating from local blood vessels.

The development of this *acute inflammatory exudate* involves three main phenomena:

- **vascular dilatation** leading to engorgement of tissue with blood (*hyperaemia*)
- **increased capillary permeability** enabling plasma proteins to pass into tissues
- **neutrophil migration** from the blood into the area of injured tissue.

Acute inflammation occurs in response to tissue damage by virtually every harmful agent; it is an energy dependent process and each component is carefully controlled by inter-dependent chemical mediators.

The stages in the evolution of acute inflammation leading to the formation of an acute inflammatory exudate are illustrated in Figures 2.2 and 2.3, and an example of a disease where acute inflammation is the main feature is illustrated by lobar pneumonia (Fig. 2.4).

Mediators of acute inflammation

The events of acute inflammation are mediated by a number of factors derived from the injured tissue, leucocytes, plasma and microorganisms summarised below in Figure 2.1. The vascular phenomena and certain of the mediators are responsible for the clinical features of acute inflammation known as the *cardinal signs of Celsus*:

- **redness** (*rubor*) due to hyperaemia
- **swelling** (*tumor*) due to fluid exudation and hyperaemia
- **heat** (*calor*) due to hyperaemia
- **pain** (*dolor*) resulting from release of bradykinin and PGE_2
- **loss of function** (*functio laesa*) due the combined effects of the above.

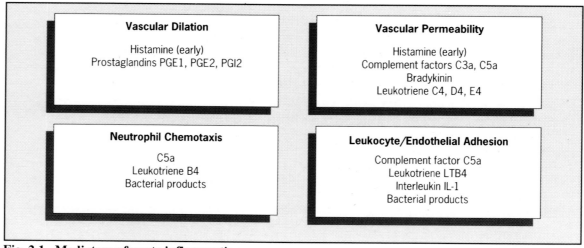

Vascular Dilation

Histamine (early)
Prostaglandins PGE1, PGE2, PGI2

Vascular Permeability

Histamine (early)
Complement factors C3a, C5a
Bradykinin
Leukotriene C4, D4, E4

Neutrophil Chemotaxis

C5a
Leukotriene B4
Bacterial products

Leukocyte/Endothelial Adhesion

Complement factor C5a
Leukotriene LTB4
Interleukin IL-1
Bacterial products

Fig. 2.1 Mediators of acute inflammation

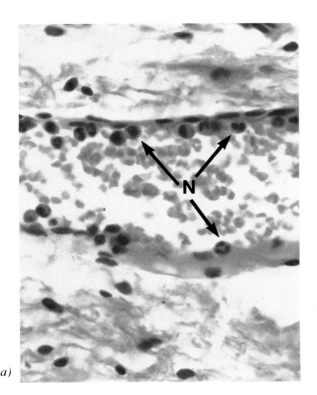

(a)

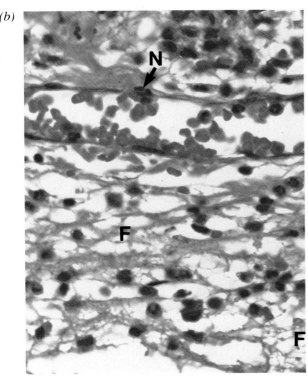

(b)

Fig. 2.2   Exudate in acute inflammation
(a) early vascular changes (HP)
(b) early formation of exudate (HP)

Shortly after tissue damage, chemical mediators cause capillaries and post-capillary venules to become dilated and blood flow within them slows. Other mediators cause increase in the permeability of the vessel walls such that there is leakage of plasma into surrounding tissues producing localised swelling *(oedema)*. The plasma fluid dilutes the injurious agents and helps to drain them away in the lymph. Plasma-derived immunoglobulins and complement help to neutralise microorganisms, attract leucocytes (chemotaxis) and promote phagocytosis (opsonisation). Neutrophils move to the periphery of the blood vessels and become adherent to the endothelium; this process is termed *margination* and is well illustrated in micrograph (a). Note that in addition to marginated neutrophils **N**, there is separation of perivascular connective tissue due to fluid exudate between collagen and cells.

Within tissues, the blood coagulation protein, fibrinogen, is converted to insoluble fibrin; this forms an interwoven meshwork of fine strands which stain bright pink on H&E staining. This is seen in micrograph (b) where fibrin strands **F** surround a dilated vessel; the fibrin may act as a physical barrier to limit invasion by microorganisms in some circumstances. As this is occurring, chemotactic agents, released from damaged tissues and plasma, cause active migration of neutrophils from the vessel lumen into the tissues *(emigration)*. In micrograph (b), a neutrophil **N** can be seen in the process of passing through the vessel wall. Once outside the vessels, neutrophils migrate to the area of tissue damage where they play an important role in phagocytosis and bacterial killing. At a later stage they are followed by monocytes and some lymphocytes.

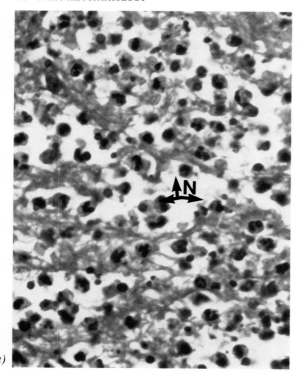

(a)

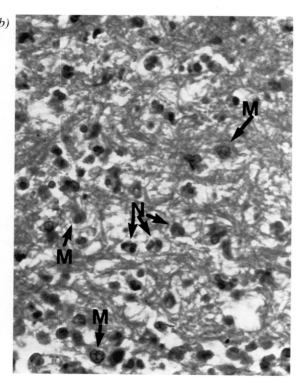

(b)

Fig. 2.3   Acute inflammatory exudate
(a) highly fluid exudate (HP)
(b) highly fibrinous exudate (HP)

The quality of an acute inflammatory exudate varies depending on the state and nature of the injured tissue and the type of noxious agent involved. These two micrographs show established acute inflammatory exudates differing from one another in the number of neutrophils **N** and amount of fibrin present; pink-staining fibrin is a much more prominent feature of micrograph (b) compared to micrograph (a).

Once in the extravascular tissues, neutrophils engulf necrotic fragments of damaged tissue, breaking them down with their lysosomal enzymes. When tissue damage has been caused by bacteria, as in lobar pneumonia (Fig. 2.4), neutrophils phagocytose and kill the causative organisms. The activity of neutrophils is limited by their inability to regenerate lysosomal enzymes, and after a burst of phagocytosis the neutrophils degenerate. Numbers of neutrophils are maintained in acute inflammation by new arrivals from the circulation, the systemic response to acute inflammation being release of neutrophils from bone marrow into the blood, resulting in a neutrophil leukocytosis. Degenerate neutrophils can be recognised by condensation (pyknosis) and fragmentation (karyorrhexis) of the nuclei and, eventually, cytoplasmic disintegration; this is best seen in micrograph (b).

Although the dominant cell type in acute inflammation is the neutrophil, small numbers of macrophages also participate, entering the damaged tissue as blood derived monocytes. Macrophages **M**, a few of which can be seen in micrograph (b), continue the phagocytic work begun by neutrophils and ultimately mop up the degenerate neutrophils and fibrin strands. Unlike neutrophils, macrophages can regenerate their lysosomal enzymes and are capable of sustained activity. The monocytes may also act as antigen presenting cells to facilitate immunological responses.

The fate of the acute inflammatory exudate depends on a variety of factors including the nature and destructibility of the injurious agent, the extent of tissue damage and the properties of the tissue in which the damage has occurred.

The process of acute inflammation terminates by one of four main processes: resolution, organisation and repair, abscess formation or chronic inflammation (described on p. 15).

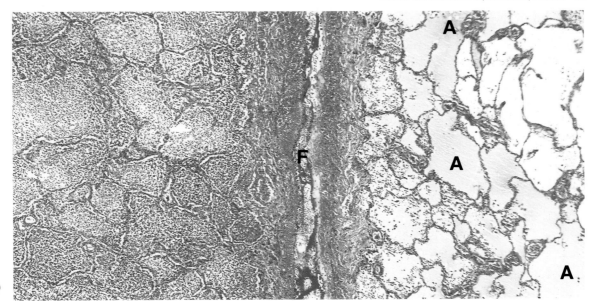

(a)

(b)

Fig. 2.4 Acute inflammation of lung: lobar pneumonia **(a)** (MP) **(b)** (HP)

A common cause of acute inflammation in the lung parenchyma is bacterial infection causing lobar pneumonia. In this case a whole lobe becomes solidified due to a massive outpouring of fluid, fibrin and neutrophils into the alveolar spaces. This pattern of pneumonia is most commonly caused by the pneumococcus *(Streptococcus pneumoniae)*.

In micrograph (a), a portion of lung is shown with an interlobar fissure **F** running vertically. The lung tissue on the left shows obliteration of alveolar spaces by purple-staining masses of inflammatory cells (mainly neutrophils) with associated fibrin; this is termed *consolidation*. Alveolar walls can just be discerned. The dense inflammatory exudate is sharply limited by the interlobar fissure. The lung on the right of the fissure shows the earliest changes of acute inflammation, with faint pink-staining serous exudate in alveoli **A** and the earliest phase of neutrophil emigration giving rise to a few scattered cells within alveolar spaces.

At higher magnification in micrograph (b), alveolar wall capillaries **C** are seen engorged with blood. The alveolar spaces are obliterated by an acute inflammatory exudate rich in neutrophils and lesser amounts of wispy pink-stained fibrin. Occasional large, rounded mononuclear cells, macrophages **M**, can also be seen, but these are few in the acute phase of the disease.

If untreated, there are three main outcomes to lobar pneumonia. Death may occur (as in this patient), there may be complete resolution (Fig. 2.9), or the exudate may become organised with consequent permanent fibrosis of the lung tissue.

Clinical nomenclature of acute inflammatory processes

The nomenclature used to describe inflammation in different tissues employs the tissue name (or its Greek or Latin equivalent) and the suffix "*-itis*", for example acute inflammation of the appendix is referred to as acute appendicitis, acute inflammation of the fallopian tube is termed acute salpingitis, and acute inflammation of the pericardium is termed acute pericarditis. While this holds true for most tissues and organs there are notable exceptions in traditional clinical usage. For example, acute inflammation of the pleura is usually termed acute pleurisy, while acute inflammation of subcutaneous tissues as a result of infection is usually termed acute cellulitis. Many examples of acute inflammatory diseases are presented in the systems pathology chapters which form the second half of this book. In addition, the nomenclature applied to common forms of acute inflammation is presented in Figure 2.5; the causes given in this table only illustrate some of the factors which may initiate each type of acute inflammatory response.

Fig. 2.5   Nomenclature and aetiology of common types of acute inflammation

Tissue	Acute inflammation	Typical causes
Meninges	Acute meningitis	Bacterial and viral infections
Brain	Acute encephalitis	Viral infections
Lung	Acute pneumonia	Bacterial infection
Pleura	Acute pleurisy	Bacterial and viral infections
Pericardium	Acute pericarditis	Bacterial and viral infections, myocardial infarction
Oesophagus	Acute oesophagitis	Gastric acid reflux, fungal infection
Stomach	Acute gastritis	Alcohol abuse
Colon	Acute colitis	Bacterial infection, 'ulcerative colitis'
Rectum	Acute proctitis	'Ulcerative colitis'
Appendix	Acute appendicitis	Faecal obstruction, bacterial infection
Liver	Acute hepatitis	Alcohol abuse, viral infections
Gallbladder	Acute cholecystitis	Bacterial infection
Pancreas	Acute pancreatitis	Pancreatic enzyme release
Urinary bladder	Acute cystitis	Bacterial infections
Bone	Acute osteomyelitis	Bacterial infections
Subcutaneous tissues	Acute cellulitis	Bacterial infections
Skin	Sunburn	UV radiation
Joints	Acute arthritis	Bacterial and viral infections, autoimmune reactions
Arteries	Acute arteritis	Autoimmune reactions

Morphological types of acute inflammation

While the basic process of acute inflammation is the same in all tissues, there are frequently qualitative differences in the inflammatory response seen under different circumstances. Terms describing these variations are widely used in clinical practice and are summarised below:

- **Suppurative inflammation (purulent inflammation)** refers to acute inflammation in which the acute inflammatory exudate is particularly rich in neutrophil leucocytes. Suppurative inflammation is most commonly seen as a result of infection by bacteria where the mixture of neutrophils (viable and dead), necrotic tissue, and tissue fluid in the acute inflammatory exudate form a semi-liquid material referred to as *pus,* from which is derived the term *purulent inflammation.* This is illustrated in Figure 2.6. Within tissues, a circumscribed collection of semi-liquid pus is termed an *abscess.*

  Bacteria which produce purulent inflammation are described as *pyogenic bacteria.* They initiate massive neutrophilic infiltration with subsequent destruction of infected tissues. Pyogenic bacteria include *Staphylococci,* some *Streptococci (S. pyogenes, S. pneumoniae), Escherichia coli* and the *Neisseriae (meningococci* and *gonococci).*

- **Fibrinous inflammation** refers to a pattern of acute inflammation where the acute inflammatory exudate has a high plasma protein content. Fibrinogen derived from plasma is converted to fibrin which is deposited in tissues. This pattern is particularly associated with membrane-lined cavities such as the pleura, pericardium, and peritoneum where the fibrin strands form a mat-like sheet causing adhesion between adjacent surfaces. This is illustrated in Figure 2.7.

- **Serous inflammation** describes a pattern of acute inflammation where the main tissue response is an outpouring of fluid with a low plasma protein and cell content. This pattern of response is most commonly seen in the skin in response to a burn.

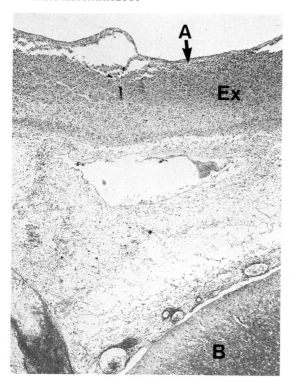

Fig. 2.6 Purulent inflammation: acute meningitis (LP)

Acute inflammation in the meninges surrounding the brain illustrates an example of an exudate in which very little fibrin is formed. In acute meningitis, the exudate is almost entirely composed of oedema fluid and neutrophils.

Acute meningitis is almost invariably caused by bacterial infection, for example *Neisseria meningitidis* or *Streptococcus pneumoniae*. The presence of pathogenic bacteria in the meninges excites an acute inflammatory exudate in the sub-arachnoid space, in which neutrophils predominate. Macroscopically, this appears as a creamy thick fluid, and the term acute purulent inflammation is often used to describe such a reaction.

In the micrograph, note the densely cellular exudate **Ex** lying between brain **B** and arachnoid **A**. A purulent exudate such as this appears blue stained because of the great cellular content (neutrophils); contrast this with the pink-staining fibrin-rich exudate shown in Figure 2.7 below.

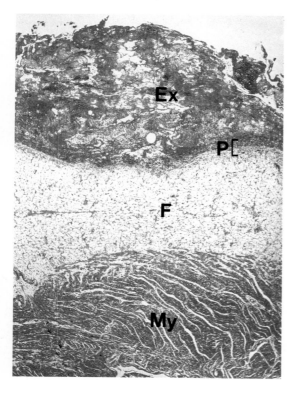

Fig. 2.7 Fibrinous inflammation: acute pericarditis (LP)

When an acute inflammatory exudate forms on a serosal surface, the exudate is usually dominated by the presence of large amounts of fibrin. Macroscopically, a shaggy layer of fibrin coats the formerly smooth surface. This is seen in acute pericarditis (as shown here) and also in acute pleurisy and acute peritonitis.

In this photomicrograph taken at low magnification, the exudate **Ex** is well established on the epicardial aspect of the pericardium **P**. At the bottom of the illustration is the myocardium **My,** and in the centre is the epicardial fat **F**. Acute pericarditis most commonly occurs secondary to death of underlying cardiac muscle (myocardial infarction). The acute inflammatory exudate is made up of dense masses of pink-staining fibrin with comparatively few neutrophils.

The usual fate of serosal exudates such as this is organisation via ingrowth of granulation tissue, and eventual formation of collagenous scar tissue binding adjacent serosal surfaces together. If this process occurs in the peritoneal cavity, then bowel loops can be obstructed by these fibrous adhesions.

Outcomes of acute inflammation

The process of acute inflammation is designed to neutralise injurious agents and to restore the tissue to useful function. There are three main outcomes of acute inflammation:

- Exudate is resorbed and tissue returns to normal, a process termed *resolution*.
- The damaged area and associated exudate are removed by phagocytic cells, and the defect is repaired by ingrowth of vascular and later fibrous tissue, processes termed *organisation* and *repair*.
- The damaging agent cannot be eliminated and the processes of organisation and repair take place concurrently often with continued tissue damage. This protracted process is termed *chronic inflammation* and is the subject of Chapter 3.

Three factors determine which of these outcomes occurs:

- the severity of tissue damage
- the capacity of specialised cells within the damaged tissue to replicate and re-grow, a process termed *regeneration*
- the type of agent which has caused the tissue damage.

Resolution involves complete restitution of normal architecture and function. This can only occur if the tissue damage has been slight and the tissue involved has the capacity to make good any loss of specialised cells (regeneration). Examples of resolution are recovery from sunburn (acute inflammatory response in the skin as a result of ultra-violet radiation exposure) and the restitution of normal lung structure and function following lobar pneumonia (see Fig. 2.9).

Regeneration of tissues can play an important part in resolution, for example re-growth of alveolar lining cells following pneumonia. Another example of regeneration is seen in the peripheral nervous system where axonal processes can re-grow following damage. This function depends on viability of the cell body of the neurone and is an example of regeneration of one part of a cell, not the formation of new cells.

Healing by repair occurs when tissue has been completely destroyed and lacks the ability to regenerate specialised cells. In these instances, dead tissues and acute inflammatory exudate are first removed from the damaged area by phagocytic cells (see Fig. 2.8), and the defect becomes filled by ingrowth of a specialised vascular connective tissue called *granulation tissue* (see Fig. 2.10). This is termed *organisation*. The granulation tissue gradually produces collagen to form a fibrous (collagenous) scar at the original site of tissue damage, constituting the process of *repair* (see Fig. 2.11). Despite the loss of some specialised cells and some architectural distortion by fibrous scar, structural integrity is re-established and function is restored. Any impairment of function is dependent on the extent of loss of specialised cells. Modified forms of repair occur in bone after a fracture when new bone is created (Fig. 2.12), and in brain with the formation of an *astrocytic scar* (Fig. 22.1).

Chronic inflammation occurs when an injurious agent persists over a prolonged period causing continued tissue destruction while at the same time acute inflammation, organisation and repair are underway. Histologically, affected tissues exhibit fibrous scarring, granulation tissue and inflammation concurrently. The qualitative characteristics of the cellular infiltrate change under these circumstances such that lymphocytes take over from neutrophils as the dominant cell participating in the inflammatory response. Chronic inflammation is discussed fully in Chapter 3.

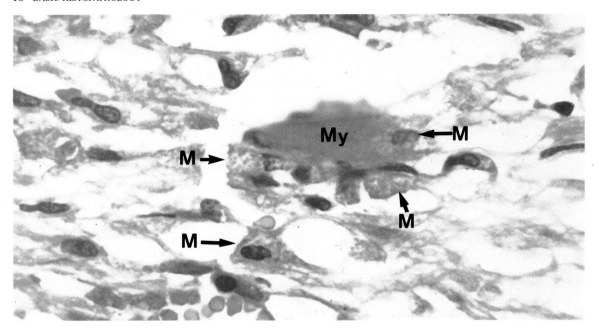

Fig. 2.8 Early outcome of acute inflammation: macrophage accumulation (HP)

Once the acute inflammatory exudate is established and the damaging agent removed or neutralised, macrophages gradually accumulate, being derived from monocytes arriving in vessels around the damaged area. Macrophages phagocytose cell debris, dead neutrophils, and fibrin. At the same time, lymphocytes begin to enter the damaged area, reflecting an immune response to any introduced antigens.

This micrograph shows an area of cardiac muscle which has undergone necrosis following cessation of its arterial supply (myocardial infarction). The acute inflammatory response has almost run its course, and the neutrophils and fibrin predominant in the earlier stages have been removed by macrophages. All that remains is a soft, loose tissue containing a few necrotic myocardial remnants **My**, one of which is shown here being engulfed by macrophages **M**. The macrophages can be identified under these circumstances by the accumulation of brownish pigmented granules in their cytoplasm which represent partly digested material in secondary lysosomes. Further details of the events following myocardial infarction are shown in Figure 9.2.

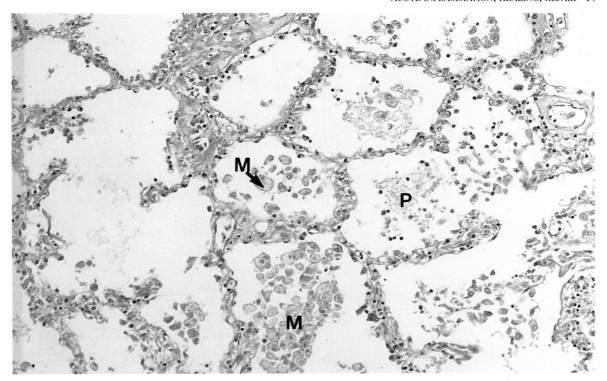

Fig. 2.9 Resolution of acute inflammation: lobar pneumonia (HP)

Occasionally, a potentially damaging stimulus may excite an acute inflammatory response even though the amount of tissue damage is minimal. In such circumstances, the process of resolution of the exudate may occur without the processes of organisation and repair thereby leaving no residual tissue scarring.

This phenomenon occurs in lobar pneumonia in which the acute inflammatory response is due to infection by a bacterium, commonly the pneumococcus (see Fig. 2.4). The alveoli of one or more lobes of the lung are filled with acute inflammatory exudate and the loss of respiratory function may be so great as to cause fatal hypoxia. This was a common cause of death in previously fit young people in the preantibiotic era.

Bacteria are engulfed by neutrophils of the inflammatory exudate, and fibrin strands are broken down by fibrinolysins derived from plasma and neutrophil lysosomes. Macrophages **M** are recruited and phagocytose necrotic neutrophils, extravasated red cells and other cell debris. Fluid and degraded proteinaceous material **P** together with the macrophages are then resorbed into the circulation via alveolar wall vessels and interstitial lymphatics or may be coughed up as brown-coloured sputum. Alveolar spaces are thus cleared of exudate and can participate in gaseous exchange. Regeneration of alveolar lining cells completes the return to normal structure and function.

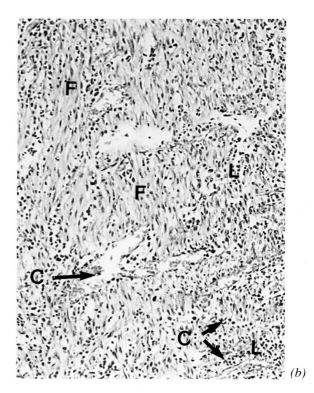

Fig. 2.10   Granulation tissue
(a) vascular granulation tissue (HP)
(b) fibrous granulation tissue (HP)

In the process of tissue repair, the former site of tissue damage and acute inflammation becomes occupied by a mixture of proliferating capillaries, fibroblasts, macrophages and lymphoid cells, termed granulation tissue.

Capillaries are derived by budding from vessels at the periphery of the damaged area and form an interconnected network **C** well shown in micrograph (a). In this early form, termed vascular granulation tissue, spaces between the capillaries are occupied by macrophages **M**, lymphocytes **L** and a few elongated spindle-shaped fibroblasts.

With time, this highly vascular pattern becomes progressively less vascular and more fibrous with migration of many of the lymphoid and macrophagic cells back into the circulation, atrophy of capillary vessels and selective proliferation of fibroblasts. The effect of this

evolution is seen in micrograph (b), where numerous plump fibroblasts **F** can be seen with a few lingering lymphoid cells **L** and relatively inconspicuous capillary vessels **C**. This is now termed fibrous granulation tissue in recognition of the predominant fibroblast population of cells.

Collagen is laid down by the fibroblasts, and the fibrous granulation tissue takes on the characteristics of an early fibrous scar as seen in Figure 2.11.

An identical form of granulation tissue is involved in healing of wounds whatever the cause and site of defect in the tissue. In the case of a simple skin incision, the wound edges may well be in apposition and the actual defect is minimal. In other situations the tissue defect will be large and filled with blood clot and a variable amount of tissue debris; in this case organisation and filling of the defect by granulation tissue take considerably longer.

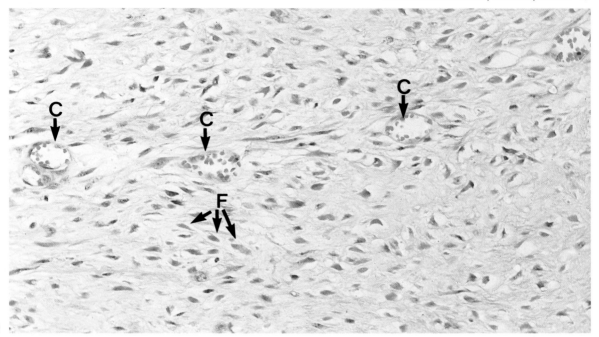

(a)

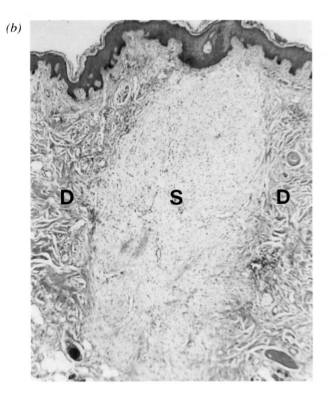

(b)

Fig. 2.11   Fibrous scar
(a) fibrous scar tissue (HP)
(b) skin scar (LP)

The deposition of collagen within fibrous granulation tissue occurs over a period of many weeks. Collagen is deposited in an appropriate orientation to withstand the tensile stresses placed on the area of repair by tissue movement and stretching. With time, the previously plump and metabolically active fibroblasts atrophy and become relatively inconspicuous as shown in micrograph (a) of a typical area of early fibrous scar. Note the condensed nuclei of inactive fibroblasts **F.** Some capillaries **C** persist accounting for the red appearance of recent scars.

Micrograph (b) illustrates at low magnification, a recent area of scarring in the skin after healing of a simple incision for biopsy of a skin tumour. Fibroblastic tissue forms a pale scar **S** which interrupts the normal pink collagen of the dermis **D** on either side. There are no skin appendages in a skin scar. During the ensuing months and years, the cellularity of the scar diminishes, there is progressive loss of capillary vessels and the scar contracts so that after many years a skin scar may be virtually undetectable macroscopically. Note that healing of skin or mucous membrane involves epithelialisation of the surface by proliferation of epithelium at the edges of the defect.

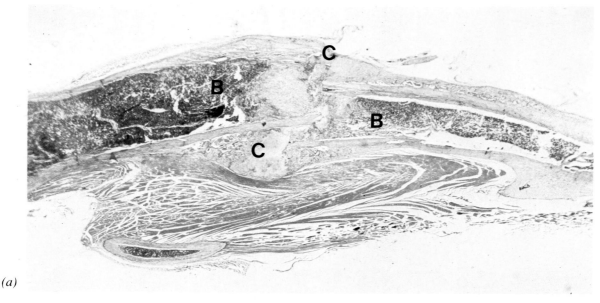

(a)

(b)

Fig. 2.12 Specialised repair: healing in bone
(a) (LP) **(b)** (HP)

In most tissues, fibrous scar forms a functionally adequate, albeit unspecialised, replacement for damaged tissues. In bone, however, the replacement of damaged tissue by fibrous scar is inadequate for restoration of function and so a specialised form of granulation tissue develops where the final product is new bone.

Following fracture there is usually bleeding in and around the fracture site resulting in a mass of coagulated blood termed a haematoma. An initial acute inflammatory response is rapidly followed by organisation of the haematoma with formation of granulation tissue in much the same way as described in Fig. 2.10. In the case of bone fracture, this granulation tissue is termed *provisional callus* **C** and forms around the ends of the bones **B** loosely uniting them; this is seen at low magnification in micrograph (a).

In contrast to normal granulation tissue, that of bone contains osteoblasts which produce osteoid, the organic matrix of bone. This is seen in micrograph (b) where typical granulation tissue **G** at the top of the field gives way to osteoblasts **O** which surround pink-staining newly formed osteoid **OS**. Osteoid then becomes mineralised to form the *bony callus* between the two fractured ends. This initial bone is haphazardly arranged and over the next few months undergoes extensive remodelling by osteoclasts and osteoblasts to form lamellar bone with trabecular architecture best suited to resist local stresses. The end result is *restitution* of normal bony architecture and function.

Fig. 2.13   Abscess formation: lung (LP)

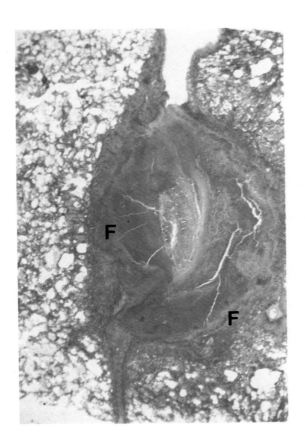

An abscess is a localised collection of pus, which usually develops following extensive tissue damage by one of the pyogenic bacteria, such as *Staphylococcus aureus*; such organisms excite an inflammatory exudate in which neutrophils predominate. In these circumstances, vast numbers of neutrophils die releasing their lysosomal enzymes and undergoing autolysis; the resulting viscous fluid, *pus*, contains dead and dying neutrophils, necrotic tissue debris and the fluid component of the acute inflammatory exudate with a little fibrin. Pyogenic bacteria often remain viable within the abscess cavity and may cause enlargement of the lesion which at this stage is described as an *acute abscess*. At an early stage, attempts are usually made to limit expansion of the lesion by the processes of organisation and repair at the margins of the abscess. Thus the abscess may become walled off, isolating the bacteria-containing pus and preventing further spread; an abscess encapsulated by granulation tissue is termed a *chronic abscess*. On the other hand, if the bacteria are highly virulent and present in large numbers, such attempts at organisation and repair may be overwhelmed, and expansion of the abscess ensues with destruction of surrounding tissue. The co-existence of active tissue damage and attempts at repair are an example of chronic inflammation (see Ch. 3).

The micrograph shows an abscess in the lung. The centre is composed of a purple-staining mass of pus. At its margin is a pink staining zone of fibrin **F**. The lung immediately adjacent shows some consolidation, but as yet there is little evidence of organisation at the margins of the abscess; this therefore represents an *acute abscess*.

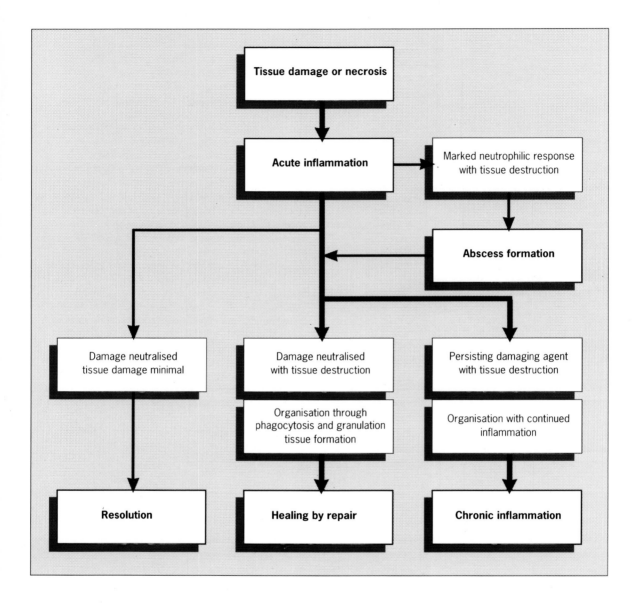

Fig. 2.14   Outcomes of acute inflammation

3. Chronic inflammation

Non-specific chronic inflammation

In the previous chapter, the sequence of events which follows an episode of tissue damage is described. The usual result of acute inflammation is organisation of the exudate and repair through the production of granulation tissue which eventually forms a fibrous scar. In most instances the agent which produced the tissue damage is destroyed or neutralised in the early stages of the acute inflammatory reaction. Sometimes, however, the damaging stimulus persists despite the presence of acute inflammation, and further tissue destruction may occur. In such circumstances, the processes of tissue damage, acute inflammation, granulation tissue formation and attempts at fibrous repair proceed concurrently instead of sequentially. The non-specific acute inflammation process then becomes supplemented by attempts to mount a specific immune response, and the damaged area comes to be infiltrated by a variety of lymphoid cells (see Fig. 3.2). This phenomenon is termed chronic inflammation.

While the histological appearances of acute inflammation are dominated by neutrophils and fibrin, the histological appearances of chronic inflammation are dominated by lymphoid cells and fibrosis. Chronic inflammation can be considered as a battle between destruction and repair. If the body defences are dominant then neutrophils are few and there is repair with shrinkage of the lesion through fibrosis; if the damaging agent dominates then there is necrosis, neutrophil infiltration and weak fibrosis limited to a small zone around the margin of an expanding lesion. This process is well illustrated by chronic ulceration of the stomach (Fig. 3.1), chronic inflammation of the bronchi (Fig. 3.3) and chronic inflammation of the colonic mucosa (Fig. 3.4).

Specific chronic inflammations

There are certain diseases in which the primary tissue response to a damaging agent involves lymphoid cells and fibrosis rather than the neutrophils and fibrin typical of the acute inflammatory response. Such damaging agents are those which are resistant to destruction by neutrophils or which fail to excite a strong acute inflammatory reaction. The commonest examples are *Mycobacteria* (the causative organism of tuberculosis and leprosy), *Treponema* (the causative organism of syphilis and yaws), certain fungi and inert foreign materials such as talc and beryllium. The tissue reactions provoked by these types of agents are collectively known as the *specific chronic inflammations,* in contrast to the term *non-specific chronic inflammation* for the case of the chronic inflammatory response which may follow acute inflammation.

Granulomatous inflammation

In some cases of specific chronic inflammation discussed above, there is a strong cytotoxic immune response (type IV hypersensitivity); this is mediated by T-lymphocytes which produce lymphokines which attract and activate macrophages. Macrophages (histiocytes) recruited in this way form clusters within the tissues which are termed *histiocytic granulomas*. Such *chronic granulomatous diseases* include tuberculosis, leprosy and sarcoidosis.

The use of the term granuloma can lead to confusion. The word granuloma was originally used to describe the mass of granulation tissue (capillaries, fibroblasts and macrophages) which forms at a site of tissue repair and is still so used by some authors. It is also still used in clinical practice to describe this type of response; for example, a dental 'apical granuloma' refers to a mass of granulation tissue at a site of non-specific chronic inflammation in association with a chronic dental abscess. Modern pathological use of the term granuloma, however, now almost exclusively refers to a tissue aggregate of histiocytic cells as part of a cell-mediated immune response.

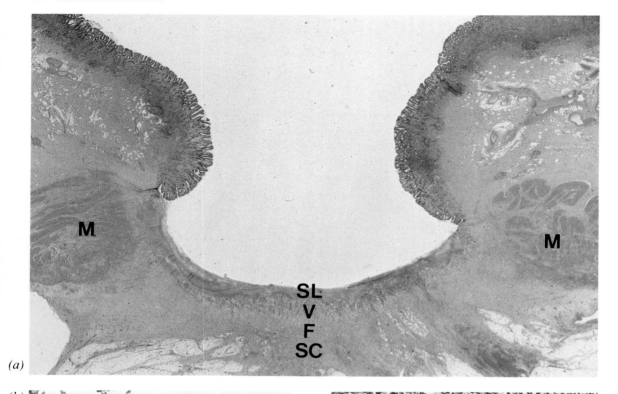

(a)

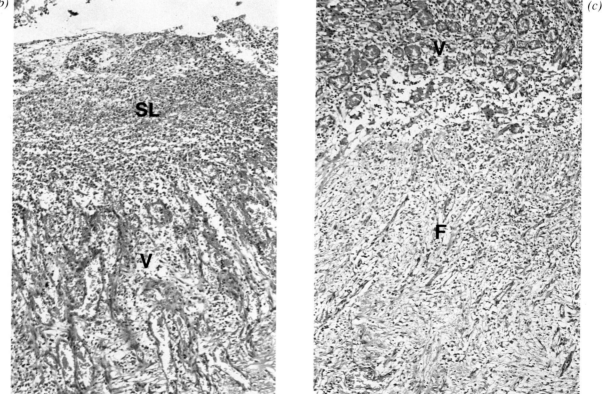

(b) *(c)*

Fig. 3.1 Chronic peptic ulcer *(caption opposite)*

Fig 3.1   Chronic peptic ulceration *(illustrations opposite)*
(a) entire ulcer (LP)   (b) surface layers of ulcer (MP)   (c) deep layers of ulcer (MP)

A common example which illustrates the principles of non-specific chronic inflammation is the localised chronic ulceration of the stomach or duodenum caused, in certain susceptible individuals, by the damaging effects of acidic gastric secretions; such lesions are collectively referred to as *chronic peptic ulcers.*

Necrosis of surface epithelium is caused by gastric acid, possibly resulting from loss of the normal protective surface mucus barrier. This allows access of irritant gastric secretions to submucosal tissues leading to the formation of an *acute ulcer*. If the process proceeds unchecked, then gastric acid can erode through the full thickness of the stomach wall leading to perforation and escape of gastric contents into the peritoneal cavity (see Fig. 12.7a). Most commonly, however, the destructive process is arrested by an acute inflammatory response which dilutes and buffers the toxic effects of gastric secretions and limits tissue damage. Tissue repair is then attempted by formation of granulation tissue; repair may be effective if conditions are favourable. Gastric acid may, however, cause continuing tissue destruction, the concurrent organisation and repair resulting in chronic inflammation. A chronic peptic ulcer reflects a dynamic balance between tissue destruction and tissue repair. If reparative responses weaken there is progression of the ulcer with the risk of perforation of the stomach wall.

A section through a chronic ulcer is shown in micrograph (a). The ulcerated surface is covered in a slough **SL** composed of a pink-staining layer of necrotic debris combined with the fibrin and neutrophils of an acute inflammatory exudate. Beneath the slough is a zone of vascular granulation tissue **V**; these features are seen at a higher magnification in micrograph (b). Beneath the layer of vascular granulation tissue is a zone of fibrous granulation tissue **F**, seen in detail in micrograph (c). Deeper still in the ulcer base, the fibrous granulation tissue becomes collagenised to form a fibrous scar **Sc**. Also in micrograph (a) note that the muscular wall **M** is completely replaced by the ulcer crater, granulation tissue and scar. A common feature of a chronic peptic ulcer is the presence of one or more large blood vessels (usually arteries) in the ulcer base; erosion of such a vessel leads to bleeding into the stomach lumen, giving rise to the classical symptoms of *haematemesis* (vomiting blood) or *melaena* (black, tar-like faeces due to the presence of altered blood).

The outcome of chronic peptic ulceration depends on whether conditions favour the damaging stimulus of the gastric acid or the reparative process of the local tissues. If healing is favoured, then fibrous tissue gradually repairs the ulcer crater and mucosa regenerates from the ulcer margins to cover the epithelial defect and protect the fibrous tissue from further damage. A healed peptic ulcer thus consists of a localised area of fibrous scarring replacing all or part of the thickness of the stomach wall. Internally, the regenerated mucosa is usually puckered due to contraction of the underlying scarred wall.

The most important single factor which favours healing of a peptic ulcer is reduction of gastric acid, for example by H2 receptor antagonist drugs or vagotomy. Factors which favour the destructive process include excessive gastric acid secretion (especially for duodenal ulceration), or reduced capacity for repair which may result from corticosteroid therapy and non-steroidal anti-inflammatory drugs.

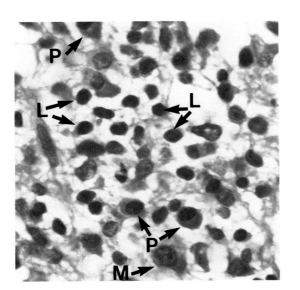

Fig. 3.2   Chronic inflammatory cells (HP)

The term chronic inflammatory cells is frequently used to indicate a cellular infiltrate composed of lymphocytes, plasma cells and macrophages. In epithelial tissues such as nasal or gastrointestinal mucosae, eosinophils are also seen.

The micrograph shows such a chronic inflammatory infiltrate at high magnification. The cells are mainly plasma cells **P** identified by their extensive basophilic cytoplasm, and small lymphocytes **L** seen as dark rounded nuclei. Macrophages **M** are smaller in number and recognisable by their much greater size. These cells reflect the immune response typical of chronic inflammation.

Populations of chronic inflammatory cells may persist in an area of previous inflammation long after the process of repair has occurred.

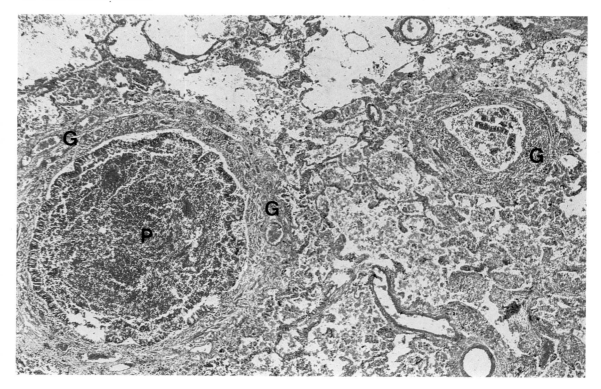

Fig. 3.3 Bronchiectasis (LP)

Bronchiectasis is a chronic inflammation of the bronchi associated with destruction of the wall and permanent dilatation.

Damage to the bronchial wall is usually the combined result of repeated episodes of infection coupled with stasis of secretions, leading to progressive destruction of the normal elastic and muscular component of the airway wall. Such damage is particularly likely to occur when airways become partially or completely obstructed. The elastic and muscular components of the bronchial wall are replaced by fibrovascular granulation tissue and later collagenous fibrous tissue. This process weakens the wall, leading to dilatation of the airway, which in turn predisposes to stagnation of secretions and further episodes of bacterial infection.

In this micrograph, two abnormal bronchi are seen with their lumina filled with pus **P**. The wall of each affected bronchus is formed of fibrovascular granulation tissue **G** in which there is a heavy infiltrate of small dark-staining cells just visible at this magnification; these cells are a mixture of plasma cells and lymphocytes.

Bronchiectasis exemplifies the concept of coexisting tissue damage and attempts at repair which are the hallmark of chronic inflammation.

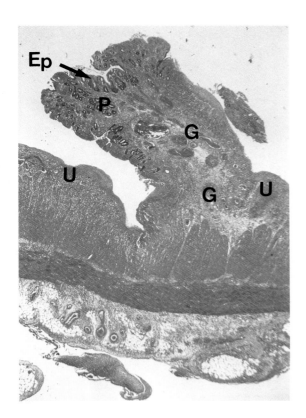

Fig. 3.4   Ulcerative colitis (LP)

Ulcerative colitis is a chronic inflammatory disorder of the colon of no known aetiology; it is characterised by phases of quiescence punctuated by acute exacerbations in which there may be extensive inflammatory destruction of the mucosa, leading to ulceration. Between acute attacks, the mucosa shows infiltration of the lamina propria by chronic inflammatory cells (Fig. 3.2). During an acute attack, confluent areas of mucosal ulceration **U** occur, leaving protruding islands of chronically inflamed mucosa and submucosa which simulate colonic polyps **P**. These so-called *pseudopolyps* bear remnants of colonic epithelium **Ep**. The submucosa becomes largely replaced by fibrovascular granulation tissue **G** with a variable chronic inflammatory cell infiltrate. This disease illustrates the balance that occurs in chronic inflammatory processes between tissue repair and active destruction. During a destructive ulcerative phase, an acute inflammatory response is the characteristic histological feature. When this subsides, the ulcerated areas may heal and the inflammatory component becomes lymphoid in nature. Ulcerative colitis is illustrated in more detail in Figure 12.13.

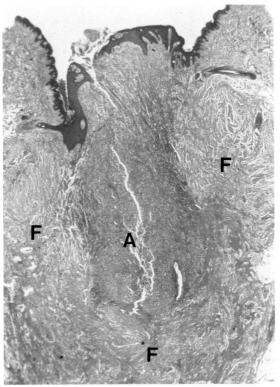

Fig. 3.5   Pilonidal sinus (LP)

A common example of a chronic abscess is the pilonidal sinus. In this condition, a chronic subcutaneous abscess forms, most commonly in the sacrococcygeal area. Hair shafts, derived from locally destroyed follicles and shed body hair, are present in the abscess and act as a focus for chronic inflammation. Successful healing and repair are hindered by the persistence of foreign material (the hairs) which is resistant to phagocytosis. Secondary infection further complicates the process. As part of the attempt at healing, epithelium migrates from the skin surface and comes to line the track leading down into the abscess cavity; such a track is known as a sinus.

In this micrograph, note the subcutaneous abscess cavity **A**, the wall of which is formed by chronic inflammatory granulation tissue heavily infiltrated by lymphocytes. There is surrounding fibrosis **F** in the dermis as a result of previous attempts at fibrous repair.

A pilonidal sinus, like any other chronic inflammatory lesion, will only heal if the source of persistent irritation is removed; surgical excision or laying open the complex of sinuses and abscess cavities is usually the only satisfactory method in this situation.

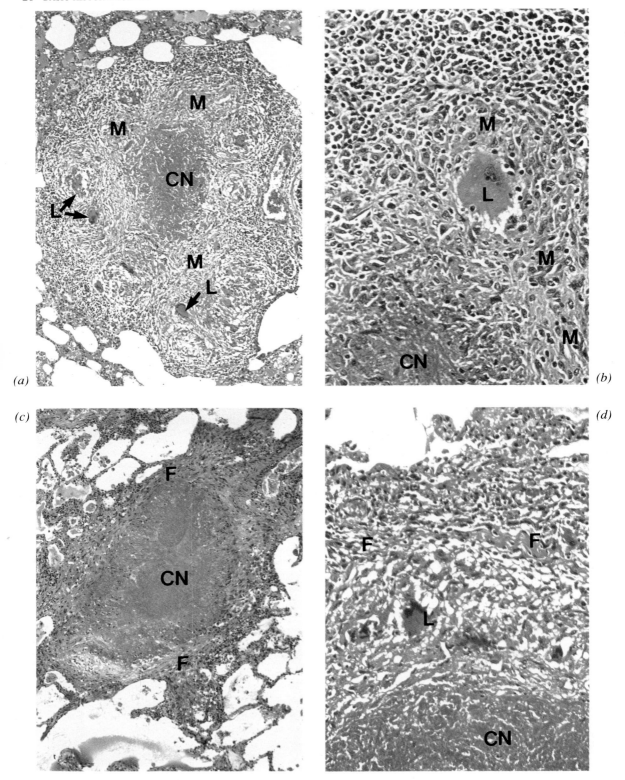

(a)

(b)

(c)

(d)

Fig. 3.6 Early pulmonary tuberculosis *(caption opposite)*

Fig. 3.6   Early pulmonary tuberculosis *(illustrations opposite)*
(a) early tubercle (MP)
(b) early tubercle (HP)
(c) later tubercle (MP)
(d) later tubercle (HP)

As described earlier, certain infecting organisms and foreign materials do not excite a full acute inflammatory reaction, but instead, almost from the outset, excite a response more typical of chronic inflammation. In this type of reaction, macrophages aggregate in the vicinity of the organisms to form a lesion traditionally called a *granuloma*. An example of this is tuberculosis, caused by the bacterium *Mycobacterium tuberculosis*; in this case the specific granuloma is known as a tubercle.

When tubercle bacilli gain access to the lungs by inhalation, they tend to localise in the periphery of the lung where they excite a transient and inconclusive neutrophil response. The organisms survive neutrophil enzyme activity, probably because of their thick and resistant glycolipid bacterial cell wall and the short life span of neutrophils. The tubercle bacilli are then ingested by macrophages where they may initially continue to divide within macrophage cytoplasm. The tubercle bacilli also antigenically stimulate some lymphocytes which thereby become 'sensitised'. The sensitised lymphocytes then produce various factors (lymphokines) which attract and 'activate' the macrophages, enhancing their ability to kill ingested tubercle bacilli. Such activated macrophages become large and develop granular eosinophilic cytoplasm; because of their supposed resemblance to epithelial cells they were formerly known as *epithelioid cells*. These cells form a major component of all granulomata including tubercles.

Micrograph (a) shows an entire tubercle at an early stage, and (b) illustrates a sector of the same tubercle at higher magnification. At the centre of the tubercle is an area of caseous necrosis **CN** containing tubercle bacilli; these can only be demonstrated by specific staining methods for acid-fast bacilli. The caseous area is surrounded by a zone of plump macrophages **M** with abundant granular eosinophilic cytoplasm (epithelioid cells). Some of the macrophages fuse to produce multinucleate giant cells called *Langhans' giant cells* **L**; a typical Langhans' giant cell is shown in more detail in Figure 3.7. Peripheral to the macrophages, aggregation of lymphocytes occurs, indication of the involvement of immune mechanisms in the granulomatous response.

Progressive central caseous necrosis results in enlargement of the tubercle; the zone of peripheral macrophages and lymphocytes becomes relatively thinner. These changes can be observed by comparing micrograph (a) with micrograph (c) which shows a more advanced tubercle. With further development, spindle-shaped fibroblasts **F** appear in the peripheral lymphocytic zone of the tubercle where they begin to lay down collagen in the extracellular tissue; this process is evident in micrograph (c) and at higher magnification in (d).

At this stage, further changes in the tubercle can occur in one of two ways. If the tubercle bacilli are virulent and present in large numbers, and particularly if the body's resistance is low (as for example in a debilitated or immunosuppressed patient), then the tubercle rapidly enlarges due to increasing caseous necrosis. The macrophage-lymphocyte-fibroblast defensive reaction is overwhelmed, failing to confine the infection; an example is seen in Figure 3.10. On the other hand, if the balance of resistance and attack is reversed, the macrophage-lymphocyte-fibroblast barrier resists enlargement of the tubercle, and proliferation of fibroblasts produces a firm shell confining the infection. Production of collagen by these fibroblasts further strengthens this capsule, imprisoning the necrotic tissue and its contained tubercle bacilli, and isolating the organisms from other susceptible tissue (see Fig. 3.8). Calcium salts may become deposited in the collagenous shell and necrotic centre. In the lung, carbon is also taken up by the macrophages of the granuloma.

In children, the initial tubercle in the lung is known as a *Ghon focus* and is usually situated in the subpleural area in the middle zone of the lung. This lesion rarely attains a large size and undergoes the process of fibrosis described above. Before the lung lesion is walled off, however, tubercle bacilli pass via lymphatics to regional lymph nodes in the lung hilum where tubercles develop in a manner identical to the Ghon focus in the lung. The outcome of the infection depends on what happens to this tuberculous infection of the hilar lymph nodes; possible outcomes are discussed in Figures 3.8 to 3.17.

In adults where previous exposure has afforded partial immunity, the pattern of infection is somewhat different. The initial lung lesion is usually located at the apex of the lung where it is known as an *Assmann focus*, and tends to enlarge and produce a cavitating abscess from whence further infection of the rest of the lungs may occur; regional lymph nodes are rarely involved. If host resistance is high, healing occurs by fibrosis in the same way as described above.

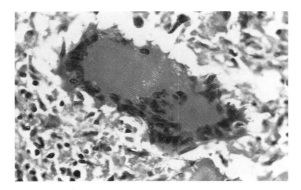

Fig. 3.7 Langhans' giant cell (HP)

This micrograph illustrates a typical Langhans' giant cell formed by fusion of macrophages in a tuberculous granuloma. A ring of peripherally arranged nuclei characteristically encircles a faintly granular eosinophilic cytoplasm.

Although prominent in tuberculosis, similar multinucleate giant cells occur in other chronic inflammatory conditions such as leprosy and in response to the presence of certain non-lysable foreign bodies. In such conditions, the nonspecific term *foreign body giant cell* is usually applied.

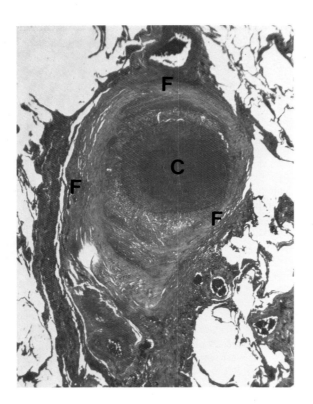

Fig. 3.8 Fibrocaseous tuberculous nodule (LP)

In favourable circumstances, healing of tubercles occurs by proliferation of peripheral fibroblasts and deposition of an encircling wall of dense collagen (see Fig. 3.6). If the healing process is initiated at an early stage of tubercle formation as frequently occurs with a Ghon focus, then all that later remains is a small fibrous nodule often heavily calcified and containing little or no central caseous material. If the healing process supervenes at a later stage in tubercle development, then the fibrous shell often surrounds a mass of caseous material. Such a structure is called a *fibrocaseous tuberculous nodule* and is most frequently seen in healed, adult-pattern pulmonary tuberculosis where such nodules are usually located at the lung apices. Viable tubercle bacilli may remain dormant within the sequestered caseous material from which they may reinfect adjacent lung tissue should the restricting fibrous wall break down. This phenomenon, known as *reactivated fibrocaseous tuberculosis*, may occur many years later when a patient becomes debilitated by age, malnutrition or immunosuppressive therapy.

The fibrocaseous nodule illustrated here was taken from the lung apex of an adult whose pulmonary tuberculosis had been successfully treated by chemotherapy. A strong fibrous wall **F** completely encircles a mass of caseous necrotic material **C**. In this case there has been little calcium deposition.

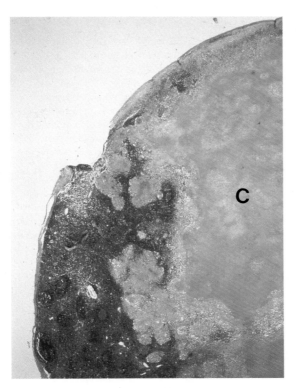

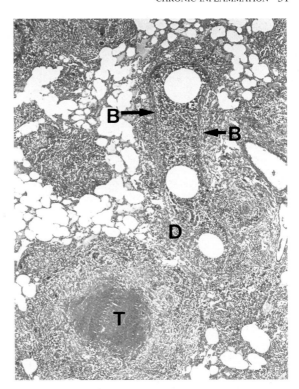

Fig. 3.9 Tuberculous lymph node (LP)

With the formation of a Ghon focus in a child's lung, tubercle bacilli may pass via lung lymphatics to regional lymph nodes where they initiate caseous necrosis and tubercle formation similar to that in the lung. The combination of a Ghon focus in the lung and tuberculous regional (peribronchial) lymph nodes is called a *primary complex.*

The outcome of infection in a child depends on the fate of the lymph node lesion. If the child's defences are strong, healing of all the tubercles occurs by fibrosis as described previously; all that remains is a small fibrocalcific nodule in the lung periphery and similar lesions in the regional lymph nodes. On the other hand, if the patient's defence mechanisms are poor, the lymph node tubercle enlarges as a result of extensive caseous necrosis, tending to overwhelm the surrounding macrophage-lymphocyte-fibroblast reactions. The lymph node enlarges until its capsule is breached, then ruptures discharging caseous material, heavily populated by tubercle bacilli, into surrounding tissues. The enlarging node may ulcerate through nearby bronchial walls (see Fig. 3.10) or blood vessels (see Fig. 3.11), leading to extensive spread of the tubercle bacilli.

In this micrograph, the tubercle has greatly enlarged so that the lymph node has almost been destroyed by caseous necrosis **C,** and the zone of cellular reaction around it is very thin and insignificant. The necrosis has almost reached the lymph node capsule; rupture is imminent.

Fig. 3.10 Tuberculous bronchopneumonia (MP)

When the wall of a bronchus is eroded by an enlarging tuberculous node or an apical Assmann focus, tubercle bacilli pass into the bronchial lumen from which they may be spread in various ways. If coughed up in sputum, the infection may be transmitted to other susceptible persons by droplet infection, sometimes infecting the patient's larynx *(tuberculous laryngitis)* on the way. Infected sputum may be swallowed and subsequently produce *tuberculous oesophagitis* or *ileitis.* Infected sputum may also gravitate to lower areas of the same or opposite lung where, by destruction of a bronchiolar wall, the organism may invade peribronchial lung tissue to form further caseating tubercles. This is called *tuberculous bronchopneumonia.*

In this example of an early lesion in tuberculous bronchopneumonia, note a segment of bronchiole containing infected material; the walls of the bronchiole are indicated by the arrows marked **B**. A segment of the bronchiolar wall has been destroyed **D**, permitting access of bacilli which have initiated a caseating tubercle **T** in the nearby lung parenchyma. Large numbers of such lesions may form, merging with one another to produce a wide area of rapidly enlarging caseation, usually in the lower lobes of the lungs. This is the pathogenesis of the once dreaded 'galloping consumption'.

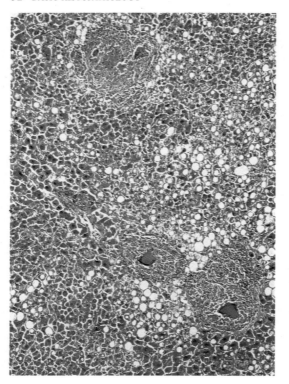

Fig. 3.11 Miliary tuberculosis (MP)

If a ruptured tuberculous lymph node (or a rapidly enlarging Assmann focus in an adult) erodes a blood vessel wall, masses of tubercle bacilli are discharged into the circulation and are carried along in the blood until they lodge in the microcirculation. When the eroded vessel is a branch of the pulmonary artery, the organisms are passed to other areas of the lung; when a pulmonary venous tributary is involved they are spread in the systemic circulation to many organs, notably the liver, kidney and spleen. In this way, vast numbers of new tubercles may be produced throughout the body. Such multiple lesions rarely attain any great size because this occurrence usually produces rapid clinical deterioration and death; because the gross appearance of individual lesions resembles millet seeds, this condition is known as *miliary tuberculosis*.

In this illustration are three miliary tubercles in the liver, recently formed as a result of blood-borne spread from pulmonary tuberculosis. The centre of two of the new tubercles is formed by a Langhans' giant cell, and the third shows early central caseous necrosis.

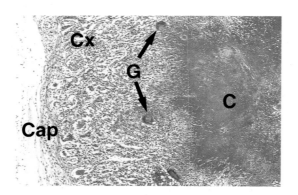

Fig. 3.12 Adrenal tuberculosis (MP)

The adrenal glands are a common site of blood-borne dissemination of tuberculosis, and bilateral caseous destruction of the adrenal cortex may be so extensive that the patient develops the clinical syndrome known as *Addison's disease* (adrenocortical insufficiency). This micrograph illustrates part of an adrenal gland in which caseous material **C** occupies most of the cortex leaving only small surviving areas of cortical tissue **Cx** beneath the capsule **Cap**. Note the Langhans' giant cells **G** which are mainly seen near the margins of the lesion.

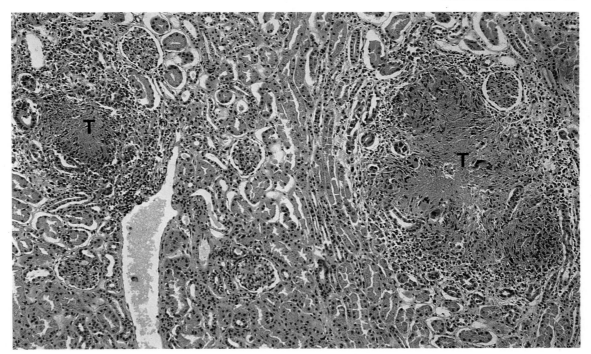

Fig. 3.13 **Renal tuberculosis** (MP)

Most episodes of pulmonary tuberculous infection are well enough contained by local and systemic defence mechanisms such that gross, blood-borne (miliary) tuberculosis is a relatively uncommon outcome. Nevertheless, it appears that a relatively small number of organisms can be disseminated by the blood stream to a variety of other organs.

For many reasons, probably including low bacterial virulence and high host resistance, most of these blood-borne bacilli are neutralised without initiating the formation of significant lesions in the organs in which they lodge. It seems that in certain tissues, some organisms remain viable but quiescent, only to become reactivated at a later date when the host's immune status is temporarily or permanently impaired; this is often long after the initial pulmonary lesion has healed. Active tuberculosis, with the formation of characteristic caseating granulomata, may then reappear in tissues remote from the original lesion and often many years later. This phenomenon is known as *metastatic* or *isolated organ tuberculosis* and most commonly involves the kidneys, adrenals, meninges, bone, Fallopian tubes, endometrium and epididymis.

This micrograph illustrates renal involvement with the formation of small tubercles **T** in the renal cortex. The granulomata exhibit the classical central caseation of tuberculosis, with larger tubercles tending to become confluent with adjacent lesions. Continuation of this process results in destruction of much of the renal cortex and medulla, with eventual rupture of large confluent tubercles into the pelvicalyceal system which becomes distended with caseous material; this condition is known *tuberculous pyonephrosis*. In more advanced cases, the infection spreads to involve the ureter and bladder. Renal tuberculosis is frequently bilateral and may result in renal failure.

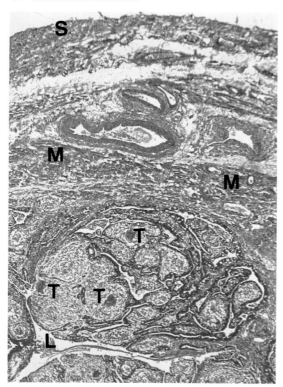

Fig. 3.14 Tuberculous salpingitis (MP)

Tuberculous involvement of the Fallopian tubes is a common complication of pulmonary tuberculosis, particularly if this is contracted during adolescence. Tuberculous granulomata **T** develop in the mucosa of the Fallopian tube, producing gross thickening of the mucosa and encroachment upon the lumen **L**; the muscular wall **M** and serosa **S** in this example are relatively uninvolved. With healing, subsequent scarring often leads to distortion of the tube and obliteration of the tubal lumen, and tubal tuberculosis is thus an important cause of female infertility in countries where tuberculosis is endemic.

Tuberculous salpingitis is frequently accompanied by involvement of the endometrium and adjacent myometrium, although tuberculous endometritis may also occur in isolation from salpingitis.

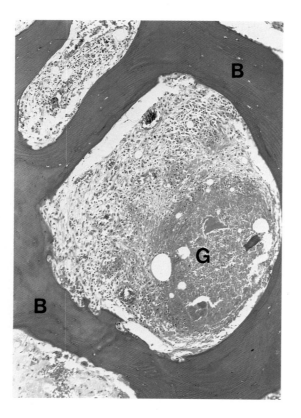

Fig. 3.15 Tuberculosis of bone (MP)

Bone tuberculosis *(tuberculous osteomyelitis)* most frequently affects the long bones and associated joints, and the vertebrae; involvement of vertebrae often leads to spontaneous collapse and is known as *Pott's disease*. In long bones, the infection may produce a localised, painful, tumour-like swelling which may drain to the skin to form a chronic sinus. Joint involvement *(tuberculous arthritis)* is most common in children and often affects the hips or joints associated with the vertebrae *(tuberculous spondylitis)* as part of Pott's disease of the spine.

As in other tissues, the characteristic tuberculous lesions are caseating granulomata **G** which cause progressive destruction of the bony trabeculae **B**. The infection tends to spread extensively in the cancellous medullary bone, leading to necrosis of surrounding cortical bone.

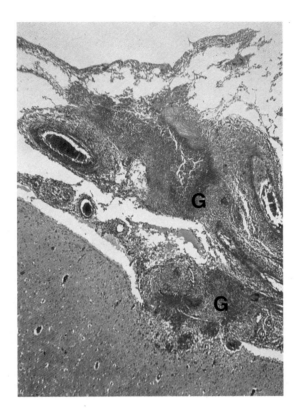

Fig. 3.16 Tuberculous meningitis (MP)

Meningitis is a fatal, although uncommon complication of pulmonary tuberculosis. Most commonly involved are the meninges around the base of the brain and spinal cord.

Tuberculous granulomata **G** with characteristic central areas of caseation develop in the leptomeninges and adjacent brain tissue where they may damage cranial and spinal nerves.

Langhans' giant cells are relatively sparse in the granulomata, but a heavy infiltrate of lymphocytes is almost always present. The presence of numerous lymphocytes in CSF obtained from lumbar puncture is useful in distinguishing tuberculous meningitis from purulent (bacterial) meningitis; in the latter, neutrophils are predominant.

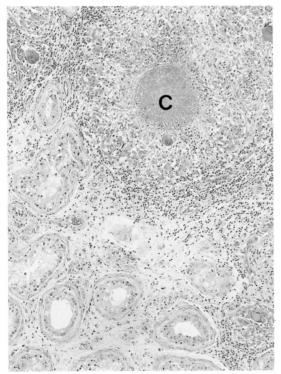

Fig. 3.17 Tuberculous epididymo-orchitis (LP)

The male genital tract may also be infected by blood-borne spread of pulmonary tuberculosis; the epididymis is the most common initial site involved.

Enlargement of miliary tubercles leads to extensive areas of confluent caseation **C** with destruction and atrophy of epididymal tubules.

If untreated, epididymal infection may spread to involve the adjacent area of the testis *(orchitis)* as here. Tuberculous epididymo-orchitis is also sometimes associated with tuberculous infection of the prostate and seminal vesicles. Infection of these glands is, however, more usually the result of spread from renal and urinary tract tuberculosis; even in this event it is a rare complication.

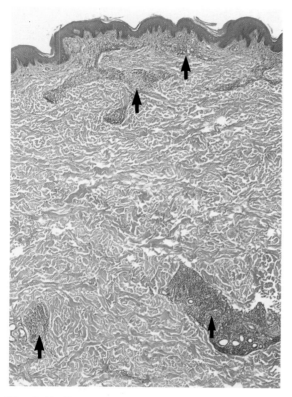

(a)

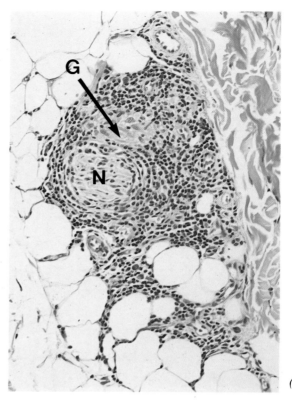

(b)

Fig. 3.18 Leprosy
(a) dermal infiltration (LP) (b) nerve involvement (HP)

Leprosy is a disease caused by infection with *Myco-bacterium leprae*. The tissue reaction to the bacillus depends on the immune response of the infected person. In the tuberculoid form of the disease, there is an active cell-mediated immune response and granulomas are formed in tissues similar to those seen in tuberculosis but without evidence of caseation. In the lepromatous form, there is no effective cell-mediated immune response and tissues are infiltrated with macrophages colonised by large numbers of bacteria. Intermediate forms of leprosy exist with both tuberculoid and lepromatous features.

Clinically, people with the lepromatous form of the disease have nodular dermal and subcutaneous deposits of macrophages filled with bacteria and lipid. The disease affects the face, ears, arms, knees and buttocks, as bacteria require cooler areas of the body for proliferation. In contrast, the tuberculoid form of the disease gives rise to macular or plaque-like skin lesions and in addition causes extensive inflammatory destruction of peripheral nerves, giving rise to anaesthesia in limbs which become prone to damage through repeated non-perceived injury.

Micrograph (a) is from the skin of a person with tuberculoid leprosy. Histiocytic granulomata are present at all layers throughout the dermis (arrows) but particularly in relation to small nerves; this is seen in the higher magnification micrograph (b) where a small nerve **N** is seen surrounded by lymphoid cells with an associated granuloma **G**. Special stains typically show very few bacilli in the tuberculoid form of the disease.

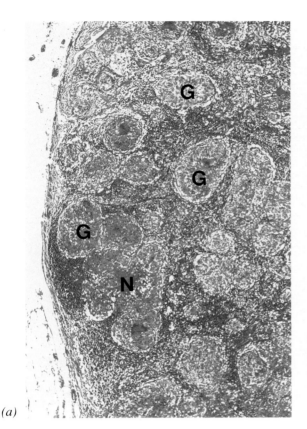

(a)

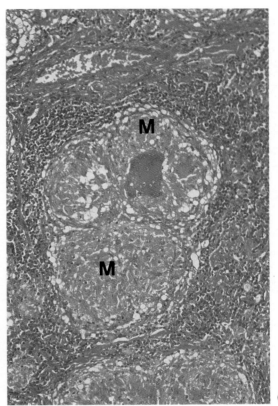

(b)

Fig 3.19   Sarcoidosis
(a) sarcoidosis in a lymph node (MP)   **(b) sarcoid granulomata** (HP)

Sarcoidosis is a chronic granulomatous inflammation of unknown aetiology characterised by the formation of multiple discrete granulomata similar in many respects to those of tuberculosis. In marked distinction to tuberculous granulomata, those of sarcoidosis do not typically undergo central caseation, although small foci of necrosis may be seen in large granulomata.

The sarcoid granuloma is largely composed of a broad zone of macrophages, but multinucleate giant cells are a feature of most of the granulomata. The cytoplasm of sarcoid giant cells may contain inclusion bodies of two types: star-shaped *asteroid bodies* or small, laminated calcified concretions called *Schaumann's bodies*. In practice, these inclusion bodies are rarely seen. Although characteristic of sarcoid giant cells, such inclusion bodies are occasionally found in other chronic inflammatory granulomata.

Sarcoidosis may occur in any organ or tissue, notably the spleen, liver, skin and lymph nodes, but frequently also involves the lungs which may be peppered with numerous granulomata. In most cases of pulmonary sarcoidosis, the hilar lymph nodes are also grossly enlarged by masses of granulomata; such

massive nodes are a useful diagnostic feature when visible on a chest radiograph.

Micrograph (a) illustrates part of a typical lymph node. Note the scattered non-caseating granulomata **G**; one larger granuloma exhibits a small area of necrosis **N**. Since there is no central mass of caseation, the sarcoid granuloma differs from the tuberculous granuloma by having a much broader zone of epithelioid macrophages. As in tuberculosis, sarcoid granulomata are surrounded by a zone of lymphocytic infiltration, although this feature is much less obvious in sarcoid lesions.

Micrograph (b) shows a typical sarcoid granuloma at high magnification. Note the broad zone of epithelioid macrophages **M** and prominent multinucleate giant cells.

Sarcoidosis is most commonly a chronic remitting disease, often exhibiting no symptoms; in persistent cases, the granulomata undergo progressive fibrosis although some giant cells still remain. In pulmonary sarcoidosis, the diffuse fibrosis may lead to chronic respiratory failure.

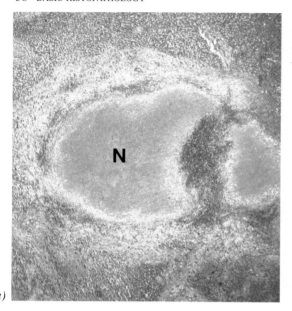

(a)

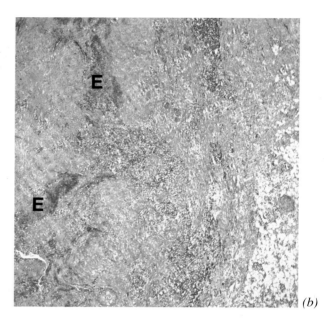

(b)

Fig. 3.20 Syphilis (a) syphilitic gumma of the liver (LP) **(b) syphilitic aortitis** (MP)

Although now relatively uncommon, late stage syphilis is still regarded as one of the classic examples of specific chronic inflammation. The infecting organism, the spiral-shaped *Treponema pallidum*, resists usual tissue defences and excites a progression of fascinating pathological and clinical phenomena which represent typical chronic inflammatory responses with superimposed hypersensitivity reactions mounted by the immune system. Classically, the condition proceeds through three stages extending over a long period.

In brief, the organism usually gains access to the body by penetrating the genital mucosa where it produces a single, small primary lesion known as a *chancre*. The chancre is a raised, reddened nodule caused by an intense local accumulation of plasma cells and lymphocytes in the sub-epithelial connective tissue. The chancre may ulcerate at this stage, but it is often painless and may easily pass unnoticed. By the time the chancre has developed, the organism has multiplied extensively and has been disseminated via local lymphatics to regional lymph nodes and thence into the bloodstream causing a generalised bacteraemia. The chancre and concomitant bacteraemia (*primary syphilis*) are followed some weeks or months later by a transient *secondary stage* characterised by a widespread variable skin rash often with moist warty genital lesions and ulceration of the oral mucosa. These various mucosal lesions are histologically similar to the primary chancre and are full of spirochaetes. The syphilis is now at its most contagious, yet the patient usually feels well and the only other evidence of a generalised infection is a widespread lymphadenopathy and positive serological findings.

In most untreated cases, the infection is effectively resolved by body defences, and in many of these even serological evidence of previous infection disappears. Unfortunately, a proportion of untreated cases proceed from the secondary stage to the formation of *tertiary syphilis* after a variable interval of from one to many years. The lesions of tertiary syphilis may be either focal or diffuse, and it is the focal lesion of tertiary syphilis, known as the *gumma,* which exhibits many of the features of a granulomatous inflammation. Tertiary lesions may occur in almost any organ or tissue, and the clinical consequences vary enormously. The diffuse form of tertiary syphilis most notably involves the cardiovascular system, particularly the aorta, and less commonly the central nervous system; the well known *tabes dorsalis* and *general paralysis of the insane* are two of the manifestations of diffuse neurosyphilis. In the focal form of tertiary syphilis, gummata may develop in the liver, bone, testes and other sites, the clinical outcome depending on the nature and extent of local tissue destruction.

Micrograph (a) illustrates the classical appearance of a gumma. The active gumma has a central area of homogeneous coagulative necrosis **N** surrounded by a zone of cells typical of chronic granulomatous inflammation, namely 'epithelioid' macrophages, lymphocytes, plasma cells and plump fibroblasts. Fibrous healing of liver gummata may produce a pattern of coarse deep scars dividing the liver surface into numerous irregular lobules; this condition is known as *hepar lobatum.*

Micrograph (b) illustrates *syphilitic aortitis,* the most common form of diffuse tertiary syphilitic lesion. The characteristic feature of diffuse tertiary syphilis, and also of primary and secondary syphilitic lesions, is a low grade chronic vasculitis of small vessels which exhibit thickening of the wall and a perivascular cuff of lymphocytes and plasma cells. In the aorta, the vasculitis affects the vasa vasorum of the tunica adventitia and their smaller branches which extend into the tunica media; the blue stained areas in the tunica media represent lymphocytic cuffing around numerous small vessels. The smooth muscle and elastic fibres of the media degenerate, probably due to ischaemia, and the aortic wall is replaced by collagen. Residual elastin can be seen as deep pink stained areas **E**. The loss of elasticity and contractility in the aortic wall allows progressive stretching with the formation of an *aortic aneurysm*, usually in the ascending aorta or aortic arch.

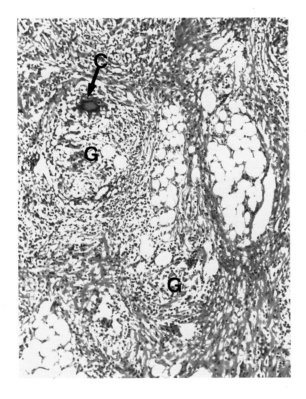

Fig. 3.21 Granulomatous inflammation due to foreign material (MP)

The presence of certain nonlysable foreign materials in the tissues may excite a chronic granulomatous inflammatory response similar to that seen in sarcoidosis. Common examples of such *foreign body reactions* are those produced by talc and starch (introduced into the tissues as glove powder during surgical procedures), suture material, wood, metal or glass splinters, and inorganic materials such as silica and beryllium inhaled deep into the lungs during industrial dust exposure. Inhaled materials are of particular clinical importance because of their tendency to produce progressive pulmonary fibrosis similar to that which may occur in sarcoidosis. Many of these foreign bodies are refractile when viewed with polarized light and can be identified within the granulomata or giant cells.

This micrograph illustrates granulomata **G** formed in the peritoneum in response to the introduction of talc particles during surgery. Foreign body giant cells **C** are a characteristic feature; the actual talc particles are too small to be seen. This trivial lesion was an incidental finding at autopsy.

Fate of chronic inflammation

As the term implies, a central feature of chronic inflammation is its prolonged course, reflecting a state of dynamic balance between recurrent tissue damage on the one hand, and continued attempts at repair on the other. The outcome of chronic inflammation depends on whether local or systemic factors favour the injurious agent or the process of healing. Factors which impair healing include poor nutrition, immunosuppression, retained foreign material or sequestered dead tissue, and poor blood supply. Factors which aid resolution of chronic inflammation include administration of appropriate antibiotics, surgical removal of foreign material or sequestered dead tissue, and general attempts to improve nutrition, for example by administration of vitamins.

In summary, chronic inflammation is marked by continuing tissue damage, acute inflammatory exudation, organisation and fibrous repair occurring concurrently rather than sequentially; the process is prolonged and is overlaid by immunological responses. It may be a result of inconclusive acute inflammation or may be a direct reaction to certain specific microorganisms or foreign bodies.

4. Amyloidosis

Introduction

Amyloidosis is a condition characterised by the extracellular deposition of an abnormal fibrillar protein, termed amyloid, in a wide variety of tissues and organs. Amyloid proteins have three unusual features:

- A peculiar molecular conformation in their secondary peptide folding termed a β-pleated sheet; this renders them resistant to degradation once formed in tissues.

- Several different types of peptide can form this sort of secondary protein structure and are said to be precursors of amyloid proteins.

- When deposited in tissues, amyloid proteins have a characteristic quaternary protein structure where the β-pleated sheet elements line up to form rigid straight fibrils 10-15 nm in diameter.

It is the physical and three dimensional molecular structure of a protein which makes it an amyloid, rather than any specific peptide sequence. It is thought that cells of the mononuclear-phagocyte system are responsible for processing a precursor peptide to form amyloid fibrils, however, the reasons for this are unclear. In certain types of amyloid the precursor protein has been shown to have undergone amino-acid substitutions, rendering it abnormal and possibly accounting for a predisposition to form a β-pleated sheet structure.

Despite uncertainty about why amyloid is formed, there are well characterised associations between particular diseases and the deposition of amyloid. In each case there is accumulation of a precursor peptide which becomes processed to an amyloid protein. In some of these diseases there is an identifiable reason for the accumulation of the precursor peptide, and the amyloid is termed *secondary amyloid*. In other cases the cause of the accumulation of a precursor peptide is not known and the amyloid is termed *primary amyloid*. In addition, there are several inherited disorders, the *heredo-familial amyloidoses*.

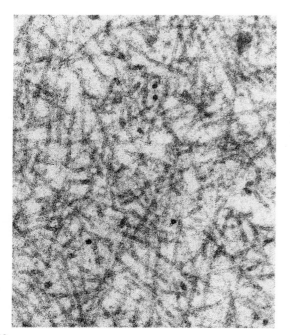

Fig. 4.1 Amyloid ultrastructure (EM)

Electron microscopy is a useful method for the detection of amyloid in tissues, particularly when it is in small quantities and hence does not show up with special stains. This electron micrograph shows amyloid which had been deposited in a renal glomerulus and resulted in proteinuria (excess protein leaking into the urine). A renal biopsy was performed and at light microscopy this revealed thickening of the basement membrane of the glomeruli. Ultrastructural examination of a portion of the thickened basement membrane revealed the deposition of amyloid.

The amyloid is seen to have a fibrillar ultrastructure, each fibril being composed of the precursor peptide arranged as finer filaments of a β-pleated sheet.

In this instance, the amyloid was deposited as a result of longstanding rheumatoid disease and was presumably of the serum amyloid A protein type (see Fig. 4.2).

Distribution of amyloid

Amyloid is deposited in the extracellular compartment of tissues, and in H&E preparation is seen as uniformly eosinophilic (pink-staining) material. It can be highlighted in histological sections by use of special stains such as Sirius red and Congo red. Congo red staining is commonly used for diagnostic purposes, amyloid staining orange in colour and exhibiting a green colouration when viewed with polarised light.

Amyloidosis may involve many tissues in the body but most commonly affects kidneys, spleen, liver, adrenals and heart. It has a particular predilection for deposition in blood vessel walls and basement membranes. The progressive accumulation of amyloid leads to cellular dysfunction, either by preventing normal diffusion through extracellular tissues or by physical compression of functioning parenchymal cells. In some diseases amyloidosis is a systemic process affecting many organs simultaneously *(systemic amyloid)*; there is also a group of conditions in which amyloid only affects one organ or tissue *(localised amyloid)*.

Classification of amyloid

Amino-acid sequencing of amyloid proteins in different disease states has enabled a classification of amyloid to be made on biochemical grounds (Fig. 4.2).

Fig 4.2 Classification of amyloid

Localisation	Clinical association	Precursor protein
Systemic amyloid	Plasma cell tumours	Immunoglobulin light chain
	Chronic inflammation	Serum amyloid A protein
	Familial Mediterranean fever	Serum amyloid A protein
	Familial neuropathy	Transthyretin (prealbumen)
	Dialysis associated	β-2-microglobulin
Localised amyloid	Senile cardiac amyloid	Transthyretin (prealbumen)
	Medullary carcinoma	Calcitonin
	Alzheimer's disease	β protein (A4 protein)
	Cerebral angiopathy	β protein (A4 protein)

Amyloid associated with abnormal proliferation of plasma cells is made up of immunoglobulin light chains; examples of diseases leading to such amyloid deposition include myeloma, plasmacytoma and non-Hodgkin's lymphoma.

Reactive amyloid occurs in rare instances associated with chronic inflammatory processes. The end result is deposition of amyloid derived from serum amyloid A protein, an acute phase protein of unknown function which is manufactured in response to inflammatory processes and circulates in the serum. Examples of diseases leading to this type of secondary amyloid include tuberculosis, rheumatoid arthritis, bronchiectasis and chronic osteomyelitis.

Certain familial types of amyloid involve the deposition of transthyretin-derived amyloid (transthyretin is so named as it transports thyroxine and retinol in plasma –this was formerly termed pre-albumen). Transthyretin amyloids in the familial types are associated with amino acid substitutions in the protein which in some way predispose to the formation of the amyloid structure.

Tumours of peptide-secreting endocrine cells may form amyloid from the hormone peptide. A well known example is the localised deposition of calcitonin-derived amyloid in medullary carcinoma of the thyroid. This is an example of a localised amyloid.

The central nervous system provides perhaps the commonest example of localised amyloid deposition in *Alzheimer's disease* (Fig. 22.6) derived from a peptide termed β-protein (also called A4 protein) related to a secreted protease inhibitor. It is also deposited in cerebral blood vessels in *congophilic angiopathy*.

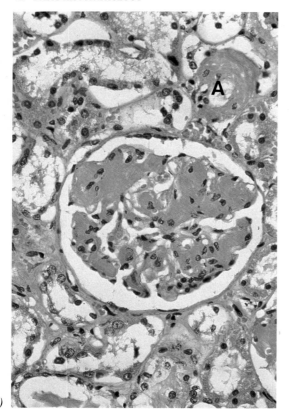

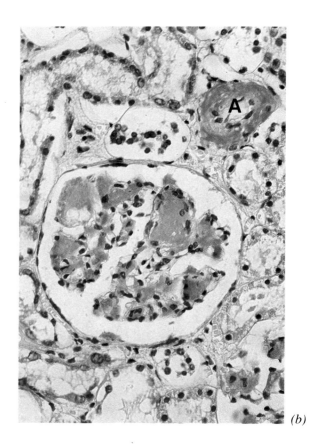

(a)   *(b)*

Fig. 4.3   Renal amyloidosis (a) H&E (HP)   **(b) Sirius red** (HP)

The kidneys are the organs most commonly involved by systemic amyloidosis, and renal failure is one of the most serious clinical complications, accounting for the majority of deaths from the disease. These sections from the same glomerulus are from an autopsy specimen taken from a 58 year old woman with a 20-year history of rheumatoid arthritis; the sections have been stained with contrasting histological methods to illustrate the principal features.

Amyloid deposition usually begins in the glomerular mesangium and around capillary basement membranes, leading to progressive obliteration of capillary lumina, destruction of glomerular endothelial, mesangial and podocyte cells, and eventually complete replacement of the glomerulus by a confluent mass of amyloid. Concurrently, the walls of renal arterioles and arteries **A** may become infiltrated by amyloid, causing impairment of the blood supply to the glomeruli. Interstitial spaces between renal tubules may also become infiltrated, further compromising tubular function. With H&E staining, amyloid appears as a homogeneous eosinophilic (pink) material, difficult to distinguish from normal structures. Staining methods such as Congo red or Sirius red, as in micrograph (b), readily distinguish amyloid which stands out as red-stained material, in this case in the glomerulus and an affected afferent arteriole.

Amyloid of the kidney usually presents with proteinuria, often severe enough to produce the nephrotic syndrome. As increasing amyloid deposition leads to glomerular ischaemia and tubular atrophy, chronic renal failure supervenes.

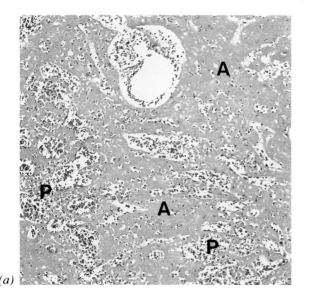

(a)

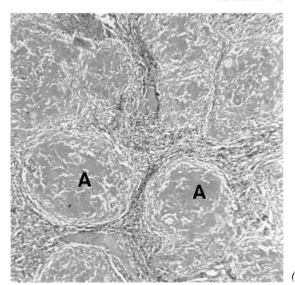

(b)

Fig. 4.4   Splenic amyloidosis   (a) diffuse type (MP) (b) nodular type (MP)

There are two patterns of amyloid deposition seen in the spleen, described as either diffuse or nodular.

Micrograph (a) shows the more common diffuse pattern. Splenic amyloidosis most commonly begins with deposition in the walls of splenic sinuses progressing until the deposits coalesce to form large diffuse masses **A**; little red pulp **P** and lymphoid tissue (white pulp, not seen in this specimen) remains. This form is sometimes termed 'lardaceous' because of the waxy firmness of the spleen when the specimen is cut.

Less commonly, amyloid deposition results in the formation of the so-called 'sago' spleen as illustrated in micrograph (b). In this pattern the amyloid **A** becomes deposited in the periarteriolar lymphoid sheaths (white pulp), giving the appearance of discrete deposits on the cut surface of the gross specimen. Note the small vessels in the centre of the pink-staining nodular amyloid deposits.

Amyloid deposition in the spleen can give rise to clinically palpable splenic enlargement.

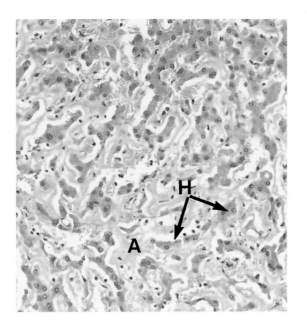

Fig. 4.5   Hepatic amyloidosis (HP)

In the liver, amyloid is deposited in the space between sinusoidal lining cells and hepatocytes. With progressive deposition, hepatocytes become compressed by sheets of amyloid and undergo atrophy.

Amyloid is visible as ribbon-like pink staining deposits **A** within hepatic sinusoids. Hepatocytes **H** have become compressed and are atrophic.

Clinically, hepatic amyloidosis may be a cause of hepatomegaly (enlargement of the liver). However, even when liver involvement is severe, there is rarely significant clinical evidence of impaired liver function.

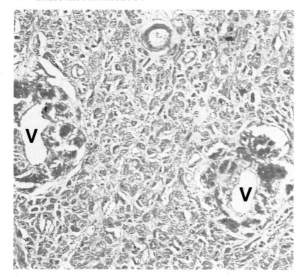

Fig. 4.6 Cardiac amyloid (MP)

Amyloid involvement of the heart may be an incidental finding at autopsy in the elderly, and in such cases is usually a manifestation of *senile cardiac amyloid* derived from transthyretin (pre-albumen).

The most severe form of cardiac amyloid is seen in systemic heredo-familial amyloidosis derived from serum amyloid A protein, e.g. in familial Mediterranean fever. Cardiac involvement may also occur in cases of secondary amyloidosis.

Myocardial amyloidosis leads to intractable cardiac failure with enlargement of the heart; subendocardial deposition of amyloid may interfere with the conducting system resulting in cardiac arrhythmias.

In the case illustrated here, amyloid has accumulated in the walls of myocardial vessels **V** and is extending to form masses within the myocardium.

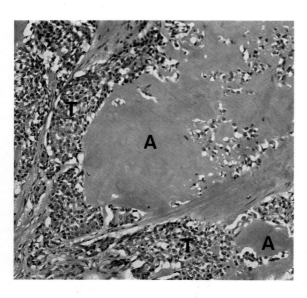

Fig. 4.7 Localised amyloid: medullary carcinoma of the thyroid (MP)

An example of localised amyloid is seen in tumours derived from the calcitonin-secreting cells of the thyroid, medullary carcinomas. Large islands of pink-stained amyloid **A** are present in between zones of tumour cells **T**. The amyloid is derived from pro-calcitonin secreted by the tumour. Amyloid is present only within the tumour and is not systematised. Another example of localised amyloid is seen with insulin-derived polypeptide in tumours, arising from the islets of Langerhans in the pancreas, termed insulinomas.

In contrast, systemic amyloidosis may occur in association with certain tumours in particular Hodgkin's disease and renal adenocarcinomas (derived from serum amyloid A protein) and myeloma (derived from immunoglobulin light chain).

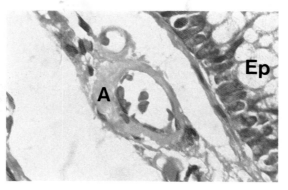

Fig. 4.8 Vessel amyloid in rectal biopsy (HP)

The diagnosis of systemic amyloidosis can only be confirmed by tissue biopsy, and the rectum is the commonest biopsied site.

In rectal biopsies, amyloid can be detected in the submucosal vessels in 60-70% of cases of generalised amyloidosis. This photomicrograph, taken at very high magnification, shows rectal glandular epithelium **Ep** with a small blood vessel in the adjacent lamina propria. The vessel wall is thickened by homogeneous pink-staining amyloid **A**. Amyloid in small vessels such as this may be subtle, and it is usual to confirm the diagnosis by a special stain such as Congo red.

5. Disorders of growth

Introduction

Cells respond to environmental changes in several fundamentally different ways depending on the nature of the stimulus. As briefly discussed in Chapter 1, if the stimulus is overwhelming then the cells undergo degeneration or cell death. However, many less noxious stimuli cause cells to adapt by altering their pattern of growth. This may occur in three main ways:

- change in the size of cells
- change in the differentiation of cells
- change in the rate of cell division.

In an organ composed of different types of cell, only one of the cell types may be affected leading to a marked change in tissue appearance and function.

The normal pattern of cell growth in an organ depends both on factors inherent in the cells as well as extrinsic environmental factors. Intrinsically, cells may be divided into three types by their capacity for cell division:

- cells which divide and *replicate continuously*, such as squamous cells in the epidermis
- cells which do not normally replicate but which are capable of cell division in response to certain demands such as hepatocytes after partial hepatectomy *(facultative dividers)*
- cells which are incapable of cell division *(non-replicators)*; these are typified by neurones and cardiac muscle cells – the heart and brain have no capacity for regeneration.

Extrinsic to the cell, factors such as blood supply, innervation, hormonal stimulation, physical stress or biochemical alterations will determine the normal pattern of cell growth in an organ or tissue. Depending on the intrinsic characteristics of a particular cell type, a change in environment may result in a change in the growth pattern. Such responses are now recognised as being under the control of various growth factors which act upon specific cell-surface receptors. Alterations in the concentrations of growth factors or the expression of growth-factor receptors will result in altered cell growth.

Increased cell mass

Certain organs may respond to environmental stimulation by an increase in functional cell mass. There are two mechanisms by which this occurs:

- increase in cell number as a consequence of cell division; this is termed *hyperplasia*
- increase in the size of existing cells; this is termed *hypertrophy.*

In practice, increase in functional cell mass is more often due to a combination of both hyperplasia and hypertrophy, as seen in the myometrium in pregnancy (Fig. 5.3). Hypertrophy also occurs in the muscle of a viscus which is obstructed, such as small bowel proximal to an obstructing tumour (Fig. 5.1).

A pathological example of hyperplasia is the response of the parathyroid gland to a low serum calcium. The thickening of the skin which occurs with prolonged local trauma is due to hyperplasia of the squamous epithelium. Hyperplasia occurs most commonly in response to endocrine stimuli, a classic example being endometrial proliferation during the menstrual cycle (Fig. 5.2).

For poorly understood reasons, the process of hyperplasia may not be uniform throughout an organ or tissue, and in these instances, nodules of excessive cell growth arise in between areas of unaltered cell growth. This phenomenon, known as *nodular hyperplasia*, is seen in the thyroid gland (see Fig. 19.4), the adrenal gland (Fig. 19.7), the prostate gland (Fig. 18.7) and the breast (Fig. 17.2).

A cardinal feature of the forms of increased cell mass described above is that following removal of the environmental stimulus, the altered pattern of growth ceases and usually the tissue reverts to its former state. Hypertrophy and hyperplasia can in many circumstances be regarded as normal physiological adaptations, as exemplified by exercise-induced skeletal muscle hypertrophy, and hyperplasia and hypertrophy of the myometrium during pregnancy. Many pathological stimuli, on the other hand, may also invoke the responses of hypertrophy and hyperplasia.

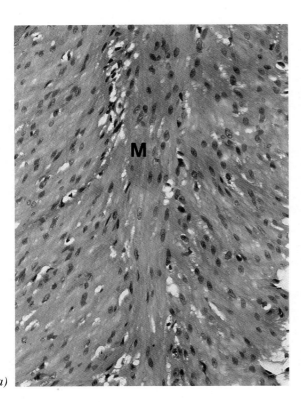

(a)

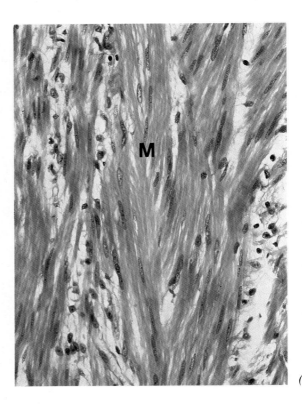

(b)

Fig. 5.1 Hypertrophy
(a) normal small bowel muscle (HP)   (b) hypertrophy of muscle of bowel wall (HP)

Pure hypertrophy without coexisting hyperplasia is virtually only seen in muscle where the stimulus is an increased demand for work. Taken at the same magnification, micrograph (a) shows the muscle **M** of normal small bowel, whilst micrograph (b) shows a portion of thickened muscle in small bowel proximal to an intestinal obstruction. To overcome the obstruction, peristaltic activity must be increased and this is achieved by increasing muscle cell mass by hypertrophy. Note that the individual cells in micrograph (b) are larger than in the normal bowel (a).

A similar type of change is seen in myocardial muscle when there is an increased demand on cardiac function caused by obstructed or incompetent valves, or by systemic hypertension. Likewise, skeletal muscle increases in bulk by hypertrophy in response to regular exercise. Prostatic obstruction of the bladder neck is followed by hypertrophy of the muscle of the bladder wall. In all the foregoing examples, when the stimulus for hypertrophy is removed, the muscle cells will slowly return to their normal size.

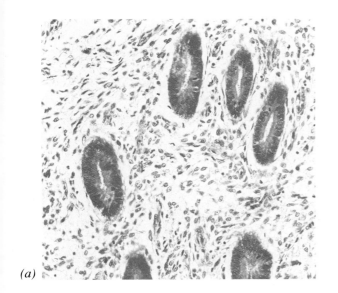
(a)

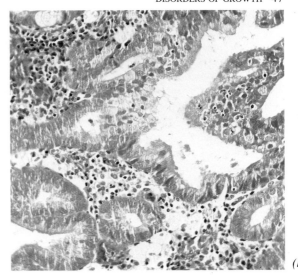
(b)

Fig. 5.2 Hyperplasia
(a) normal late proliferative endometrium (HP) (b) hyperplasia of endometrium (HP)

Endometrial hyperplasia occurs when there is abnormal oestrogenic stimulation. Micrograph (a) shows the degree of endometrial hyperplasia which occurs under normal ovarian oestrogenic stimulation. In contrast, in micrograph (b), the endometrial glands are markedly hyperplastic and continued increase in the number of cells in each gland has resulted in a few showing some degree of cystic dilatation. This example is from a woman taking an oestrogen-containing preparation on a long term basis, the result

being persisting growth of the endometrium; similar changes may also be seen in the endometrium of women with oestrogen-secreting ovarian tumours.

In such examples, removal of the abnormal oestrogenic stimulation restores the normal pattern of endometrial growth. The menstrual cycle can be regarded as a classic example of physiological endocrine-induced hyperplasia which normally occurs on a monthly cyclical basis under the control of ovarian hormones.

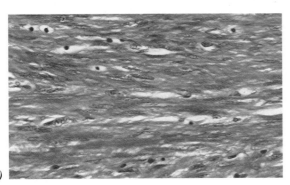
(a)

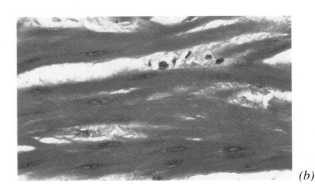
(b)

Fig. 5.3 Hyperplasia with hypertrophy
(a) normal myometrium (HP) (b) hyperplasia and hypertrophy in pregnant myometrium (HP)

Hypertrophy and hyperplasia commonly occur together in response to increased functional requirements. When compared to the normal myometrial fibres seen in micrograph (a), the fibres of the pregnant uterus (b), at the same magnification, are greatly enlarged; their larger nuclei reflect increased protein synthesis.

Within the uterus as a whole, the number of cells is

increased by hyperplasia. Occasionally in the uterus a mitotic figure may be seen where a myometrial cell is in the process of cell division.

Following pregnancy, the uterus returns to normal size by physiological atrophy which by convention is termed *involution*.

Reduction in functional cell mass

When the mass of functioning cells in a tissue is reduced, the tissue is then said to have undergone *atrophy*. The mechanisms of atrophy may involve reduction in cell volume or in cell number, both leading to a reduction in functional capacity. Grossly, the appearance of the tissue depends on whether the functional cell loss is replaced by other tissue. Commonly, when atrophy occurs, the lost cells are replaced by either adipose or fibrous tissue, often maintaining the overall size of the organ; when adipose or fibrous replacement does not occur, then the overall size of the organ is reduced. Examples are the testis in the elderly (Fig. 5.4) and the adrenal gland when suppressed by exogenous steroid administration (Fig. 19.7b). Atrophy may occur as a physiological event, when it is usually termed *involution*. An example is the normal involution of the thymus gland during adolescence.

Atrophy must be distinguished from *hypoplasia,* a condition where there is incomplete growth of an organ, and *agenesis,* where there is complete failure of growth of an organ during embryological development. In general, conditions opposite to those causing hypertrophy or hyperplasia result in atrophy. Thus disuse of skeletal muscle will result in a loss of cell mass. Removal of endocrine stimulation causes atrophy in target organs. Reduction in blood supply to a tissue may result in loss of functional cells; this is termed *ischaemic atrophy* and is seen commonly in the kidney.

In many atrophic tissues, a brown pigment called *lipofuscin* accumulates within the shrunken cells. This is thought to represent degenerate lipid material in secondary lysosomes produced by breakdown of the cell membranes and organelles. Lipofuscin accumulates particularly in the atrophic myocardial fibres of the hearts of elderly people and gives rise to the term *brown atrophy*.

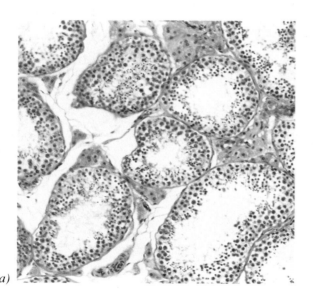 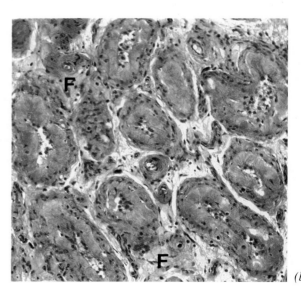

(a)   (b)

Fig. 5.4   Atrophy (a) normal testis (HP)   **(b) atrophic testis** (HP)

Micrograph (b) illustrates atrophy of the testis in a man aged 94; reduced secretion of trophic hormones may be responsible. When compared with the normal testis in micrograph (a), the seminiferous tubules of the atrophic testis show minimal spermatogenic activity. The tubular walls are thickened and pink-stained, a process known as *hyalinization*. The interstitial tissue shows an increased deposition of fibrous tissue **F**.

Hyaline is a term used to describe replacement of tissue by an amorphous pink-staining material similar to basement membrane matrix; it is a common end result of atrophy or cell damage, being frequently accompanied by fibrosis. It is a feature of end-stage kidney (Fig. 14.2).

Change in cell differentiation

When cells adapt to a change in environment by altering their morphological appearance, this is termed *metaplasia*. Metaplasia is thought to be an adaptive response which produces cells better equipped to withstand a new environment. For example, in the bronchi, the respiratory epithelium may be replaced by squamous epithelium under the influence of chronic irritation by cigarette smoke *(squamous metaplasia)*. Similarly, in the bladder, the normal transitional epithelium may be replaced by squamous epithelium in response to chronic irritation by, for example, bladder stones (Fig. 5.5). Metaplasia may coexist with hyperplasia and hypertrophy.

Metaplasia most commonly occurs in epithelial tissues but may also be seen in mesodermal tissues; for example, areas of fibrous tissue exposed to chronic trauma may form bone *(osseous metaplasia)*. A key feature of metaplastic transformation is that one mature, fully differentiated cell type takes on the morphology of a totally different, fully differentiated cell type.

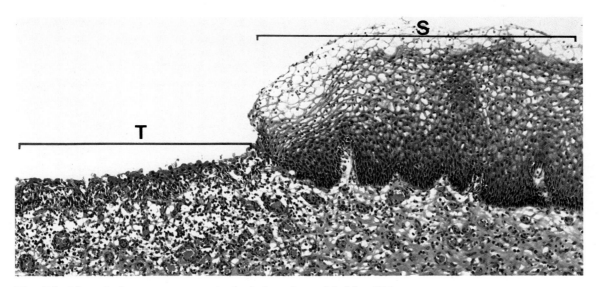

Fig. 5.5 Metaplasia: squamous metaplasia in urinary bladder (HP)

This micrograph illustrates the effects of chronic irritation upon the bladder mucosa by a bladder stone. The transitional epithelium **T** is inflamed and degenerate, and squamous metaplasia has occurred in one area with the replacement of the native transitional epithelium by stratified squamous epithelium **S**. Note the coexisting acute and chronic inflammatory change in the underlying supporting connective tissue. Squamous metaplasia also occurs in the bladder in chronic irritation by the parasitic infection, schistosomiasis.

An important example of squamous metaplasia is seen in the respiratory tract epithelium of the bronchi in response to exposure to cigarette smoke. In these examples, the squamous epithelium is better suited to withstand the irritating environment than the native ciliated columnar epithelium

Dysplasia

Cells may undergo a morphological transformation in which an increased rate of cell division is coupled with incomplete maturation of the resultant cells. This change is known as *dysplasia*. The cells of dysplastic tissues tend to exhibit a high nuclear to cytoplasmic ratio and there is an increased rate of mitotic cell division. The incomplete cellular maturation is often reflected by partial or complete loss of certain specialised cellular structures normally seen in that cell type, such as cilia or mucin vacuoles; this is a feature termed *failure of differentiation*. Dysplastic tissues may also show loss of the normal architectural relationships between cells.

Like metaplasia, dysplasia is most frequently seen in epithelia subject to chronic irritation. Dysplasia is present to some degree in the regenerating epithelia of damaged tissues, and in these instances it is associated with concomitant inflammatory and reparatory changes. In other instances, dysplasia occurs in the absence of obvious tissue damage or repair, and in such cases the cytological features of the dysplastic tissue may merge with those seen in neoplastic conditions (described later in Ch. 6). In many clinical situations malignant neoplastic change follows pre-existing dysplastic change. Dysplasia *per se* is not a neoplastic condition, and removal of the adverse environmental stimulus may cause restoration of the normal cell growth pattern.

Dysplastic change may be seen in the squamous epithelium at the squamo-columnar junction of the uterine cervix and in the epidermis of sun-exposed skin (see below). Dysplastic changes in colonic and gastric mucosa are associated with chronic colitis and chronic gastritis respectively.

Because of the sinister association of dysplasia with the development of neoplasia, treatment of dysplastic conditions is undertaken to minimise the risk of subsequent development of a malignancy. Recognition of dysplastic changes by cytological examination of cervical smears (PAP smears) forms the basis of screening for cancer of the cervix (Fig. 16.5).

Fig. 5.6 Dysplasia *(illustrations opposite)*
(a) normal cervix (HP)   **(b) dysplasia in the cervix** (HP)
(c) normal skin (HP)   **(d) dysplastic skin** (HP)

Dysplasia is a morphological feature characterised by increased cellular proliferation with incomplete maturation of cells. It occurs commonly at the uterine cervix and in the skin, and in both cases is thought to predispose to neoplastic change.

Micrograph (a) illustrates normal stratified squamous epithelium from the cervix. Cellular proliferation is confined to the basal layer **B** where the cells are small, uniform and darkly stained. As the cells migrate through various strata towards the surface, their cytoplasm expands and becomes more eosinophilic (pink stained). Near the surface the cells become progressively flattened; the ratio of nucleus to cytoplasm diminishes as the cells pass from basal to surface layers. In contrast, micrograph (b) shows dysplastic cervical epithelium where there is disruption of the normal orderly maturation sequence. Cells in the mid strata now exhibit very large nuclei with prominent nucleoli, and mitotic figures may be seen above the basal layer. Cells near the surface now show a higher ratio of nucleus to cytoplasm than in the normal state. It is the presence of such surface cells with large nuclei which alert the cytologist to underlying dysplasia in a cervical smear.

Micrographs (c) and (d) demonstrate similar differences between normal and dysplastic skin respectively. Note how the normal cellular stratification is disrupted in the dysplastic specimen by cells with large, darkly staining nuclei extending far up into the middle strata. In addition, a disturbed pattern of maturation is reflected in the development of a thick layer of keratin which contains purple-stained nuclear remnants. It is this keratin layer which becomes clinically evident as thickening and scaling of the skin over such areas of dysplasia.

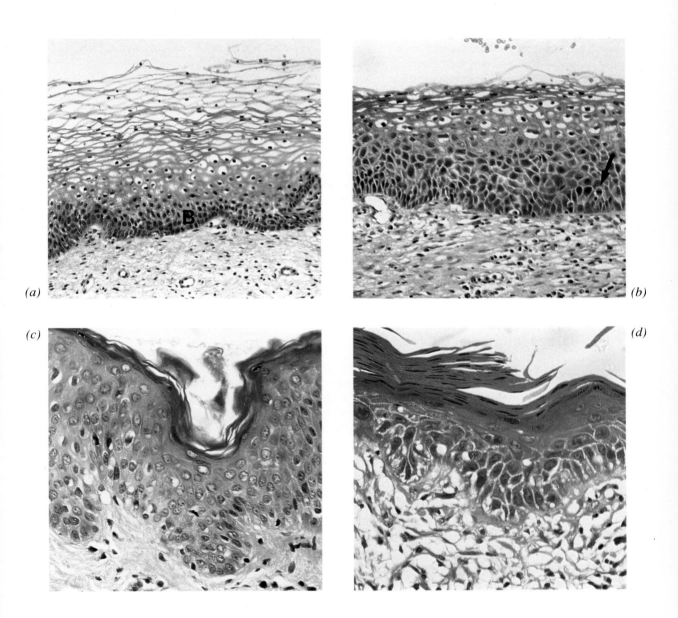

Fig. 5.6 Dysplasia *(caption opposite)*

6. Neoplasia

Introduction

In a neoplastic state, cellular proliferation and growth occur in the absence of any continuing external stimulus. The term neoplasia therefore describes a state of poorly regulated cell division, and the abnormal mass of cells that results is termed a *neoplasm*. In neoplastic cells and tissues there is a failure of the mechanisms which control cellular proliferation and maturation. These abnormalities arise out of changes in genetic material which are transmitted to each new generation of cells within the neoplasm. The state of neoplastic growth contrasts with hyperplasia, discussed in the preceding chapter, where although there is abnormal proliferation of cells, this ceases with removal of the causative stimulus.

Several factors are known to induce neoplastic transformation of cells including irradiation, chemical agents and certain viruses. Although causally related factors are known for several human neoplasms, most are poorly understood and the majority unknown. Some neoplasms develop in the setting of another disturbed pattern of growth such as hyperplasia, metaplasia or dysplasia.

By convention, a neoplastic mass of cells is termed a *tumour;* the Latin derivation used to refer to any tissue swelling, although this literal use has largely gone out of fashion.

General characteristics of neoplasms

Neoplasms may be divided into two broad groups according to their behaviour:

- If the margins of the tumour are well-defined and cell growth is entirely local, then the neoplasm is termed *benign.*
- If the margins of the neoplasm are poorly defined and the neoplastic cells extend into and destroy surrounding tissues, then the neoplasm is termed *malignant.*

The property whereby a malignant tumour can grow into and at the expense of surrounding tissue is termed *invasion*. A further property of malignant neoplasms is distant spread of neoplastic cells away from the main neoplasm (termed the *primary tumour*) to form subpopulations of neoplastic cells which are not in continuity with the primary tumour. These detached neoplastic masses are termed *secondary tumours*. The property of distant spread of tumour is termed *metastasis;* the secondary tumours which result are often termed *metastases.*

In general terms, a benign tumour will behave in a relatively innocuous manner, and a malignant tumour will have deleterious effects often leading to death. There are, however, exceptions to these generalisations, and factors other than the biological growth pattern of a tumour may be important in influencing the outcome, most notably the location of the tumour; for example a benign tumour of the brain stem may lead to rapid death, whereas a malignant tumour of the skin may progress slowly over many years.

Systemic symptoms such as weight loss, loss of appetite, fever and general malaise frequently accompany malignant tumours; in most cases the pathophysiology is poorly understood but includes effects of secreted cytokines such as tumour necrosis factor. Some tumours, benign and malignant, retain the function of their organ of origin, and if this happens to be an endocrine function then the tumour may exert harmful effects by secretion of excess hormone.

As well as abnormal cell proliferation, neoplasia is characterised by abnormal maturation of cells. A feature of normal tissue growth is the maturation of constituent cells into a form adapted to a specific function; this adaptation may involve the acquisition of specialised structures such as mucin vacuoles, neurosecretory granules, microvilli or cilia. This process of structural and functional maturation is termed *differentiation*. A fully mature cell of any particular cell line is said to be highly differentiated, whereas its primitive precursor cells are described as being relatively undifferentiated. In any given tissue, the normal cells have a characteristic state of differentiation; in contrast, neoplastic cells exhibit variable states of differentiation and commonly fail to achieve a highly differentiated state. In general, the cells of benign neoplasms are differentiated to a degree which fairly closely corresponds to that of the cells from which they were derived. In the case of malignant neoplasms there is a variable degree of differentiation. At one end of the spectrum, the constituent cells may closely resemble the tissue of origin, in which case the tumour is described as being a *well-differentiated* malignant neoplasm; alternatively, the constituent cells may bear little resemblance to the tissue of origin, in which case the neoplasm is described as being *poorly differentiated*. At the extreme end of the spectrum, neoplasms which exhibit no evidence of differentiation are termed *anaplastic* neoplasms; in such poorly differentiated tumours it is not possible to identify the cell of origin on morphological grounds alone. On the basis of clinical observation and pathological investigation, it has been shown that the degree of differentiation of a neoplasm is generally related to its behaviour. A poorly differentiated neoplasm tends to be more invasive and more aggressive than a well-differentiated neoplasm.

Histological assessment of neoplasms

Histological examination of a neoplasm provides a useful guide to tumour behaviour and provides a basis for rational treatment. The principal features to be established are:

- The proportion of cells undergoing mitosis (mitotic figures). This is known as the *mitotic index* and provides an indication of the rate of cell proliferation. This is generally high in more malignant tumours and low in differentiated tumours.
- The degree of differentiation of tumour cells. This takes into account the morphology of tumour cells as well as the overall architecture of the tissues compared to the tissue of origin (Fig. 6.2).
- Variation in size and shape of constituent cells of the tumour. The degree of variation *(pleomorphism)* increases with failure of differentiation (Fig. 6.3).
- Evidence of invasion of surrounding tissues including vascular and lymphatic spread (Figs. 6.4-6.8).

The histological features which distinguish benign and malignant tumours are summarised below in Figure 6.1.

Fig. 6.1 Histological features of neoplasms

	Benign	Malignant
Behaviour	Expansile growth only; grows locally	Expansile and invasive growth; may metastasise
Histology	Resembles cell of origin (well-differentiated)	May show failure of cellular differentiation
	Few mitoses	Many mitoses, some of which are abnormal forms
	Normal or slight increase in ratio of nucleus to cytoplasm	High nuclear to cytoplasmic ratio
	Cells are uniform through the tumour	Cells vary in shape and size (cellular pleomorphism) or nuclei vary in shape and size (nuclear pleomorphism)

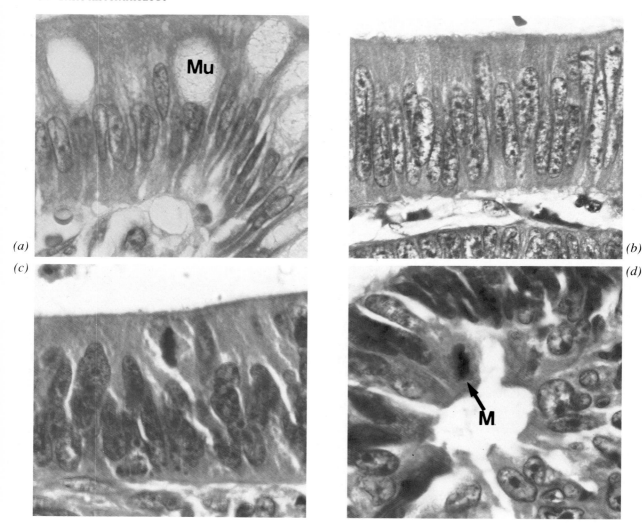

Fig. 6.2 Degrees of tumour differentiation

(a) normal colonic mucosa (HP)

(b) benign colonic neoplasm (HP)

(c) well-differentiated malignant colonic neoplasm (HP)

(d) poorly differentiated colonic neoplasm (HP)

This series of micrographs demonstrates the variable degree of differentiation that may be seen in tumours arising from the same cell of origin, in this case the mucus-secreting columnar epithelium of the colon.

Note the similarity between normal colonic mucosa in micrograph (a) and a benign colonic neoplasm in micrograph (b); in both cases the epithelial cells are tall, columnar and regular in form. The main points of difference are that the cells of the benign neoplasm contain no mucin **Mu** and their nuclei are more prominent. Note also that the nuclei of the benign neoplasm are more intensely stained with haematoxylin, a feature termed *hyperchromatism*.

The cells of the well-differentiated malignant colonic neoplasm shown in micrograph (c) are also tall and columnar, but the nuclei are irregular in shape and arrangement and are hyperchromatic; there is no mucin secretion, most of the cell being occupied by nucleus, i.e. there is a high nuclear-cytoplasmic ratio. Despite these cytological changes, the cells still retain a reasonable semblance of the normal columnar arrangement.

In contrast, in the poorly differentiated colonic neoplasm shown in micrograph (d), the cells and their organisation bear less resemblance to the tissue of origin having lost most semblance of a columnar pattern. The cells show a great variability in size and nuclear shape; mitoses **M** are seen, and there is no evidence of mucin secretion.

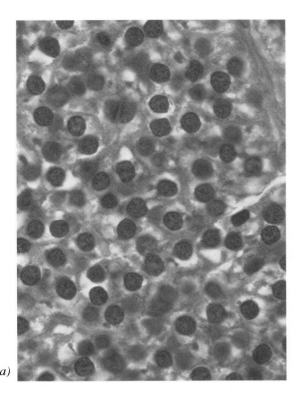

(a)

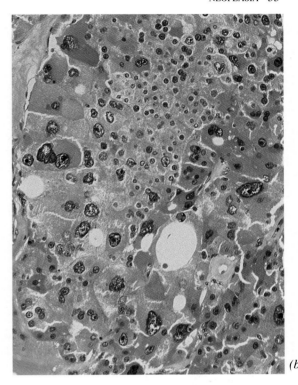

(b)

(c)

Fig. 6.3 Pleomorphism, nuclear hyperchromicity and abnormal mitoses
(a) benign neoplasm (HP)
(b) malignant neoplasm (HP)
(c) malignant neoplasm (HP)

Pleomorphism, nuclear hyperchromicity and abnormal mitotic activity are features of malignant neoplasms and are not usually seen in benign neoplasms. In the benign neoplasm in (a), note the uniformity of cell and nuclear size and shape, and the regular nuclear staining. The malignant tumour illustrated in (b) shows remarkable variation in cell size and shape (cellular pleomorphism) and nuclear size and shape (nuclear pleomorphism); in addition, many nuclei are very darkly stained (nuclear hyperchromatism). Increased numbers of cells in mitosis are seen in many conditions in which there is excess cellular proliferation (e.g. hyperplasia), but in malignant neoplasms many of the mitotic figures are abnormal; micrograph (c) shows an abnormal tripolar mitosis in a poorly differentiated malignant neoplasm.

Modes of spread of malignant neoplasms

There are four main modes of tumour spread:

- **Local invasion**. Invasive tumours tend to spread into surrounding tissues by the most direct route (Figs 6.4 and 6.5). Some tumours, however, spread along lines of least resistance such as naturally occurring tissue planes, e.g. around and along nerve bundles.

- **Lymphatic spread**. Tumour may spread via lymphatic vessels draining the site of the primary tumour; neoplastic cells are conducted to local lymph nodes where they become trapped and set up secondary tumours (Figs. 6.7 and 6.8).

- **Vascular spread**. Tumour can spread via the venules and veins draining the primary site; gut tumours tend to be conducted via the portal vein to the liver where secondary tumours are very frequently established. In the systemic circulation, neoplastic cells may be trapped in the capillaries of the lung to form pulmonary metastases (Fig. 6.6).

- **Trans-coelomic spread**. Certain tumours can spread directly across coelomic spaces, e.g. across the peritoneal or pleural cavities.

In situ neoplasia

Occasionally, a neoplasm exhibits cytological features of malignancy, i.e. cellular pleomorphism and increased mitotic activity, but is seen not to be invasive. This phenomenon is found commonly in epithelial tissues, particularly in the squamous epithelium of the cervix (see Fig. 16.6) and the skin (see Fig. 20.17). This type of lesion is termed *carcinoma in situ* since the cytological features are of a malignant epithelial neoplasm yet the basement membrane is not breached and there is no local invasion or distant metastasis. Other examples of this phenomenon are seen in the breast where cytologically malignant cells may be confined within ducts (intraduct carcinoma) or within lobules (intralobular carcinoma, see Fig. 17.6). The diagnosis of in situ neoplasia is important as such lesions may progress to become invasive, while early detection and treatment at this pre-invasive stage is often completely curative.

Staging of malignant tumours

The extent of local, regional and distant tumour spread is an important determinant of tumour management and prognosis. A number of systems have been devised for defining these characteristics in a standardised fashion; this is known as *staging* of a tumour. The *TNM system* is the most widely used method and involves scoring the extent of local **T**umour spread, regional lymph **N**ode involvement and the presence of distant **M**etastases. Despite advances in diagnostic techniques, the stage of a tumour is generally a very good indicator of likely prognosis. Tumour stage assessment is also important in planning therapy; tumours at an advanced stage (extensive spread) may require aggressive treatment, while early stage tumours (localised) can be treatable by relatively conservative measures.

The TNM method of breast cancer staging is illustrated as follows:

T0 =	breast free of tumour	N0 =	no axillary nodes involved
T1 =	local lesion < 2 cm in size	N1 =	mobile nodes involved
T2 =	lesion 2-5 cm	N2 =	fixed nodes involved
T3 =	skin and/or chest wall involved		

M0 = no metastases,   M1 = demonstrable metastases,   MX = suspected metastases.

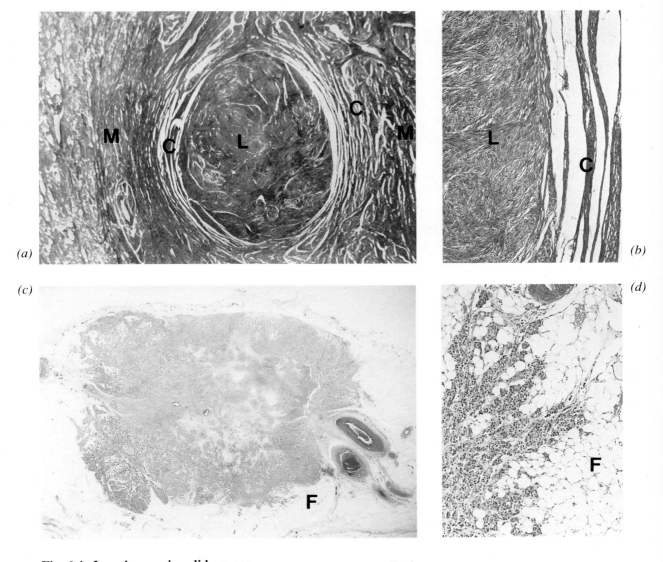

Fig. 6.4 Invasiveness in solid organs
(a) benign neoplasm of myometrium (LP)   **(b) margin of lesion in (a)** (MP)
(c) malignant neoplasm of breast (LP)   **(d) margin of lesion in (c)** (MP)

These micrographs compare the invasive behaviour of benign and malignant neoplasms within solid organs. Micrograph (a) shows a benign neoplasm of the uterine smooth muscle, a leiomyoma **L**, surrounded by normal myometrium **M**. The tumour margin is shown at higher magnification in micrograph (b). Note that the neoplasm is well circumscribed and shows no evidence of local invasion. This neoplasm has expanded symmetrically and compressed the supporting stroma of the myometrium to form a pseudocapsule **C**.

Micrograph (c) illustrates a malignant neoplasm of female breast epithelium; note that the neoplasm has an irregular outline with tongues of neoplastic cells invading the fatty tissue **F** of the breast. There is no tendency to form a capsule. The ill-defined tumour margin is illustrated in micrograph (d) in which dark-staining malignant cells can be seen infiltrating the surrounding adipose tissue.

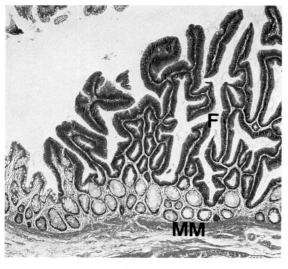

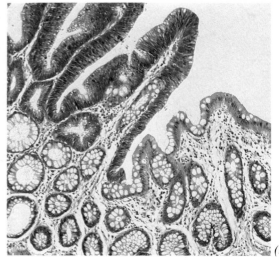

(a)

(b)

(c)

(d)

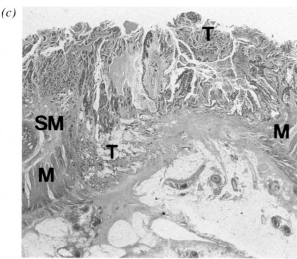

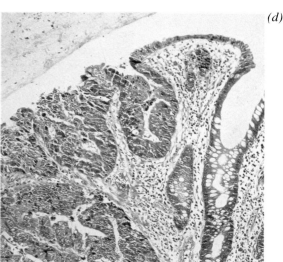

Fig. 6.5 Invasive characteristics of surface neoplasms
(a) non-invasive (benign) neoplasm of surface epithelium (MP)   **(b) same lesion as in (a)** (HP)
(c) invasive (malignant) neoplasm of surface epithelium (LP)   **(d) same lesion as in (c)** (HP)

Benign neoplasms of surface epithelia usually grow in the form of warty, papillary or nodular outgrowths from the surface and show no tendency to infiltrate downward into the subepithelial connective tissue or submucosa. Micrograph (a) shows one form of benign neoplasm occurring in the colon; note that this benign epithelial tumour has grown into the lumen in the form of papillary fronds **F**. The underlying muscularis mucosae **MM** is intact and there is no downward invasion by the tumour; at higher magnification in micrograph (b), the differences between the normal and benign neoplastic epithelium are more readily seen.

Malignant neoplasms of surface epithelium not only grow outward, but also infiltrate across the epithelial basement membrane to spread into subepithelial tissues and further. In micrographs (c) and (d) of a malignant neoplasm of the colon, note that the tumour cells **T** have grown outward into the lumen and have also broken through the epithelial basement membrane invading muscularis mucosae, submucosa **SM** and the muscle **M** of the colon wall. Compare the cytological characteristics of the benign and malignant tumour cells in micrographs (b) and (d) respectively . The malignant cells are disorganised, crowded together and are less differentiated than are the cells of the benign neoplasm.

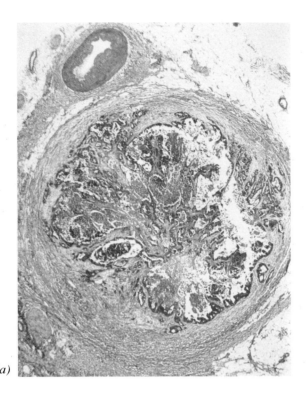

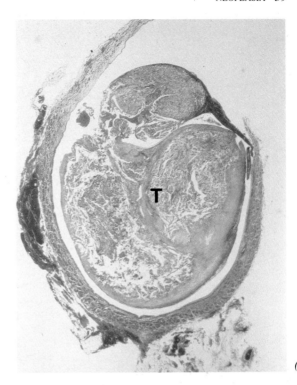

T

(a)

(b)

Fig. 6.6   Blood stream spread of malignant neoplasms
(a) venous spread of malignant colonic neoplasm (MP)
(b) venous spread of malignant renal neoplasm (LP)

The vascular system provides a ready means of spread for many types of malignant tumour *(haematogenous spread)*. Malignant cells gain access to the bloodstream usually through the thin-walled vessels of the venous system; invasion of arterial vessels is rare and tends to result in severe haemorrhage or infarction rather than tumour spread. After infiltrating through the vessel walls, malignant cells may grow along veins in solid cores from which fragments may break off to form *tumour emboli*. Such emboli tend to lodge in the first capillary beds encountered; in the case of most malignancies, these are the pulmonary capillaries, but in the case of gut malignancies, they are the capillaries of the liver. The lungs and liver are therefore frequent sites of metastatic deposition. Small clumps of tumour cells may also pass through liver and lung capillaries and are then distributed by the arterial system throughout the entire body. Brain and bone marrow thus become other common sites for metastatic deposits.

Micrograph (a) provides an example of venous invasion and is taken from the serosa of a colon in which there was an extensive malignant neoplasm. It shows a large serosal vein, the lumen of which contains a solid mass of blue-staining tumour which is growing along the vessel lumen; the site of invasion of the vessel wall was proximal to this section and therefore cannot be seen.

Venous invasion and permeation are particularly common in malignant neoplasms of the kidney, as in micrograph (b). In this case, vessel invasion begins at the thin-walled venous tributaries within the renal parenchyma, but the tumour then rapidly grows as a solid core along the lumina of increasingly large renal vein tributaries until, as shown here, the main renal vein itself becomes filled with tumour **T**. From the renal vein, the tumour may even extend into the inferior vena cava.

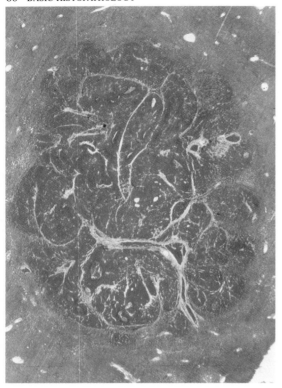

(a)

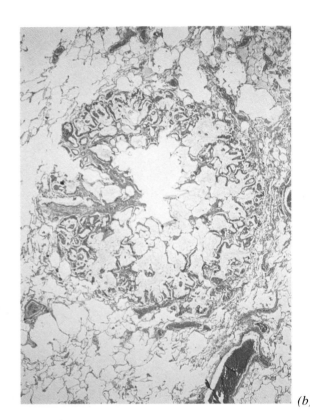

(b)

Fig. 6.7   Metastatic tumour deposits in solid organs
(a) metastatic deposit in liver (LP)
(b) metastatic deposit in lung (LP)

Metastatic deposits of tumour are frequently encountered in liver, lung, bone marrow and brain as a result of haematogenous spread of malignant cells. Other tissues in the body are, by comparison, infrequent sites for deposition of metastatic tumour - for example the heart or skeletal muscle. Certain types of tumour have characteristic patterns of spread; for example malignant tumours of the prostate gland have a propensity to spread to bone. It is thought that the malignant cells and the target organ must express mutually compatible receptors and cell-surface adhesion molecules which facilitate cellular anchorage and subsequent growth promotion; presumably such compatibility is an infrequent occurrence in heart and skeletal muscle.

Micrographs (a) and (b) show examples of hepatic and pulmonary blood-borne metastases respectively. Hepatic metastases often arise from organs drained by the portal system; the lesion in micrograph (a) is from a poorly differentiated primary neoplasm in the stomach. Lung metastases on the other hand arise from tumour emboli from the systemic venous circulation, and micrograph (b) is an example of secondary spread from an ovarian primary lesion.

Metastasis to bone is most commonly seen with malignant epithelial tumours from the breast, bronchus, prostate, kidney and thyroid.

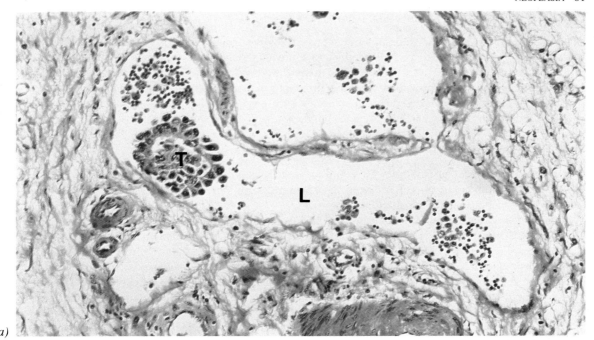

(a)

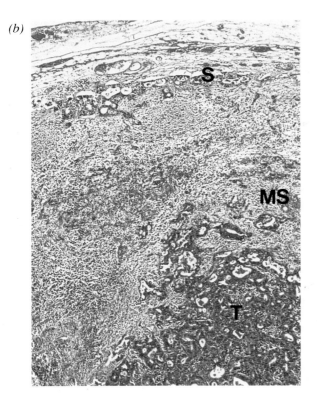

(b)

Fig. 6.8 Lymphatic spread of malignant neoplasm
(a) tumour in lymphatic vessel (HP)
(b) metastasis in a lymph node (MP)

Malignant tumours may invade through the walls of lymphatics, and tumour may then spread along lymphatic channels either by growth of solid cores along the lymphatic lumina, or by fragments breaking off the intralymphatic tumour mass to form emboli which pass in the lymph drainage to regional lymph nodes. Micrograph (a) illustrates a large, valved lymphatic **L** containing an embolic clump of malignant tumour cells **T** *en route* to a lymph node. Tumour embolisation via lymphatics to regional lymph nodes is a very common mode of spread in malignant tumours of epithelial origin. Micrograph (b) shows a lymph node draining a primary malignant tumour of the colon. Having arrived via afferent tributaries, tumour cells have impacted in the subcapsular sinus **S** where they have proliferated to some extent. From here, malignant cells have passed down a medullary sinus **MS** in one area and a small deposit of metastatic tumour **T** is beginning to grow in a new location deep within the node.

Tumour nomenclature and classification

The classification and nomenclature of neoplasia has developed from gross morphological, histological and behavioural observation. Ideally, the name given to a tumour should convey information about the cell of origin and the likely behaviour (either benign or malignant). While this is so for the majority of tumours of epithelial and connective tissues, there are many tumours which are given eponymous or semidescriptive names out of either poor understanding of pathogenesis or long established tradition. Some tumours have several different names which are synonymous but derive from different classifications.

Tumours of epithelial origin

- Benign neoplasms of surface epithelia, e.g. skin, are termed *papillomata* (singular *papilloma*). This term is prefixed by the cell of origin, e.g. squamous papilloma of skin, transitional-cell papilloma of bladder, squamous papilloma of larynx.
- Benign neoplasms of both solid and surface glandular epithelium are termed *adenomata* (singular *adenoma*). This is prefixed by the tissue of origin e.g. thyroid adenoma, salivary gland adenoma. Frequently a benign tumour of surface glandular epithelium (almost always in the large bowel) assumes a papillary growth pattern when it is termed a *villous adenoma*.
- A malignant tumour of any epithelial origin is termed a *carcinoma*. Tumours of glandular epithelium (including that lining the gut) are termed *adenocarcinomas*. Tumours of other epithelia are prefixed by the cell type of origin e.g. squamous cell carcinoma, transitional cell carcinoma. To classify a carcinoma further, the tissue of origin is added, e.g. adenocarcinoma of prostate, adenocarcinoma of breast, squamous carcinoma of larynx.

A more detailed summary of the nomenclature of epithelial tumours is given below in Figure 6.9.

Fig. 6.9 Nomenclature of epithelial tumours

Tissue of origin	Benign	Malignant
Surface epithelium	Papilloma	Carcinoma
Examples		
Squamous	Squamous cell papilloma	Squamous cell carcinoma
Glandular	Adenoma	Adenocarcinoma
(columnar)	(villous or tubular)	
Transitional	Transitional cell papilloma	Transitional cell carcinoma
Solid glandular epithelium	Adenoma	Adenocarcinoma
Examples		
Thyroid	Thyroid adenoma	Thyroid adenocarcinoma
Kidney	Renal adenoma	Renal adenocarcinoma
Liver	Hepatic adenoma	Hepatic adenocarcinoma

Tumours of connective tissue origin

In connective tissues there is a simpler and more descriptive classification of neoplasia. Firstly, the tissue of origin is designated, with the addition of the suffix *-oma* for a benign tumour, or *-sarcoma* for a malignant tumour. As an example, a benign tumour of adipose tissue is termed a lipoma, whilst a malignant tumour of the same origin is termed a liposarcoma. A detailed summary of other connective tissue tumours is shown in Figure 6.10.

Fig. 6.10 Nomenclature of connective tissue tumours

Tissue of origin	Benign	Malignant
Fibrous	Fibroma	Fibrosarcoma
Bone	Osteoma	Osteosarcoma
Cartilage	Chondroma	Chondrosarcoma
Adipose	Lipoma	Liposarcoma
Smooth muscle	Leiomyoma	Leiomyosarcoma
Skeletal muscle	Rhabdomyoma	Rhabdomyosarcoma

Nomenclature of other tumours

There are a variety of other neoplasms which do not fit into either the epithelial or the connective tissue category described above and these are grouped according to their tissue of origin. The main categories are as follows:

- **Lymphomas:** tumours of the lymphoid system (see Ch. 15).

- **Leukaemias:** tumours derived from haemopoietic elements which circulate in the blood and only rarely form tumour masses (see Ch. 15).

- **Embryonal tumours:** tumours of childhood which are believed to derive from primitive embryonal 'blastic' tissue; the most common are nephroblastoma of the kidney (Fig. 14.15) and neuroblastoma of the adrenal medulla (Fig. 19.10).

- **Gliomas:** tumours derived from the non-neural support tissues of the brain (Ch. 22).

- **Germ cell tumours**: tumours derived from germ cells in the gonads (Chs. 16 and 18).

- **Teratomas:** tumours which contain elements of all three embryological germ cell layers –ectoderm, endoderm, and mesoderm; these are most commonly found in the testis and ovary. They vary in malignancy from benign to extremely malignant and are commonest in young people. Teratomas represent complex forms of germ cell tumours.

- **Neuroendocrine tumours**: tumours derived from cells of the neuroendocrine system and which secrete polypeptide hormones or active amines. Examples include phaeochromocytoma of the adrenal medulla (Fig. 19.9), carcinoid tumour of the appendix (Fig. 12.10) and medullary carcinoma of the thyroid (Fig. 4.7). Certain of these tumours are grouped under the term APUD tumours in recognition of functional amine precursor uptake and decarboxylation.

In addition to the system described above, individual tumours may also be known by other names according to function (e.g. insulinoma), histological appearance (e.g. oat cell carcinoma), or by an eponym (e.g. Hodgkin's disease).

Finally, there is a group of tumour-like lesions known as *hamartomas* which represent non-neoplastic overgrowths of tissues indigenous to the site of their occurrence. These are thought to be developmental abnormalities. A common example is the 'port-wine stain' of the skin composed of blood vessels and known as a haemangioma; note that the suffix –oma erroneously implies that this is a benign neoplasm. An example of a haemangioma in the liver is shown in Figure 10.12.

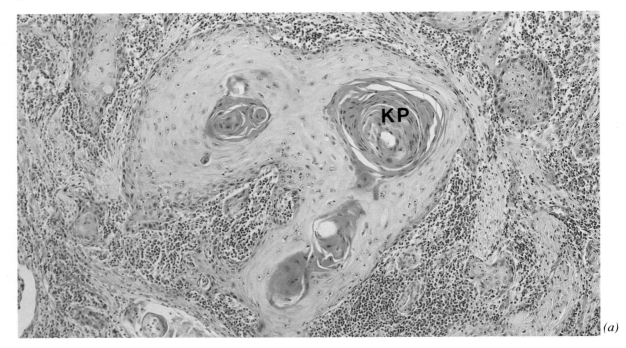

(a)

Fig. 6.11 Squamous cell carcinoma
(a) well-differentiated (HP)
(b) poorly differentiated (HP)

Squamous cell carcinomas may arise in any site of native stratified squamous epithelium, e.g. skin, oesophagus or tongue. They may also arise in stratified squamous epithelium which has formed by the process of metaplasia, e.g. bronchus or urinary bladder.

The degree of differentiation varies widely. Well-differentiated tumours as seen in micrograph (a) have cytological features similar to the prickle cell layer of normal stratified squamous epithelium; the cells are large and slightly fusiform in shape. The nuclei exhibit a moderate degree of pleomorphism, and mitotic figures are not very abundant. The cells are commonly arranged in broad sheets and large clumps, and at very high magnification intercellular bridges (typical of normal prickle cells) may be visible. The most characteristic feature of well-differentiated squamous carcinomas is the formation of keratin which may be seen within individual cells but more often forms lamellated pink-stained masses known as *keratin pearls* **KP**.

In contrast, poorly differentiated squamous carcinomas (b), lose most of their resemblance to normal prickle cells and have a high nucleus-cytoplasmic ratio. Keratin pearl formation is not seen, although individual cell keratinisation **K** may be present. In the most anaplastic squamous carcinomas, the only evidence of cell of origin may be intercellular bridges only visible at high magnification after careful search.

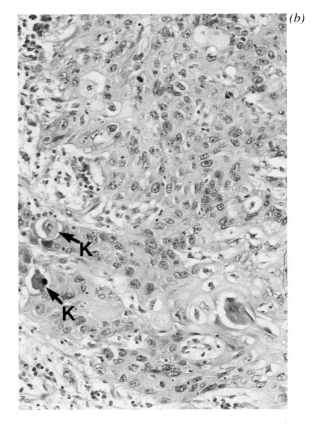

(b)

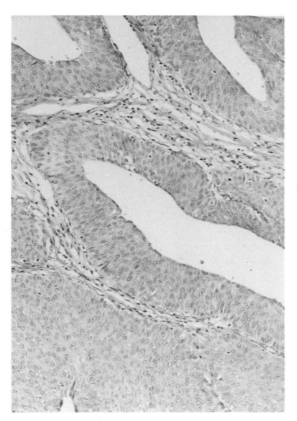

(a)

Fig. 6.12   Transitional cell carcinoma
(a) well-differentiated (papillary) (HP)
(b) poorly differentiated (HP)

These tumours arise almost exclusively from native transitional epithelium in the urinary tract.

The well-differentiated lesions usually adopt a papillary growth pattern (see Fig. 14.16) and the cytological features are almost indistinguishable from those of normal transitional epithelium. Micrograph (a) shows a papillary tumour resembling normal urothelium but with slight nuclear pleomorphism and minimal evidence of mitotic activity.

As the tumours become less differentiated, the growth pattern becomes more solid, and nuclear pleomorphism becomes more marked. In anaplastic tumours it may not be possible to determine the tissue of origin except by knowing that the tumour has arisen in the urinary tract. Micrograph (b) shows a poorly differentiated solid tumour from the bladder wall; note the nests of highly pleomorphic tumour cells **T** invading between bundles of smooth muscle **M**.

(b)

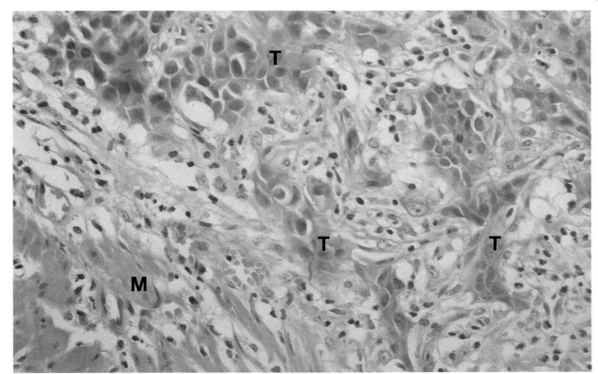

Fig 6.13 Adenocarcinoma
(a) well-differentiated colonic (HP)
(b) poorly differentiated colonic (HP)

Carcinomas which derive from surface glandular epithelium such as large bowel and stomach tend to exhibit a glandular pattern of growth, and such tumours are known as *adenocarcinomas*. The same is true of carcinomas arising in solid glandular tissues such as kidney, breast and prostate, and of tumours of the liver (which in embryological terms develops as an outgrowth of primitive gut epithelium).

Micrograph (a) illustrates a typical well-differentiated adenocarcinoma from the colon. Although it is a carcinoma, it still exhibits a well-formed glandular pattern **G** reminiscent of normal colon; the cells are, however, hyperchromatic, have a high nuclear-cytoplasmic ratio and numerous mitoses **M** are seen. Unlike the normal colon, the glandular pattern is irregular and there is little evidence of mucin secretion.

Poorly differentiated adenocarcinoma, shown in micrograph (b) displays no tendency to form a glandular pattern and the cells are extremely pleomorphic. The only evidence of its glandular origin is the presence of occasional cells with a secretory vacuole **V** containing mucin. In these cells, the nucleus is displaced to one side giving rise to the term *signet cells* from their supposed resemblance to signet rings. Signet cells from gastric carcinoma are illustrated in Figure 12.8 (c and d).

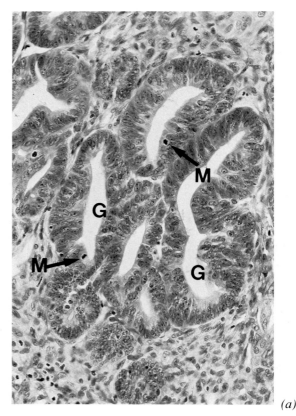

(a)

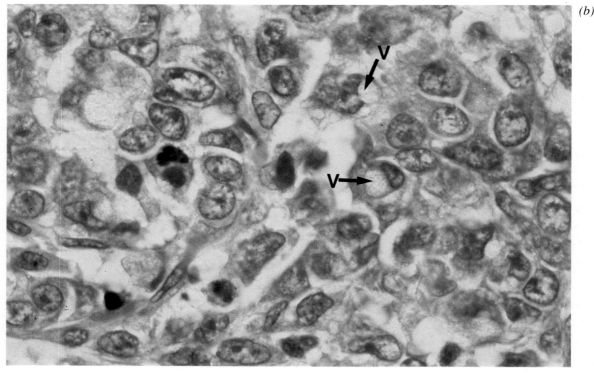

(b)

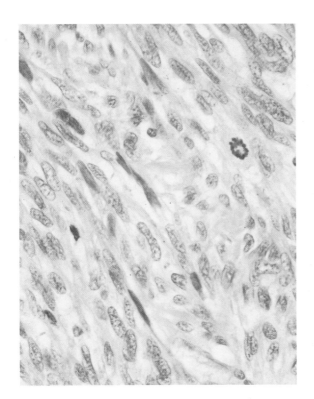

Fig. 6.14 Sarcoma (HP)

Sarcomas are malignant tumours derived from connective tissues including adipose tissue, bone, cartilage and smooth muscle. Many sarcomas resemble the tissue of origin either cytologically, structurally or by producing characteristic extracellular materials such as collagen and ground substance. For example, fibrosarcomas produce collagen; liposarcomas have intracellular lipid vacuoles and chondrosarcomas produce cartilagenous ground substance.

Poorly differentiated sarcomas may not show any evidence of tissue of origin and consist of pleomorphic, spindle-shaped cells with numerous mitotic figures. Such tumours are termed *spindle cell sarcomas* or *undifferentiated sarcomas*. Immunohistochemistry and electron microscopy are frequently used in attempts to ascertain the cell of origin in poorly differentiated sarcomas.

This micrograph shows a sarcoma derived from uterine smooth muscle. The tumour cells are spindle-shaped and resemble normal smooth muscle cells. However, they have large pleomorphic nuclei with evident mitoses; this is thus a *leiomyosarcoma*.

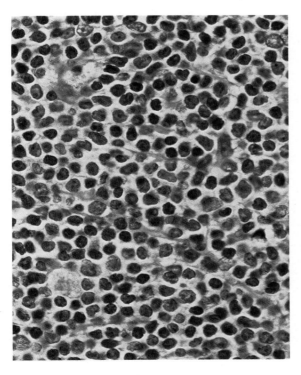

Fig. 6.15 Lymphoma (HP)

Lymphomas are a group of solid tumours derived from cells of the lymphoreticular system. They tend to be confined to lymphoid organs such as lymph nodes, spleen and bone marrow, but may spread to other tissues particularly the skin, liver and CNS; occasionally primary lymphomas arise from specialised lymphoid tissue such as in the gastrointestinal tract or salivary gland.

Histologically, lymphomas consist of sheets of lymphoid cells arranged either diffusely or in a follicular pattern. These neoplasms can be divided into good-prognosis and poor-prognosis types on the basis of cell proliferation rate and differentiation. Lymphomas are discussed in detail in Chapter 15.

This micrograph illustrates a poor-prognosis malignant lymphoma composed of diffuse sheets of large lymphoid cells with no evidence of follicular formation. Such tumours may have a rapidly progressive clinical course and respond poorly to treatment.

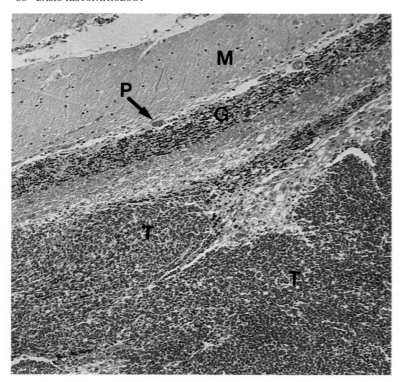

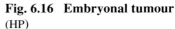

Fig. 6.16 Embryonal tumour (HP)

Embryonal tumours are derived from cells similar to those of various primitive embryonal tissues. They usually present in childhood, are rapidly growing and many are highly malignant. The tumour cells are small with blue-staining nuclei and very little cytoplasm whatever the organ of origin, giving rise to the term *small blue-cell tumour*.

This micrograph shows such a primitive tumour (termed a *medullo-blastoma*) arising in the cerebellum. The tumour **T** is composed of sheets of very small cells; note the inner granular **G** and outer molecular layers **M** of the cerebellum with normal intervening Purkinje cells **P**.

Other examples are the *nephro-blastoma* (Wilms' tumour) of the kidney (see Fig. 14.15) and *neuroblastoma* of the adrenal gland (see Fig. 19.10).

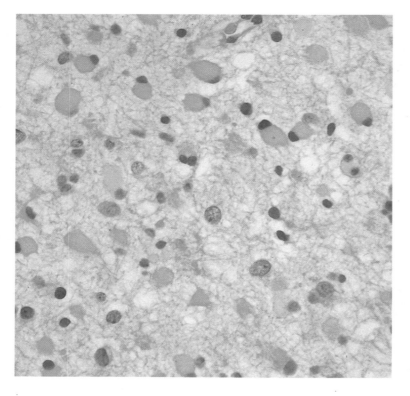

Fig. 6.17 Glioma (HP)

Tumours derived from CNS support cells are known as *gliomas* and are classified according to the cell of origin, e.g. astrocytes or oligodendro-cytes. Like tumours elsewhere, gliomas exhibit varying degrees of differentiation which correspond to prognosis.

Well-differentiated gliomas closely resemble normal glial cells, while poorly differentiated gliomas show cellular pleomorphism and necrosis. Gliomas spread by diffuse infiltration of brain tissues and may also grow into the meninges: metastasis from gliomas to tissues outside the CNS is very rare.

This micrograph shows an *astrocytoma* composed of large pink-staining neoplastic astrocytes which have replaced an area of white matter in the brain. This is a moderately well -differentiated glioma. Other gliomas are shown in Figures 22.9 to 22.11.

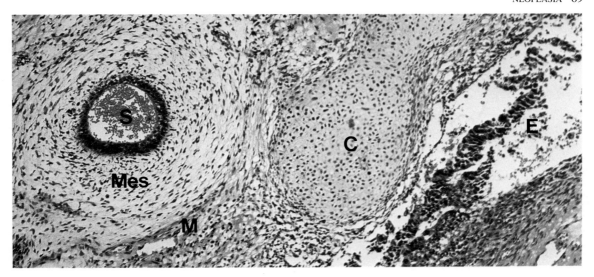

Fig 6.18   Teratoma (HP)

Teratomas are tumours derived from germ cells and most commonly arise in the testis or ovary. The tumours contain neoplastic tissues derived from all of the three germ cell layers, endoderm, mesoderm and ectoderm (including neurectoderm) and thus can contain tissues as diverse as skin, teeth, thyroid, brain and muscle. The tumours range from benign to highly malignant.

A malignant teratoma of the testis is shown in this micrograph. Respiratory type epithelium has formed a cystic space **S** into which haemorrhage has occurred. This is surrounded by pale mesenchyme-like tissue **Mes**. There is also immature cartilage **C** and bands of smooth muscle **M**. An area of desquamated epithelium **E** of indeterminate type is also seen. When a malignant teratoma metastasises, all these tissue elements may be present in the secondary deposits.

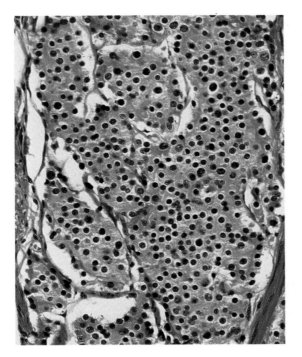

Fig. 6.19   Neuroendocrine tumour (HP)

The neuroendocrine cell system is composed of a diverse group of cells which synthesise and secrete peptide and amine hormones. Neoplasms in this group of tissues are known as *neuroendocrine tumours* and many are considered tumours of *APUD* type. They may be benign or malignant and mainly arise in the gastrointestinal tract, the pancreas, adrenal and thyroid glands. A functional classification is applied where the secretory product can be identified, e.g. *insulinoma, gastrinoma* and *glucagon-oma*, however, many neuroendocrine tumours have no identifiable secretory product. By long usage, the neuro-endocrine cell tumours which secrete 5-hydroxy-tryptamine are termed *carcinoid tumours*.

Neuroendocrine tumours have certain common histological features. As shown in this micrograph, the cells are relatively small and uniform with prominent, round nuclei and characteristic granular cytoplasm due to the presence of secretory granules; these may be demon-strated using special stains as in Figure 12.10 (b) or immunohistochemistry. Electron microscopy may also be used to identify cells according to the ultrastructural features of the secretory granules.

7. Atherosclerosis

Introduction

The walls of arterial vessels are composed of smooth muscle, elastin and collagen which together make up a resilient system for maintaining vascular tone. Alterations in the relative amounts of these specialised elements leads to hardening, thickening and loss of elasticity of vessel walls and is a major cause of illness and death, particularly in affluent societies. The term *arteriosclerosis* is often used as a general descriptive term for such diseases.

The commonest type of arteriosclerosis is that affecting large and medium sized arteries in which the underlying histopathological lesion is *atheroma;* this form of arteriosclerosis is thus known as *atherosclerosis.* Other forms of arteriosclerosis occur, such as thickening of the walls of arterioles in association with hypertension (Figs. 10.6 and 10.7); from a histopathological and clinical point of view, however, atherosclerosis is the condition of overwhelming importance.

To some extent, atherosclerotic changes can be demonstrated in large and medium-sized arteries in almost all adults, however, pathological consequences mainly occur in association with severe atherosclerosis. The factors predisposing to severe lesions with a high incidence of complications are now well recognized and can be divided into constitutional factors, those which have a major effect on atheroma formation (hard risk factors) and those with a weaker association with the development of atheroma (soft risk factors); these are summarised in Figure 7.1. In addition to epidemiological risk factors, many of the cellular pathogenic mechanisms giving rise to arterial wall disease have now been determined.

Fig. 7.1 Risk factors in atherosclerosis

Constitutional risk factors

Age	Incidence of severe disease rises with each decade up to 85 years
Sex	Higher in males up to the age of 75
Genetic	Some families have increased risk independent from other risk factors

Hard risk factors   (Large contribution to incidence; potentially avoidable or treatable)

Hyperlipidaemia	Particularly hypercholesterolaemia
Hypertension	Especially after the age of 45
Smoking	Predominant atherogenic effects in the aorta and coronary vessels
Diabetes	Particularly in coronary, cerebral, and peripheral arteries

Soft risk factors   (Small contribution to incidence in statistical studies)

Lack of regular exercise

Obesity

Stressful lifestyle

Pathology of atheroma

The normal arterial intima is a delicate layer of fibroelastic connective tissue lined on its luminal aspect by a layer of endothelial cells. In elastic arteries (such as the aorta and carotid arteries), the intima is bounded externally by the interspersed layers of elastic tissue and smooth muscle which make up the media, whereas in muscular arteries (such as the coronary and tibial arteries), the intima is separated from the muscular tunica media by a discrete internal elastic lamina. The intima contains scattered spindle-shaped cells termed *myointimal cells* which can adopt a variety of different functions including collagen and elastin synthesis as a form of fibroblast, contractility as a form of smooth muscle cell and phagocytic activity as a form of histiocytic cell.

In outline, the atheromatous lesion first begins in the intima by the accumulation of lipids in the myointimal cells, many of which become vacuolated and are termed *foam cells*. This stage is represented macroscopically by the *fatty streak*. While it is likely that most fatty streaks do not progress further, this is most likely to be the early lesion of atheroma. Lesions progressively enlarge by further accumulation of intracellular lipid which also becomes extracellular following death and breakdown of some myointimal cells. The endothelial layer becomes ulcerated over these lipid accumulations and further lipid is derived from *blood platelets* which adhere to exposed intimal collagen and become incorporated into the atheromatous lesion. At this stage the lesion is termed a *lipid plaque*. Platelet-derived growth factors facilitate the proliferation of myointimal cells which produce collagen. Smooth muscle cells also migrate from the medial layer into the intimal layer with fragmentation of the internal elastic lamina. At this stage the atheromatous lesion is represented macroscopically by the raised *fibrous plaque*. Further development of the atheromatous plaque is accompanied by endothelial ulceration and incorporation of organised thrombus into the lesion with further fibrosis and lipid accumulation. The media of the vessel undergoes atrophy and specialised elastic tissue and smooth muscle is replaced by collagen. Calcification and haemorrhage may also occur in the developed atheromatous plaque. These form so-called *complicated atheromatous plaques* which characterise the advanced form of atherosclerosis. The structure of an atheromatous plaque is shown diagrammatically in Figure 7.2 and illustrated in Figures 7.3 and 7.4.

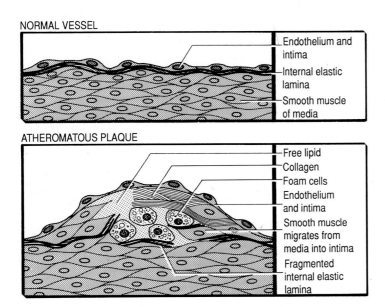

Fig. 7.2 Components of an atheromatous plaque

Consequences of atheroma

Atherosclerosis may affect all arterial vessels but the aorta, cerebral, carotid and ilio-femoral arteries are those that tend to be most severely affected and those which result in significant clinical disease.

The most important pathological and clinical sequelae of atherosclerosis are:

- **Occlusion**: narrowing of the arterial lumen produces partial or complete obstruction to blood flow; this may result in ischaemia and infarction of the tissue supplied by the atheromatous vessel (Chapter 9).

- **Thrombosis**: endothelial ulceration stimulates formation of an overlying thrombus (blood clot). This may occlude the vessel at the site of thrombosis or fragments may become detached to forms an embolus which blocks one or more smaller vessels distally (Chapter 8).

- **Aneurysm**: loss of muscle and elastin from the media causes weakening of the vessel wall, predisposing to a localised area of dilatation; such a dilatation is known as an aneurysm. Rupture of the weakened and aneurysmally dilated artery wall is a further serious complication and is seen most commonly in the abdominal aorta.

The main histopathological complications are shown in Figures 7.5 to 7.8.

Fig. 7.3   Early atheromatous lesions (*illustrations opposite*)
(a) early atheromatous plaque (LP)
(b) foam cells and lipid (HP)

These two micrographs show the early changes of atheroma in the aorta. Micrograph (a) shows a pale-staining area of thickening in the intima **I** representing an early atheromatous lesion. It consists of aggregated myointimal cells containing lipid, and some intimal fibrous tissue. Because such lesions appear macroscopically as slightly raised flat areas, they are termed *atheromatous plaques*. Note that the medial layer of the vessel **M** is uniform and appears normal at this stage; early atheroma is a disease confined to the intima.

At higher power, a detail of the intimal thickening is shown in micrograph (b). Foam cells **F** filled with lipid appear as large, pale-staining cells with very vacuolated cytoplasm. These cells are products of both myointimal cells and macrophages. As the lesion progresses, some of the foam cells break down and liberate free lipid into the intima where it is represented by non-staining angular clefts **C.** The presence of free lipid appears to induce a fibrous reaction in the surrounding tissues which appear eosinophilic (pink-staining) due to the presence of increased amounts of collagen.

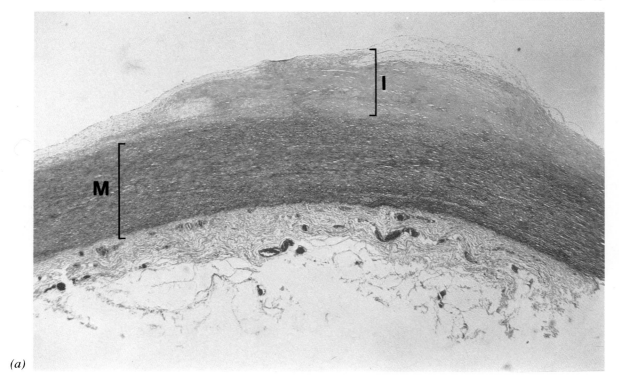

(a)

(b)

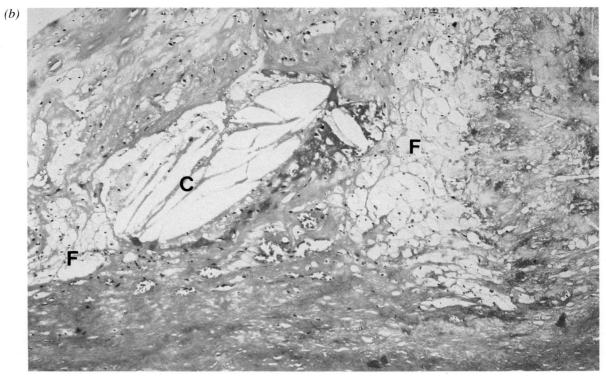

Fig. 7.3 Early atheromatous lesions *(caption opposite)*

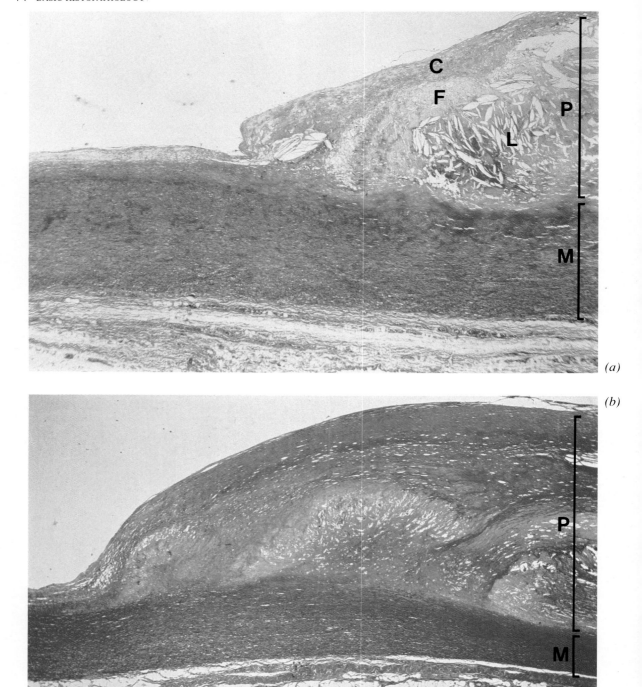

Fig. 7.4   Fibrous atheromatous plaques *(caption opposite)*

Fig. 7.4 Fibrous atheromatous plaques *(illustrations opposite)*
(a) fibrolipid plaque (LP)
(b) fibrous plaque (LP)

Early intimal atheromatous lesions enlarge by further accumulation of lipid in foam cells and also free within the extracellular intimal tissue. This is associated with a more marked fibrotic response in the intima leading to increased thickening of the plaque. Once a more significant degree of fibrous tissue develops in an atheromatous lesion, it is termed a fibrolipid plaque.

Micrograph (a) shows a section of aorta with part of a fibrolipid plaque **P**. Note the areas of nonstaining lipid **L** surrounded by pink-staining fibrous tissue **F**, making up the thickened intima. A zone of denser, more intensely stained fibrous tissue, sometimes termed a fibrous cap **C**, runs between the endothelial surface and the underlying

fibrolipid aggregate. With progression of the lesion, the fibrous cap thickens and the intimal lesion becomes larger and more raised. Micrograph (b) shows such a plaque **P**, being composed mostly of fibrous tissue. Note in both micrographs that there is early thinning of the tunica media **M** beneath the plaque compared to the adjacent normal vessel wall. This is the result of loss of supporting elastic tissue, atrophy of smooth muscle cells and progressive medial fibrosis. With time, the medial fibrous tissue stretches due to loss of elastic recoil in the vessel wall, and the vessel dilates. This dilatation is the basis of the formation of an *atheromatous aneurysm*.

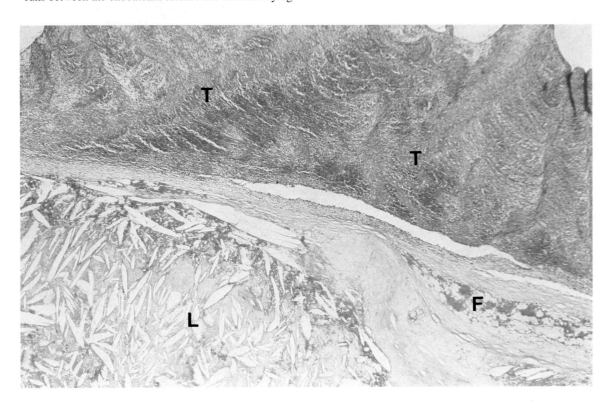

Fig. 7.5 Complicated atheroma (MP)

As an atheromatous plaque enlarges it may become very thick relative to the normal thickness of the vessel wall, and in addition to lipid, foam cells and fibrous tissue, calcium may be deposited in the lesion. With thickening and fibrosis, the blood supply to the abnormal intima may become insufficient and the lesion may undergo necrosis and surface ulceration; this is then described as a *complicated atheromatous lesion*. The normal smooth endothelial lining having gone, the collagen and lipid of

the atheromatous lesion are exposed directly to the blood flow. The coagulation sequence is thus activated and thrombus is formed on the vessel wall at the site of ulcerated atheroma (see Ch. 8).

This micrograph shows the top of an atheromatous plaque with foam cells **F** and lipid **L**. The surface has ulcerated and is encrusted with thrombus **T** composed of fibrin, platelets and entrapped blood cells. In a small vessel, such a thrombus can occlude the lumen.

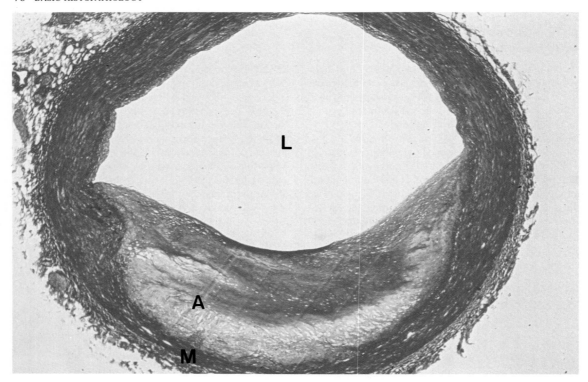

Fig. 7.6   Arterial narrowing by atheroma (LP)

The formation of a large plaque of atheroma **A** in the intima of a small or medium-sized artery, such as the coronary artery branch shown here, can greatly reduce the size of the lumen **L**. The consequent reduction in blood flow leads to ischaemia of the tissues supplied, in this case the myocardium. Note that the media **M** underlying the thickest mass of atheroma is markedly thinned. Such partly occlusive atheroma is very frequent in the coronary arteries of cigarette-smoking males, particularly in the region of the bifurcation of the left coronary artery. A frequent symptom of this arterial narrowing is the condition known as *angina pectoris*, a gripping pain in the chest particularly experienced on exertion, and settling with rest. This pain is a manifestation of ischaemia of the myocardium, and patients with long-standing angina often show replacement of small areas of myocardial muscle by fibrous scar tissue, the end result of anoxic necrosis of muscle fibres.

   Luminal narrowing by atheroma occurs similarly in many other arteries. In the leg arteries, such changes can produce severe calf pain on walking *(intermittent claudication)* and may eventually lead to the development of gangrene of the lower leg. In the vertebrobasilar arterial system which supplies the cerebellum and brain stem, severe atheroma can produce transient ischaemia manifest clinically as dizziness, loss of balance and occasional unconsciousness *(vertebro-basilar syndrome)*.

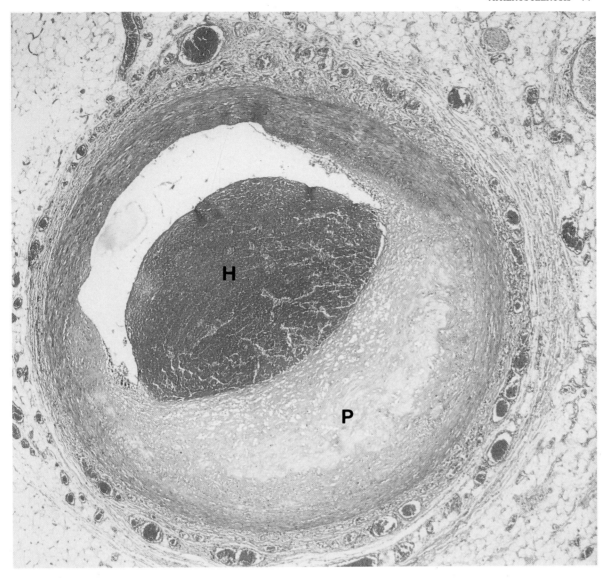

Fig. 7.7   Haemorrhage into atheromatous plaque (LP)

There are two possible mechanisms for the development of haemorrhage in an atheromatous plaque. Firstly, the rigid fibrotic plaque may split under the constant trauma of pulsatile movements and allow blood from the vessel lumen to greatly expand the plaque lesion; such a process is termed *plaque fissuring*. Alternatively, small capillary vessels which develop in established plaques may rupture and lead to haemorrhage. Whatever the mechanism, because of the confined space in which such apparently trivial haemorrhage occurs, the consequences can be disproportionately devastating. In this micrograph, a small haemorrhage **H** has occurred in the superficial area of fibrolipid atheromatous plaque **P**; the accumulated blood

has tracked beneath the non-ulcerated endothelium, causing it to bulge markedly into the artery. This has led to even greater narrowing of a lumen already reduced to about half its normal size by the pre-existing atheromatous plaque. Such an abrupt reduction in arterial flow leads to acute ischaemia in the supplied tissues.

In this patient, the lesion was situated in the anterior descending branch of the left coronary artery and resulted in a substantial area of the anterior wall of the left ventricle and the anterior half of the interventricular septum becoming acutely ischaemic. Necrosis of heart muscle ensued, a process known as *myocardial infarction*, resulting in this patient's death (Fig. 9.2).

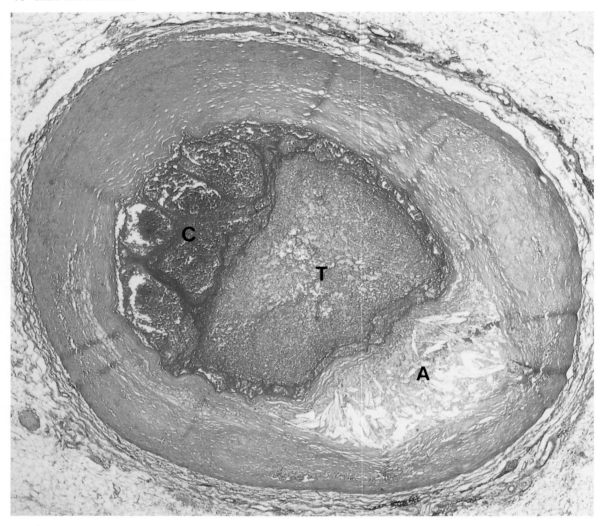

Fig 7.8   Thrombus formation on atheroma (LP)

The most important complication of atheroma in small and medium-sized arteries is the development of a thrombus on the surface of an atheromatous plaque; the process of thrombus formation is discussed in detail in Chapter 8. Thrombus, which consists of a mass of platelets and insoluble fibrin, tends, in the arterial system, to form on any intimal surface which is damaged and roughened. Endothelial ulceration over an atheromatous plaque is the commonest cause of intimal roughening in the arterial system, although plaque fissuring as discussed in Figure 7.7 can also initiate thrombosis.

This micrograph of a coronary artery shows an ulcerated atheromatous plaque **A** which has already significantly constricted the arterial lumen. A thrombus **T** has then developed on the ulcerated surface, largely obliterating the remaining lumen. The thrombus is deep pink in colour, and is composed of fibrin and platelets. The residual lumen is occupied by bright red postmortem blood coagulum **C** composed entirely of tightly packed red blood cells. The naked eye distinction between genuine antemortem thrombus and postmortem coagulum is important; thrombus is pinkish red, granular and firm, whereas coagulum is predominantly dark red, shiny and jelly-like.

When thrombus formation occurs on an atheromatous lesion in a large diameter artery, such as the aorta or carotid arteries, the thrombus may be small and cause little significant obstruction to blood flow at the site. Fragments of thrombus may, however, become detached and pass into the peripheral circulation to block a smaller vessel and cause ischaemia or infarction in its area of distribution. This phenomenon is known as thrombo-embolism and is described more fully in Chapter 8.

8. Thrombosis and embolism

Thrombosis

The vascular system normally contains fluid blood, however, it is often necessary for blood to coagulate to prevent bleeding following injury to vessel walls. To facilitate haemostasis, there are systems which either promote or inhibit the process of blood coagulation. Under certain pathological circumstances, these dynamics may be disrupted leading to the formation of a solid mass of blood products in a vessel lumen; this process is known as *thrombosis,* and the mass of blood products is referred to as a *thrombus*. It is important to distinguish thrombosis, a dynamic process occurring in flowing blood, from coagulation which is a process which takes place in static blood and involves coagulation factors only.

Thrombus consists of aggregations of platelets bound together by fibrin strands with variable numbers of erythrocytes and leucocytes trapped in the tangled mass and contributing to the bulk of the thrombus. Thrombosis may occur in any part of the circulation but most particularly in large veins, large arteries, in the heart chambers and on heart valves. Three major factors, alone or in combination, predispose to thrombosis. These are often referred to as *Virchoff's triad*.

- Damage to the vessel wall, particularly the endothelium, is the main cause of arterial and intra-cardiac thrombosis; in arteries it is due to atheroma, in the heart by endocardial damage (Fig.8.3).
- Disordered blood flow. Stasis is important in initiating thrombus in slow-flowing blood such as in veins. Turbulent blood flow predisposes to thrombus formation in arterial vessels and the heart.
- Abnormally enhanced haemostatic properties of the blood. Increased platelet concentration or stickiness, or factors promoting blood clotting or diminished fibrinolysis contribute to both arterial and venous thrombosis. Changes in blood viscosity such as occur in dehydration, major illness, carcinomatosis and the postoperative state are included in this category.

Unlike a blood clot formed in vitro or post-mortem, a thrombus has a defined architecture and consistency which reflects the manner and stages of its formation and the nature of blood flow in the vicinity. For example, thrombus formed in an artery is usually dense and composed mainly of aggregated platelets and fibrin, whereas thrombus formed in slowed or static blood more closely resembles clotted blood in that it contains masses of erythrocytes and leucocytes. The initial events in thrombus formation are shown diagrammatically in Figure 8.1.and histological appearances in Figure 8.2

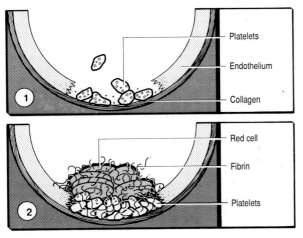

Fig. 8.1 Early thrombogenesis

(1) Following endothelial injury, platelets adhere to exposed subendothelial collagen, mediated via von Willebrand factor, and become activated, liberating ADP and thromboxane A2 which mediate further platelet aggregation.

(2) Platelets undergo degranulation and their products, together with released tissue factors, activate the coagulation cascade. This results in generation of thrombin which converts fibrinogen to fibrin. Red cells become passively entrapped in the generated fibrin-platelet mesh, the number depending on the circumstances of thrombus formation; in arteries there are few red cells and more platelets and fibrin, whereas in veins there are generally many more red cells.

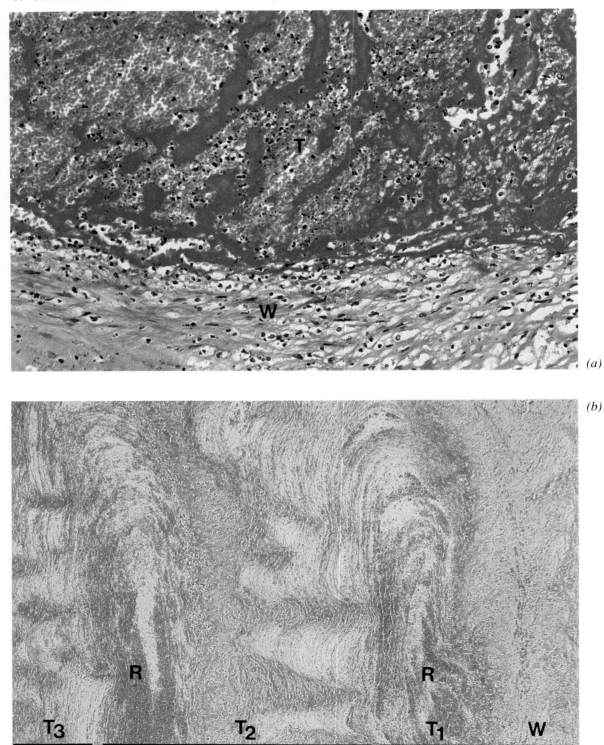

(a)

(b)

Fig. 8.2 Thrombus formation *(caption opposite)*

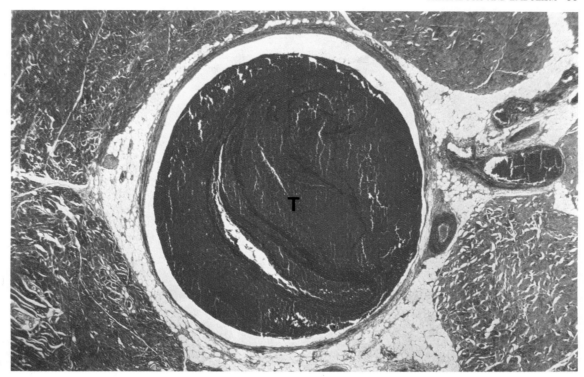

(c)

Fig. 8.2 Thrombus formation *(illustrations (a) and (b) opposite)*
(a) early thrombus (HP)
(b) enlargement of thrombus (MP)
(c) thrombosis in a vein (LP)

Damage of a vessel wall usually involves damage to the endothelial lining and exposure of intimal collagen resulting in first adherence, and then aggregation, of platelets at the site of damage. Tissue damage and collagen exposure also activate the extrinsic and intrinsic blood clotting systems respectively, the latter system also depending on release of platelet factor 3 from aggregated platelets. The result is activation of prothrombin to thrombin, which in turn catalyses the conversion of soluble plasma fibrinogen into insoluble fibrin. Thus the flimsy platelet aggregates become bound together into a solid resilient mass, the thrombus.

Micrograph (a) illustrates an arterial wall **W** damaged by atheroma. The endothelium has become ulcerated with the formation of thrombus **T** at the site of injury. This thrombus consists of platelet aggregates within a meshwork of eosinophilic fibrin; entrapped erythrocytes and leucocytes are present, but are not themselves involved in the specific haemostatic processes.

Small areas of thrombus formed on vessel walls may be resolved completely by fibrinolytic mechanisms; however, under appropriate conditions, the thrombus continues to enlarge. Micrograph (b) illustrates this process. The abnormal vessel wall **W** has become coated by a thin layer of fibrin and platelet thrombus T_1, with entrapped red cells **R**. This has formed the basis for the deposition of another layer of fibrin-platelet thrombus T_2, again with entrapped red cells. A third layer T_3 can be seen forming at the left of the picture. Thus thrombi enlarge by the successive deposition of a number of layers, a feature which is apparent to the naked eye in the laminated cut surface seen in an established thrombus *(lines of Zahn)*.

In the arterial system , damage to the intimal layer is the most common predisposing factor in thrombus formation, but in the venous system the most important factor is the rate of blood flow; reduced flow rates increase susceptibility to thrombus formation.

Micrograph (c) shows venous thrombosis **T** completely occluding the lumen of a vein in a neurovascular bundle from the muscle of the calf. This is known as *deep vein thrombosis* (DVT) and is most frequently seen in postoperative patients who are confined to bed.

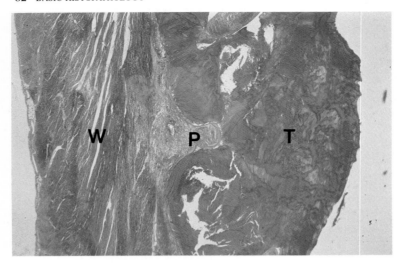

Fig. 8.3 Left ventricular mural thrombus (LP)

Thrombus within the heart chambers most commonly occurs upon endocardium damaged by myocardial infarction (see Fig. 9.2). This micrograph illustrates infarcted ventricular wall **W** with mural thrombus **T** laid down on the luminal surface; the thrombus surrounds a papillary muscle **P**.

The left ventricle is the most common site of mural thrombosis after myocardial infarction.

Consequences of thrombosis

There are two main consequences of thrombosis: vascular obstruction and embolisation.

Vascular obstruction

Thrombus may partially or completely occlude a vessel lumen. This is particularly common in the deep veins of the legs in immobilised, debilitated patients, and results in obstruction of venous return from the feet and lower legs causing oedema (Fig. 8.2 c). Thrombus forming on the surface of atheroma in an artery may occlude the vessel causing ischaemic damage to tissues distal to the obstruction. This may lead to tissue death (infarction), as discussed in Chapter 9.

Embolisation

Embolism is the process in which any abnormal mass forming in, or entering, the bloodstream passes with the circulation to lodge in an organ with resulting pathological consequences; the abnormal mass is known as an *embolus*. Emboli are most commonly caused by detachment of all or part of a thrombus from its site of formation and this form of embolism, often called *thrombo-embolism*, is of the greatest clinical importance. Stasis of blood resulting from occlusion or partial obstruction of blood flow by thrombus may lead to propagation of the thrombus in the static blood. As previously outlined, thrombus formed in such conditions contains many blood cells and relatively less fibrin and is thereby much more prone to become detached to form a thrombo-embolus. For example, following deep venous thrombosis in the leg, the thrombus may propagate as far as the common iliac vein or even the inferior vena cava; such a huge thrombus may readily become detached and pass via the right side of the heart to the pulmonary arterial tree as a pulmonary embolus which is often fatal (see Fig. 8.4).

Systemic arterial thrombo-emboli most commonly arise from the heart or major arteries, in such cases the thrombus often covers only part of the luminal wall as a plaque-like structure and is known as *mural thrombus*; for example, mural thrombus may form on the ventricular endocardium following a myocardial infarct (Fig. 8.3) or in an aneurysmal dilatation or on an atheromatous lesion in the aorta (Fig. 7.5). Emboli which arise in the arterial system impact in peripheral arterial vessels where the most dramatic outcome is necrosis of the tissue supplied *(infarction)* described in detail in the next chapter.

Whilst thrombotic emboli are the most common, emboli may also arise from other sources. These include atheromatous debris, clumps of tumour cells, bacterial vegetations from infected heart valves, fat and bone marrow after bone fracture, air entering the circulation, and rarely amniotic fluid in cases of complicated pregnancy.

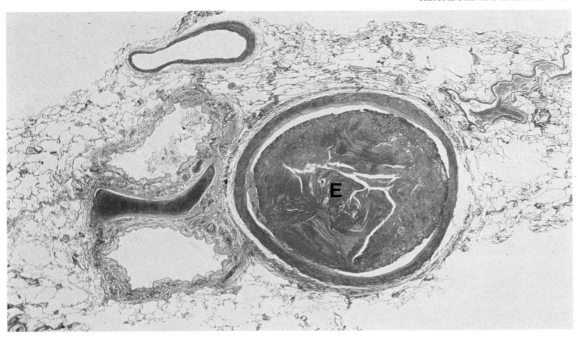

Fig. 8.4 Thrombo-embolism: pulmonary embolus (LP)

When fragments of thrombus become detached from their site of formation, they travel in the circulation (venous or arterial, according to site of origin) as thrombo-emboli. On reaching vessels of small enough calibre to prevent further passage, the thrombo-emboli impact producing sudden vascular occlusion. Depending on the size of the thrombo-embolus, the tissue or organ involved and the extent of alternative vascular supply, the result may be either inadequate blood flow for normal sustenance of the tissue (ischaemia) or frank tissue necrosis (infarction); these phenomena are described in the next chapter.

This micrograph illustrates lung tissue in which the pulmonary artery branch is occluded by an embolus **E** originating from thrombus in the deep veins of the leg.

This condition, known as pulmonary embolism, is an important cause of sudden death, especially in debilitated or immobilised patients predisposed to deep venous thrombosis.

Outcome of vascular thrombosis

Whether a thrombus arises *in situ* or by embolisation from elsewhere it may be dealt with in one of two ways:

- **Resolution.** This involves the normal physiological phenomenon of fibrinolysis as well as autolytic disintegration of the cellular elements of the clot, and the end result is complete dissolution with restoration of blood flow.

- **Organisation**. Ingrowth of granulation tissue from the vessel wall and subsequent fibrous repair occurs when fibrinolysis is ineffective in removing the thrombus. By an extraordinary mechanism, the organised thrombus may undergo *recanalisation,* a process whereby new vascular channels are formed to re-establish a patent lumen. The processes of organisation and recanalisation are illustrated over the page in Figure 8.5.

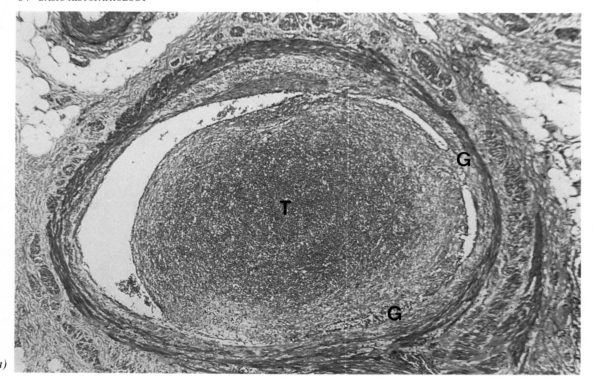

(a)

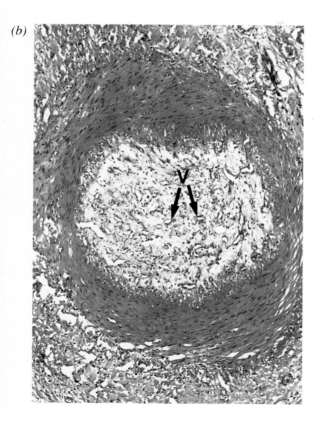

(b)

Fig. 8.5 Fate of thrombi
(a) organisation (LP)
(b) recanalisation (MP)

Following occlusion of a vessel by thrombus, there
is an initial inflammatory response in the vessel
wall. Eventually, the thrombus becomes organised
by ingrowth of granulation tissue from the intima of
the vessel wall. Micrograph (a) shows a vein
occluded by thrombus **T**. At various points,
granulation tissue **G** extends from the vessel wall
into the thrombus. This eventually results in
replacement of the thrombus by fibrovascular
granulation tissue. In some cases, larger vessels
develop within the fibrovascular granulation tissue
of the organising thrombus and may permit passage
of blood through the damaged, previously occluded
area. This occurs most commonly in arteries and is
termed *recanalisation.*

Micrograph (b) illustrates this process in an artery
which has been occluded by thrombus and is at a
later stage of organisation than in micrograph (a).
Note that the granulation tissue in the lumen
contains numerous small blood vessels **V**. These
vessels may conduct blood across the thrombosed
area and some will enlarge with time and acquire
smooth muscle walls.

9. Infarction

Introduction

Infarction occurs in any tissue when there is interruption of blood supply sufficient to cause tissue necrosis; the area of tissue involved is described as an *infarct*. Disturbance of blood supply may not always be sufficient to cause frank tissue necrosis but may instead cause temporary or permanent damage to the tissue or some of its functional elements; this situation is known as *ischaemia* and may in due course, though not necessarily, lead to infarction.

Causes of infarction

Infarction may result either from obstruction of arterial supply or, much less commonly, from obstruction of venous drainage.

- **Arterial infarction** is usually due to complete blockage of an artery by thrombosis or embolism. Arterial thrombosis is generally a complication of pre-existing atheroma (Fig. 7.8). Embolisation in the arterial system is most commonly from the heart, either mural thrombus (Fig. 8.3) or from thrombus occurring on heart valves (vegetations: see page 96); examples of infarcts from the kidney and myocardium are shown in Figures 9.1 and 9.2 respectively.

- **Venous infarction** is most commonly due to mechanical compression of the vascular supply, particularly in organs which receive their blood supply via a vascular pedicle. Such organs may become infarcted if the pedicle becomes twisted, e.g. torsion of the testis (Fig. 18.6) or constricted by becoming entrapped in a narrow space, e.g. bowel infarction due to hernial strangulation (Fig. 9.5). In such cases venous obstruction occurs as extrinsic pressure affects the thin-walled, low-pressure veins without initially compromising the arteries; tissues become massively suffused with red cells, and prolonged venous obstruction eventually causes the tissue to become ischaemic due to stasis of blood. The resulting cessation in tissue perfusion results in overt infarction. Venous infarction may also occur in the brain as a result of thrombosis of the dural venous sinuses.

Macroscopic appearance of infarcts

When infarction is due to simple cessation of arterial supply, the shape of the infarct reflects the geographical distribution of the artery involved. In most organs (e.g. kidney, spleen or brain), the infarct appears wedge-shaped on section, with the broad part of the wedge at the periphery. In contrast, infarcts in the heart are not wedge-shaped but rather involve part or full thickness of the myocardium and its overlying endocardium and/or visceral pericardium.

Like most forms of tissue damage, infarction excites an acute inflammatory response followed by replacement of necrotic tissue by granulation tissue which then undergoes fibrous repair and scarring (see Chapter 2). The naked eye and histological appearances of infarcts thus depend on how far this sequence has progressed. One important exception to this process is the brain, which does not have the capacity for the usual processes of granulation tissue formation and fibrous repair. Cerebral infarcts undergo central liquefaction with reactive gliosis at the margins of the lesion, and old infarcts are usually marked by a cystic area surrounded by a zone of gliosis; brain infarction is illustrated in Figure 22.5.

Organs in which there are extensive capillary, sinusoidal or arteriovenous anastomoses often have infarcts which in their earliest stages are dark red in colour due to congestion with blood and haemorrhage (from the Latin, *infarcire*—to stuff); important examples are the lung (Fig. 9.5) and spleen.

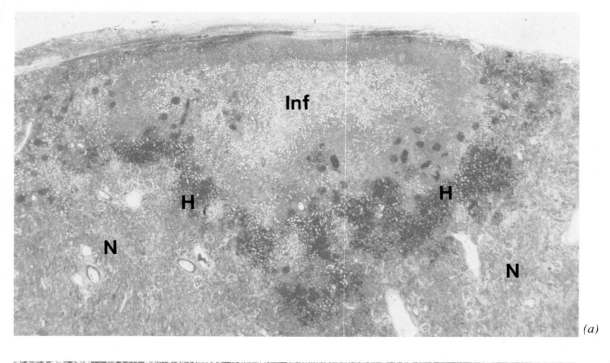

(a)

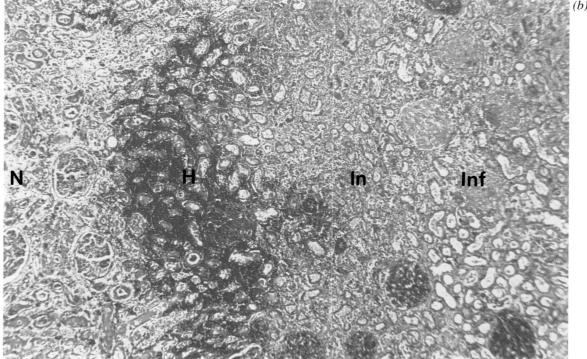

(b)

Fig. 9.1 Renal infarction *(caption opposite)*

Fig. 9.1 Renal infarction
(a) early infarct (LP) (*illustration opposite*)
(b) margin of infarct (MP) (*illustration opposite*)
(c) old renal infarct (MP)

The general features of infarction induced by thrombo-embolism are well illustrated by renal infarcts which usually result from emboli originating from thrombus in the left ventricle (e.g. mural thrombus after myocardial infarction) or the left atrial appendage (e.g. in atrial fibrillation).

In the very early stages (i.e. within 12 hours of infarction), gross examination shows the infarcted area to be ill-defined and dark, but progressively the lesion becomes paler until its wedge-shaped margins may be clearly distinguishable.

Micrograph (a) shows the histological appearance of a typical early renal infarct. The recently infarcted necrotic area **Inf** stains less intensely than the normal cortex **N**, but the general architecture of the infarct remains intact with still discernible 'ghosts' of glomeruli and renal tubules. The infarcted area has become demarcated from normal cortex by a narrow hyperaemic zone **H** representing the earliest vascular stages of a typical acute inflammatory response. Between this hyperaemic zone and the necrotic tissue is a purple-staining band containing the neutrophils of an early cellular acute inflammatory exudate.

Micrograph (b) shows, at higher magnification, the edge of the infarct in micrograph (a). Note that the normal cortical tissue **N** with its well-defined glomeruli and tubules gives way to a zone of hyperaemia **H**; next to this is a purplish band of acute inflammation **In** at the margin of the infarcted area where marked necrotic changes are evident in both glomeruli and tubules (see Fig. 1.7a). The acute inflammatory zone exhibits typically dilated and congested capillaries and an influx of small, dark-staining neutrophil polymorphs.

The necrotic tissue is progressively removed by neutrophils and macrophages and replaced by granulation tissue which eventually undergoes fibrous repair to form a small fibrous scar. This is shown in micrograph (c) which illustrates the end result of a renal infarct occurring two months previously; the infarct was of similar size to that shown in (a). All that now remains is a small, narrow, pink-staining, wedge-shaped scar **S** with its broad aspect at the capsular surface. Note that the capsular surface at the site of the scar is depressed as a result of contraction of the collagen fibres within the scar (a process known as cicatrisation; see Fig. 2.11).

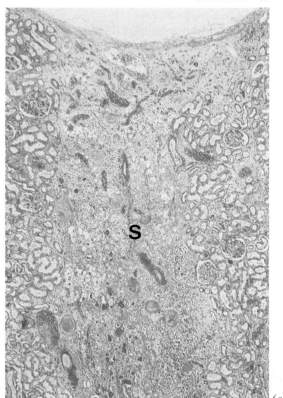

(c)

Ischaemic heart disease

Disease of cardiac muscle as a result of impaired blood supply is a major cause of death in all industrialised countries. Atherosclerosis of coronary arteries accounts for the vast majority of cases and gives rise to four main clinical syndromes: *angina pectoris* (chest pain on exertion), *acute myocardial infarction* ('heart attack' or 'coronary occlusion'), *chronic ischaemic heart disease*, and *sudden cardiac death* (immediately fatal myocardial infarct or dysrhythmia).

Acute myocardial infarction takes two main pathological forms:

- **Transmural infarction**. This involves the full thickness of a segment of the ventricular wall and is associated with complete blockage of a main coronary artery by thrombosis superimposed on an area of arteriosclerotic narrowing. As mentioned in Chapter 7, fissure or ulceration of an atheromatous plaque is the usual cause of thrombus formation.

- **Subendocardial myocardial infarction**. In this case myocardial necrosis is limited to cells in the inner third of the ventricular wall and tends to be associated with severe arteriosclerotic narrowing of both right and left coronary arteries. The pathogenesis of infarction is limitation of flow to the end arteries supplying the inner part of the ventricular wall rather than complete occlusion of the main arterial trunks.

The histological changes following infarction are illustrated in Figures 9.2 and 9.3.

Fig. 9.2 Myocardial infarction *(illustrations opposite)*
(a) 24 hour infarct (HP)
(b) 3 day infarct (HP)
(c) 10 day infarct (HP)
(d) 14 day infarct (HP)

The most common clinical example of infarction is that of the myocardium following occlusion of a coronary artery.

Using routine staining methods, the earliest histological evidence of infarction is visible some 12 to 24 hours after the onset of acute ischaemia, as illustrated in micrograph (a). The infarcted cardiac muscle fibres **In** exhibit patchy loss or blurring of cross striations and tend to become more intensely stained by eosin when compared to normal myocardial fibres **My**; there may also at this stage be some degree of early capillary engorgement and interstitial oedema, representing an incipient acute inflammatory response.

By about 2 or 3 days, as shown in micrograph (b), the infarcted fibres are intensely eosinophilic and most have lost their nuclei; there is marked infiltration by neutrophils **N** into the oedematous interstitium. The acute inflammatory process evolves during the succeeding days, during which time the necrotic myocardium undergoes autolysis and fragmentation, and the neutrophil infiltration becomes more intense.

By about the tenth day, as illustrated in micrograph (c), most of the necrotic muscle has disappeared as a result of the combined phagocytic activity of neutrophils and macrophages (see Fig. 2.8). The infarcted area is now largely occupied by residual macrophages, some lymphocytes and plasma cells, in a loose oedematous mesh in which a few capillaries and fibroblasts herald the earliest signs of granulation tissue formation.

By about the fourteenth day, the infarct is almost wholly replaced by fibrovascular granulation tissue **G**, as illustrated in micrograph (d), and the necrotic myocardium has been almost completely removed by the phagocytic activity of macrophages and neutrophils (Fig. 2.8).

Over succeeding weeks, the fibrovascular granulation tissue becomes progressively more fibrous and less vascular, leading to the formation of a highly collagenous and relatively acellular scar by about the end of the second month following infarction; examples of myocardial scars are shown in Figure 9.3.

The infarcted myocardium offers the least resistance to pressure around about the tenth day, and at this time the patient is most vulnerable to myocardial rupture. This not uncommon complication is almost invariably fatal, the ruptured ventricle wall spilling blood into the pericardial cavity *(haemopericardium)*. If the interventricular septum is involved in the infarct, there may be rupture of the septum with the sudden appearance of a systolic murmur. Similarly, rupture of an infarcted papillary muscle may lead to mitral valve incompetence with the sudden appearance of a characteristic systolic murmur.

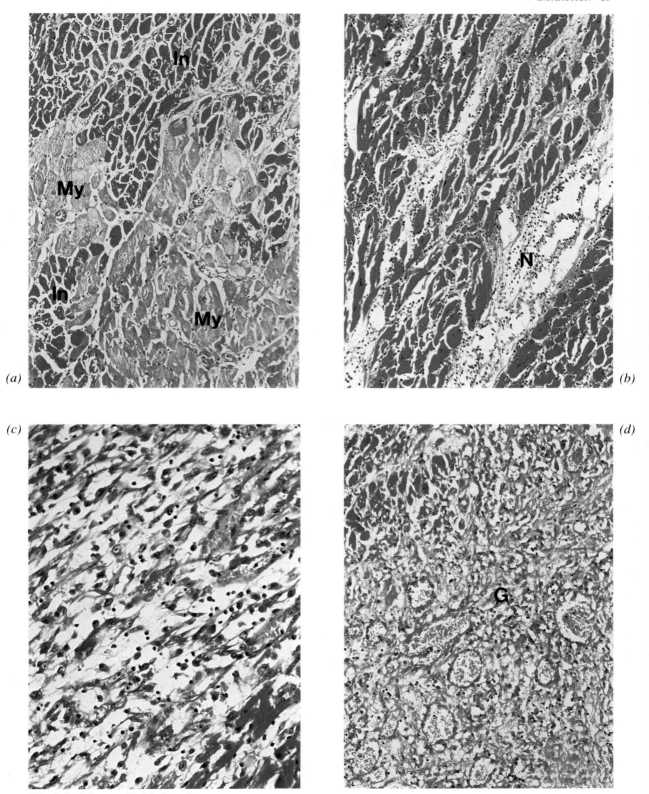

Fig. 9.2   Myocardial infarction *(caption opposite)*

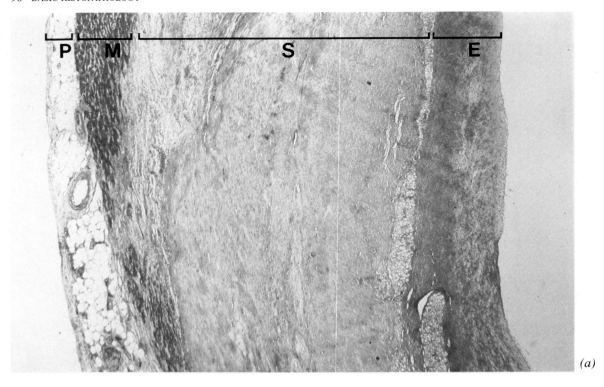

(a)

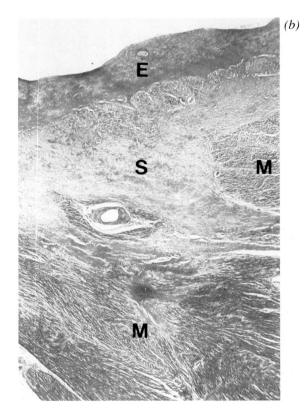

(b)

Fig. 9.3 Old myocardial infarcts
(a) full thickness scar (LP)
(b) partial thickness scar (LP)

These two micrographs show examples of myocardial
scars several months after infarction. The sites of
infarction are marked by densely collagenous pale pink-
staining scar **S**, contrasting with the more heavily
staining surviving myocardial muscle **M**. Continuing
contraction (cicatrisation) of the fibrous scar over
succeeding months leads to thinning of the infarcted area
of the ventricular wall. If the scar is inadequate to
withstand ventricular pressures (most likely after a full
thickness infarct), a *ventricular aneurysm* may develop
by ballooning of the ventricular wall. With or without
aneurysm formation, stasis in the region of the non-
contractile scar predisposes to formation of a ventricular
mural thrombus.

If the original infarct involves the endocardium **E** or
visceral pericardium **P**, or both as in some full thickness
infarcts, these normally delicate layers become markedly
thickened as a result of their involvement in the
inflammatory process and subsequent organisation and
repair.

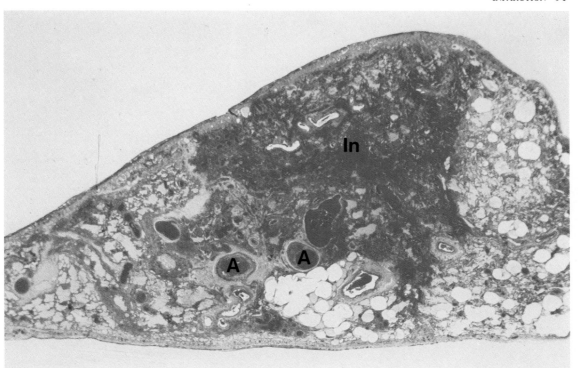

Fig. 9.4 Lung infarct (LP)

Infarcts of the lung usually result from small pulmonary emboli arising from fragments of thrombus within the veins of the legs (see Fig. 8.2c). In their early stages, lung infarcts are firm, dark red, wedge-shaped areas at the lung periphery; their firmness and colour derive from the fact that the alveolar spaces are filled with erythrocytes, partly due to leakage from damaged capillary walls and partly from blood carried by the unobstructed bronchial arterial circulation. The pleura becomes involved in the resulting acute inflammatory response; in this case, the fibrinous pleurisy results in characteristic sharp pleuritic pain and a pleural friction rub.

This micrograph illustrates the edge of a lung with a small congested infarct **In**. Note the obstructed branches of the pulmonary artery **A** and the clearly defined margins of the infarct demarcating the area supplied by this vessel.

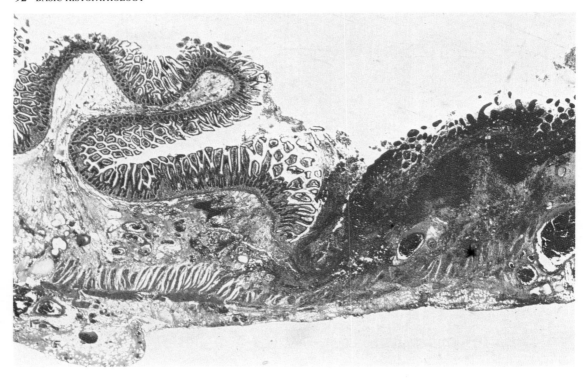

Fig. 9.5 Bowel infarction following volvulus (LP)

Bowel infarction may occur either as a result of arterial occlusion, e.g. mesenteric thrombosis or embolism, or, more commonly, as a result of venous obstruction. Venous obstruction may occur either through torsion (twisting) of a free loop of bowel around its vascular pedicle *(volvulus)*, entrapment in a tight hernial orifice (e.g. indirect inguinal hernia) or obstruction by fibrous peritoneal adhesions (e.g. following previous surgery).

 Venous obstruction initially causes the bowel to become intensely congested with blood, giving it a plum coloured appearance on gross examination; as the dammed-back blood prevents arterial inflow, the bowel becomes progressively hypoxic. Frank necrosis follows unless the venous obstruction is relieved.

 In this micrograph of a small bowel volvulus, the necrotic bowel at the right hand side of the picture is stained bright red due to massive suffusion with blood; the outline of the necrotic mucosal villi is still apparent. Note the sharp demarcation between normal and necrotic bowel, and the marked engorgement of all vessels.

PART 2

BASIC SYSTEMS PATHOLOGY

10. Cardiovascular system

Introduction

Diseases of the cardiovascular system are the commonest cause of death and serious illness in developed countries. The most common underlying cause is atherosclerosis which, because of its numerous associated disorders and complications, is the exclusive topic of one chapter (Ch. 7). Also important are the phenomena of thrombosis and embolism, which are the subject of Chapter 8, and their frequent sequel, infarction, which is described in Chapter 9.

Ischaemic heart disease

Of the diseases involving the heart, ischaemic heart disease is the most important. In almost all cases, the cause of ischaemic heart disease is atherosclerosis of the coronary arteries with or without accompanying thrombosis; coronary artery atheroma and thrombosis are illustrated in Figures 7.6 and 7.8, and the stages of myocardial infarction are shown in Figures 9.2 and 9.3.

Inflammation of the heart

This may affect the pericardium, myocardium or endocardium, either separately or concurrently. Inflammation occurs in response to a wide range of damaging stimuli but most common are ischaemia and infection. Most infections of the pericardium *(pericarditis)* and myocardium *(myocarditis)* are viral, whilst those of the endocardium *(endocarditis)* and valves *(valvulitis)* are bacterial or fungal (Figs. 10.4 and 10.5).

The main causes of pericarditis are summarised in Figure 10.1. The histological features of acute pericarditis are virtually identical whatever the cause and are illustrated and discussed in Figure 2.7; the major exceptions are tuberculous pericarditis, in which tuberculous granulomas and caseous necrosis are seen, and malignant pericarditis, in which clumps of tumour cells are often mixed with the inflammatory exudate.

The term *myocarditis* implies inflammatory damage to the myocardium and by common usage usually excludes the vigorous acute inflammatory reaction to necrotic muscle fibres seen in myocardial infarction (Fig. 9.3b). Primary myocarditis can be associated with virus infection, rheumatic fever, and exposure to certain toxins and drugs. In some cases no causative factor can be identified *(idiopathic myocarditis)*.

Endocarditis and *valvulitis* involve not only inflammation but also thrombus deposition upon the endocardium and/or valves. These are important diseases and have a high mortality rate, their clinical manifestations usually resulting from embolic phenomena.

Fig. 10.1 Important causes of pericarditis

Myocardial infarction	After transmural myocardial infarction	Common
Cardiac surgery	After surgical opening of pericardial sac	Common
Viral infections	Usually young adults. Coxackie B most common	Common
Malignancy	Local invasion or metastatic tumour deposits	Uncommon
Uraemia	Renal failure	Now uncommon
Bacterial infections	Secondary to lung infection including TB	Uncommon
Rheumatic fever	Part of rheumatic pancarditis (see Fig 10.2)	Now rare

Rheumatic fever

Rheumatic fever is a systemic inflammatory disease which, in susceptible individuals, appears to follow infection by group A *β haemolytic streptococci*; such infections commonly occur in the throat and are themselves relatively innocuous. The systemic manifestations are thought to represent a disordered immunological response resulting in inflammation of connective tissues. Connective tissues in all parts of the body may be involved, e.g. the joints and skin, with painful short term consequences. Involvement of the heart is the most important clinically, because of potentially fatal *acute myocarditis* and *endocarditis,* and the long term consequences of *chronic scarring of cardiac valves.*

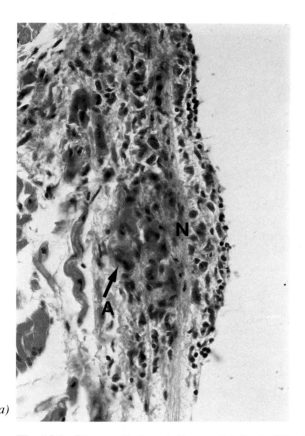

(a)

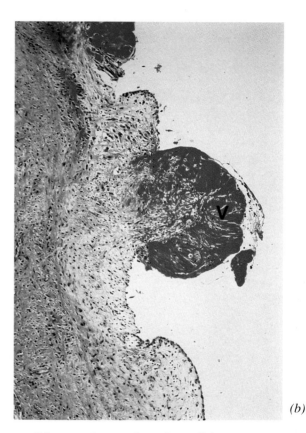

(b)

Fig. 10.2 Rheumatic heart disease (a) Aschoff body (HP) **(b) acute rheumatic endocarditis** (MP)

The characteristic acute rheumatic lesion is the *Aschoff body,* one of which is shown in micrograph (a). The fully developed Aschoff body has a central ill-defined area of degenerate material **N** surrounded by a mixture of inflammatory leucocytes. Amongst these cells can often be seen a so-called *Anitschow myocyte* **A**, recognised by its irregular, ribbon-like nucleus and extensive eosinophilic cytoplasm. Despite their name, these cells are considered to represent large modified fibro-histiocytic cells. Aschoff bodies are found in the interstitial connective tissue of the myocardium particularly near vessels, in the subepicardial fibrous tissue, and (as in this micrograph) in the subendocardial connective tissue.

The importance of endocardial involvement relates to

involvement of the heart valves where endocardial roughening induces formation of fibrin and platelet thrombi. Micrograph (b) illustrates part of a mitral valve leaflet affected by acute rheumatic endocarditis. A small thrombotic vegetation **V** has formed on the upper (atrial) surface of the valve leaflet at the site of the remnants of a large Aschoff body.

Chronic rheumatic valvular disease is the result of organisation and fibrous scarring of affected valves. This continues over many years with eventual thickening and distortion of the valve leaflets, as well as the chordae tendinae. Such distortion commonly renders affected valves stenotic or incompetent.

Valvulitis (endocarditis of valves)

The heart valves may become subject to a variety of vegetative lesions which have traditionally been described as forms of *endocarditis*. The primary phenomenon underlying all these conditions is the formation of thrombus on the valve leaflets or cusps.

As in the arterial system, roughening of the endocardial surface predisposes to thrombus formation (see Ch. 8). This may occur when valve leaflets or cusps have been previously damaged by rheumatic fever or are congenitally abnormal. Thrombus formation may also follow autoimmune valve damage in systemic lupus erythematosus *(Libman-Sachs endocarditis)* and in the acute phase of rheumatic fever (acute rheumatic carditis, see Fig. 10.2). The most frequent type of valve thrombi, however, occur in so-called *marantic endocarditis* in which warty thrombotic vegetations develop on mitral and aortic valves. This phenomenon occurs in seriously ill patients, often those with widely disseminated malignancy, and is usually associated with a state of hypercoagulability of the blood. Despite use of the term endocarditis in these conditions, inflammation itself is usually not a feature of the valve at the time of thrombus formation.

True valvular inflammation may arise, however, if these thrombotic vegetations on the valves then become infected with bacteria, fungi or other organisms, conditions collectively referred to as *infective endocarditis*. Bacterial endocarditis tends to be divided into two clinicopathological patterns. In the first, traditionally known as *subacute bacterial endocarditis*, the thrombotic vegetations develop on previously damaged valves, which then become colonised by bacteria of low virulence such as *Streptococcus viridans;* such organisms tend to reach the valves via a transient bacteraemia, e.g. following dental extraction. The major clinical consequences are those resulting from detachment of small thrombotic emboli, often infected, into the systemic circulation.

In the second type of bacterial endocarditis, known traditionally as *acute bacterial endocarditis*, thrombi form on previously normal valves and become infected by virulent organisms such as *Staphylococcus aureus*. In this case, the patient is usually already severely debilitated and septicaemic, such as from an infected urinary catheter, and the infecting organism is that which is responsible for the septicaemia. In contrast with the subacute pattern, in the acute form the fulminating infection extends into the substance of the valve causing tissue necrosis. Rapid destruction of the valve leaflet leads to valvular incompetence and acute cardiac failure is the usual clinical outcome.

Fungal endocarditis, formerly rare, is now appearing more commonly, sometimes as a complication of immunosuppressive therapy, heroin addiction, or AIDS; *Candida albicans* is the most common organism.

The incidence of the types of endocarditis just described has changed over the past few decades for many reasons, including the widespread use of broad spectrum antibiotics and decreasing incidence of rheumatic fever. Furthermore, understanding of the nature of these conditions has changed markedly in recent years, leaving behind a somewhat inappropriate terminology.

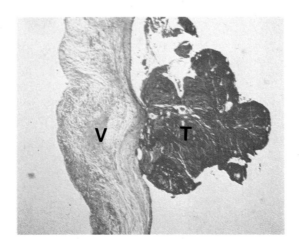

Fig. 10.3 Marantic endocarditis (LP)

Micrograph illustrates a mitral valve lesion of marantic (thrombotic, non-bacterial) endocarditis; masses of thrombus **T** have developed on the superior surface of the valve leaflet **V**. Such thrombotic masses are only loosely attached to the underlying non-inflamed valve and therefore are readily detached, leading to major embolic episodes such as cerebral, renal and splenic infarction (see Ch. 9). In practice, this type of endocarditis is rarely diagnosed in life but is a common necropsy finding.

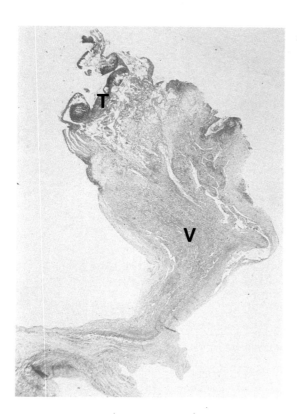

Fig. 10.4 Subacute bacterial endocarditis (LP)

The subacute form of bacterial endocarditis affecting a mitral valve is demonstrated in this micrograph. The valve leaflet **V** is covered at its tip by pink-staining thrombus **T** containing small colonies of blue-purple-staining bacteria. The underlying valve is thickened due to previous rheumatic fever, but there is no evidence of bacterial destruction and the organisms are present in relatively small numbers. Fragments of such vegetations frequently become detached giving rise to multiple small embolic episodes.

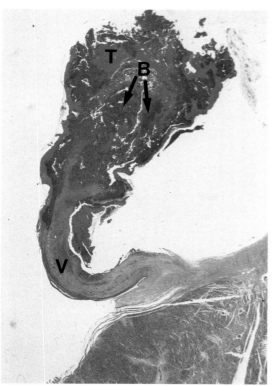

Fig. 10.5 Acute bacterial endocarditis (LP)

This micrograph shows an example of the acute form of bacterial endocarditis involving an aortic valve. The patient was septicaemic due to a fulminant local infection, in this case involving the kidney. The highly virulent bacteria **B** have settled on heart valves probably colonising small pre-existing thrombi; bacterial proliferation has then stimulated further formation of thrombus **T** forming large vegetations which have eroded and destroyed the previously normal valve **V**. Compare the huge mass of bacteria and thrombus in this case with that of the subacute form shown in Figure 10.4. Since destruction is so rapid, the clinical picture is usually of rapidly developing cardiac failure rather than thrombotic episodes.

The arterial and venous system

The most common pathological abnormality of the arterial tree is thickening and hardening of the walls, a condition known as *arteriosclerosis*. Atheroma (atherosclerosis) is the most frequent cause of arteriosclerosis and is discussed in Chapter 7.

The other important causes of arteriosclerosis are hypertension and diabetes mellitus; in both cases, however, the specific vascular changes are often superimposed upon features of the ubiquitous atherosclerosis. Some of the important arterial wall changes associated with hypertension are illustrated in this chapter in Figures 10.6 and 10.7 and in relation to the kidney in Figure 14.11. Diabetic vascular changes are illustrated in relation to their important impact on the kidney in Figure 14.12.

Aneurysms

Abnormal dilatations of arterial vessels are known as *aneurysms* and may be divided into five main types:

- **Atherosclerotic aneurysms** arise as a complication of atheroma (e.g. in abdominal aorta).

- **Syphilitic aneurysms**, usually involving the ascending aorta, result from damage inflicted upon the aortic media by the chronic inflammatory lesions of syphilitic aortitis (Fig. 3.20).

- **Dissecting aneurysms** result from idiopathic degeneration of the tunica media and usually involve the thoracic aorta; these are discussed in Figure 10.8.

- **Berry aneurysms** arise from developmental defects in the elastic layer of cerebral arteries (Fig. 10.9).

- **Microaneurysms.** Hypertensive and diabetic vascular disease predispose to aneurysm formation in small vessels of the brain and retina respectively; rupture of these microaneurysms may lead to brain haemorrhage and blindness.

The main complications of an aneurysm are rupture leading to haemorrhage, and thrombus formation leading to occlusive or embolic phenomena.

Inflammation of vessels (vasculitis)

Arterial walls become the specific target of inflammation in a group of diseases of probable autoimmune aetiology. The most common of these *arteritides* are *polyarteritis nodosa* and *giant cell arteritis,* illustrated in Figures 10.10 and 10.11 respectively. Vasculitis is also an important histological feature of organs affected by some systemic autoimmune diseases such as systemic lupus erythematosus. Small vessel vasculitis is particularly common in the skin and examples include Henoch Schönlein purpura and adverse reaction to some drugs.

The venous system

Varicose veins occur in the legs due to the hydrostatic pressure of blood in the presence of incompetent venous valves. The leg veins are an important site of thrombus formation as discussed in Chapter 8.

Tumours of blood vessel origin

Benign and malignant tumours, known as *angiomas* and *angiosarcomas* respectively, may arise from the blood or lymph vascular tissues. Most common among these are *haemangiomas* illustrated in Figure 10.12, many of which are regarded as hamartomas rather than neoplasms.

Kaposi's sarcoma is a malignant tumour of vascular tissues which is common in patients who are immunosuppressed, particularly the group of cases with AIDS. It is illustrated in Figure 10.13.

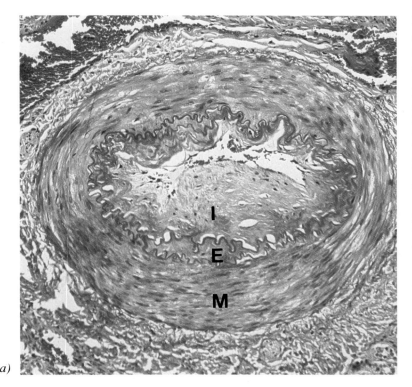

(a)

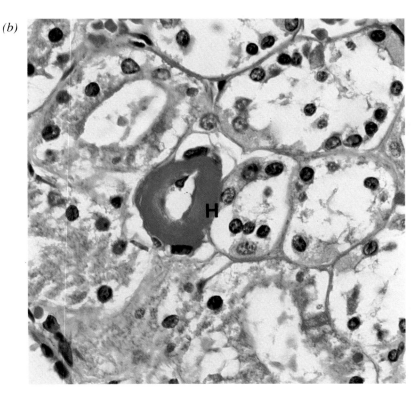

(b)

Fig. 10.6 Arterial changes in essential hypertension (a) medium sized artery (MP) **(b) arteriole** (HP)

Hypertension, whether idiopathic or secondary to known pathology, is known to be associated with concurrent changes in peripheral arterial vessels; whether such changes are part of the primary causative process, secondary, or contributory, remains unresolved.

When the increase in blood pressure is moderate and gradual in onset *(essential* or *benign hypertension)*, muscular arteries undergo progressive thickening of their walls. Three features are characteristically seen and are shown in micrograph (a): symmetrical hypertrophy of the muscular media **M**, extensive reduplication of the internal elastic lamina **E** and regular fibrotic thickening of the intima **I**. All these changes lead to reduction of luminal diameter.

Arterioles show a different type of wall thickening sometimes referred to as *hyaline arteriosclerosis* and shown in micrograph (b). The normal layers of the wall become ill defined and replaced by homogeneous eosinophilic (pink-stained) material called *hyaline* **H**, now thought to be of basement membrane-like composition. This results in reduction in size of arteriolar lumina and may contribute to further hypertension.

Fig. 10.7 Arterial changes in accelerated hypertension
(a) medium sized artery (HP)
(b) arteriole (HP)

When the increase in blood pressure is of marked degree and rapid onset *(accelerated* or *malignant hypertension)*, muscular arteries develop extensive thickening of the tunica intima **I** by proliferation of intimal cells; this gives the appearance of concentric lamellae which encroach upon the arterial lumen as seen in micrograph (a). In contrast to the findings in moderate hypertension, the tunica media **M** and internal elastic lamina **E** remain largely unchanged.

The impact of sudden and severe hypertension on arterioles is even more dramatic, as shown in micrograph (b). The intimal cells undergo rapid proliferation (as in the muscular arteries) which is often complicated by disruption of the vessel wall, with leakage of plasma proteins including fibrinogen into and beyond the arteriolar wall. This change, known inaccurately as *fibrinoid necrosis*, is characterised by obliteration of the wall by intensely eosinophilic amorphous proteinaceous material **P**; the lumen is often completely occluded.

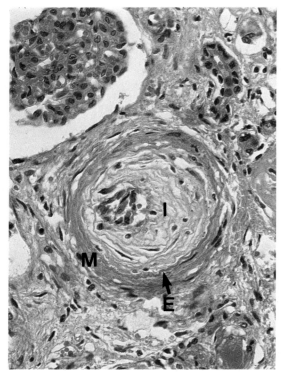

(a)

(b)

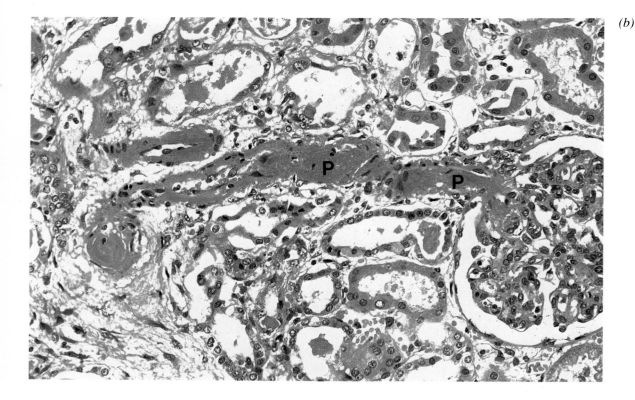

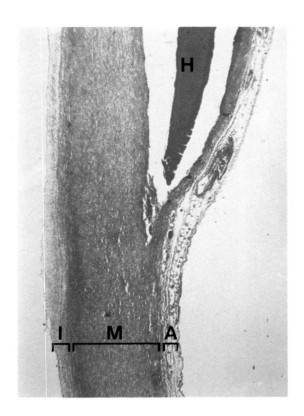

Fig. 10.8 Dissecting aneurysms of the aorta (LP)

Dissecting aneurysms most commonly affect the thoracic aorta. A laceration of the tunica intima **I** leads to tracking of blood into the tunica media **M**. The plane of cleavage (dissection) is usually between the middle and outer thirds of the media, as in this example; note that the site of intimal laceration is not included in this photographic field. The medial haematoma **H** then frequently bursts through the tunica adventitia **A** with rapidly fatal consequences.

The pathogenesis of dissecting aneurysms is poorly understood but almost all cases exhibit a peculiar type of non-inflammatory degeneration of the smooth muscle and elastic tissue of the tunica media known as *medial mucoid degeneration* or *cystic medionecrosis*. In this condition, areas of the tunica media become replaced by irregular masses of acellular polysaccharide material. Dissecting aneurysms may occur in adults at any age though they are most common in middle age, with males outnumbering females.

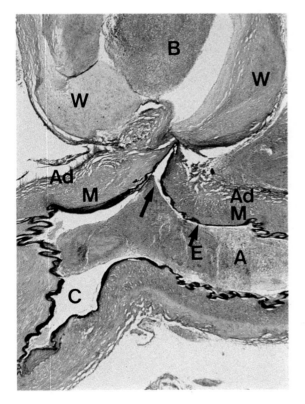

Fig. 10.9 Berry aneurysm
(Elastic van Gieson stain; LP)

Berry aneurysms are a characteristic type of aneurysm found in the cerebral circulation, particularly at junctions in the circle of Willis or at bifurcations of the major cerebral arteries (especially the middle cerebral). Berry aneurysms most often become manifest in middle age by rupturing to cause *subarachnoid haemorrhage*. These aneurysms are, however, an occasional incidental finding at all ages and are often multiple.

This micrograph illustrates a berry aneurysm **B** arising from the anterior cerebral artery **A** just proximal to the point where it gives rise to its anterior communicating branch **C**. The vessel has a normal tunica media **M**, adventitia **Ad** and internal elastic lamina **E** (elastin stains black with this staining method). Note that at the point of origin of the aneurysm, the tunica media is deficient (arrow). The wall of the aneurysm **W** is composed of loose fibrous intimal tissue and the lumen contains blood. There is no medial muscle or elastin in the aneurysm wall.

Fig. 10.10   Polyarteritis nodosa (MP)

Polyarteritis nodosa is a rare, systemic immunological disease characterised by acute inflammation of the walls of medium and small muscular arteries; the lesions are discrete and scattered and may be found in all organs but in particular the kidneys, heart, liver and gastro-intestinal tract, lungs, peripheral nerves and skin.

Histologically, the appearance is of an acute necrotising inflammation of the arterial wall with heavy infiltration of neutrophils **N** accompanied by a variable, sometimes large number of eosinophils. The vessel wall almost invariably exhibits the features of so-called *fibrinoid necrosis* **F** (see Fig. 10.6) and the lumen may become occluded by thrombus. Subsequent fibrous healing leaves the vessel wall thickened and nodular with a defective internal elastic lamina.

Apart from systemic symptoms such as fever, malaise, weakness and weight loss, the clinical presentation of this disease is extremely variable depending on which tissues become ischaemic or infarcted as a result of the arterial lesions. For example, kidney involvement may be manifest by pain, haematuria or proteinuria, heart involvement by angina, myocardial infarction or pericarditis, and skin involvement by tender subcutaneous nodules. Clinical diagnosis must usually be substantiated by tissue biopsy.

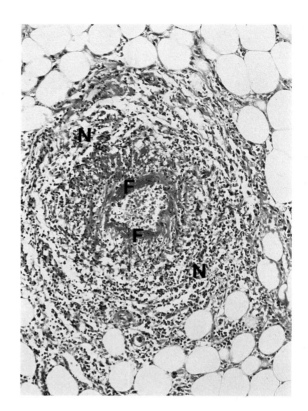

Fig. 10.11   Giant cell (cranial or temporal) arteritis (MP)

Giant cell arteritis is another systemic immunological disease of blood vessels which particularly involves medium sized arteries of the head, thereby resulting in the synonyms of *cranial* and *temporal arteritis*.

Histologically, the walls of involved vessels exhibit features more reminiscent of granulomatous than acute neutrophilic inflammation. Multinucleate giant cells **G** are the most characteristic finding and these tend to be arranged circumferentially, apparently in relation to degenerate fragments of the internal elastic lamina. Marked fibrous thickening of the intimal layer may be complicated by thrombosis, which may produce acute blindness if the ophthalmic artery is affected.

Giant cell arteritis is mainly seen in those over the age of 50. In addition to vague though often debilitating constitutional symptoms, the condition often presents as localised throbbing pain or tenderness, e.g. over the temporal artery. Alternatively it presents as more generalised pain involving the muscles of the pelvic and shoulder girdles in the condition known as *polymyalgia rheumatica.* Diagnosis of temporal arteritis is confirmed by temporal artery biopsy although results will be negative unless a discrete inflammatory lesion is included in the biopsy specimen.

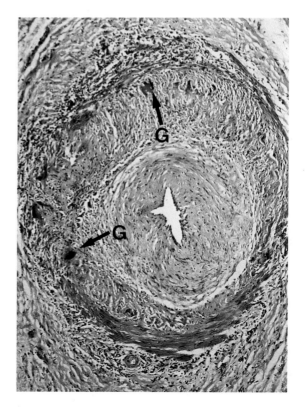

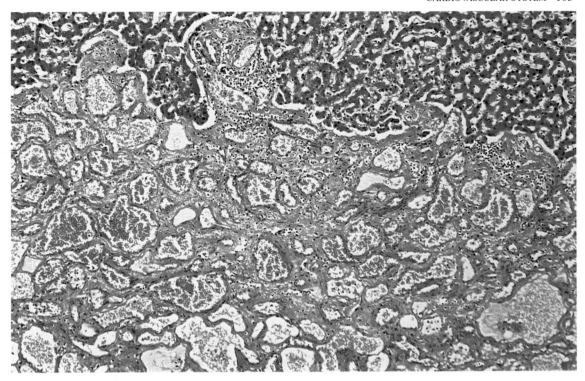

Fig. 10.12 Haemangioma (MP)

Benign tumours of vascular tissues most commonly occur in the skin and liver. The most frequent type is the simple *haemangioma* composed of blood-filled vascular spaces lined by endothelium. When large vascular spaces predominate the lesion is called a *cavernous haemangioma*, but alternatively the spaces may be small and of capillary dimensions, when the lesion is known as a *capillary haemangioma*; frequently, both forms are present in the same lesion.

This angioma was an incidental finding in the liver at necropsy.

Similar tumour-like masses of vascular tissue are found in the brain and other sites and are often regarded as *hamartomas* (see Ch. 6).

Benign tumours or hamartomas of lymphatic vessels *(lymphangiomas)* also occur but are rare. Malignant tumours of vasoformative tissue, *angiosarcomas*, are extremely rare.

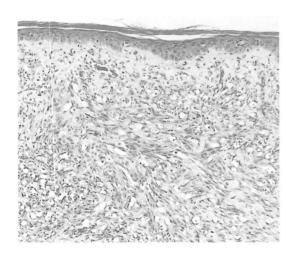

Fig. 10.13 Kaposi's sarcoma of the skin (HP)

Kaposi's sarcoma has dramatically increased in incidence as a result of AIDS (see p. 163). This tumour appears clinically as purple plaques in the skin composed of infiltrative tumour within the dermis.

Histologically, lesions have two components, an irregular system of proliferating vascular channels lined by endothelial cells which have many of the characteristics of lymphatic endothelium, and a spindle cell fibrous component; both are seen in this micrograph. In patients with AIDS these tumours spread to involve lymph nodes and viscera.

11. Respiratory system

Nose, nasopharynx and larynx

Although viral infections (coryza - the common cold) and allergic inflammation (hay fever - allergic rhinitis) commonly affect the nose, nasal sinuses and nasopharynx, there are only a few conditions of general histopathological interest in the upper respiratory tract. *Nasal polyps* (Fig. 11.1) are a common sequel of prolonged or recurrent inflammation, particularly allergic inflammation. Malignant tumours of the nasal passages and sinuses are rare but *nasopharyngeal carcinoma* (Fig. 11.2) is of special interest because of a possible viral aetiology.

   The stratified squamous epithelium of the larynx may undergo hyperplastic or dysplastic change to form benign squamous papillomata or invasive carcinoma (Fig. 11.3). Cigarette smoking and alcohol consumption predispose to the development of carcinoma of the larynx.

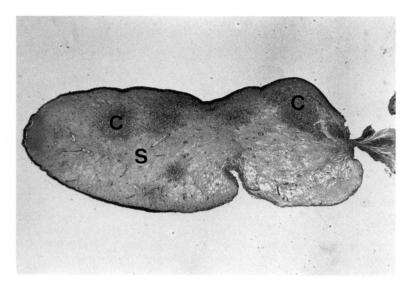

Fig. 11.1 Nasal polyp (LP)

Nasal polyps are the product of chronic inflammation of the nasal mucosa, commonly infective or allergic in nature. There is marked oedema and engorgement of mucosal connective tissue and infiltration by chronic inflammatory cells; eosinophils are prominent in allergic rhinitis.

   In this example, note the grossly oedematous stroma **S** and stretched but otherwise relatively normal covering epithelium. In this polyp, the predominant inflammatory cells present are plasma cells and eosinophils, mainly in clumps **C** at the periphery of the polyp.

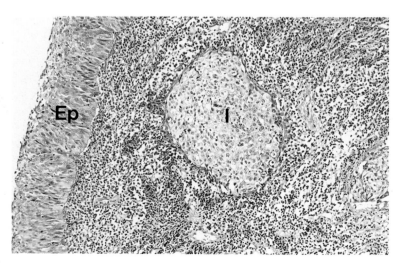

Fig. 11.2 Nasopharyngeal carcinoma (MP)

In the nasal cavities and nasopharynx, malignant tumours take the form of transitional, squamous or adenocarcinomas, although anaplastic carcinomas also occur, particularly in the nasopharynx. In this micrograph, an invasive transitional cell carcinoma of the nasal cavity is shown. A possible viral aetiology (EB virus) has been postulated for some nasopharyngeal carcinomas. Note the islands **I** of invasive carcinoma beneath the dysplastic surface transitional epithelium **Ep**.

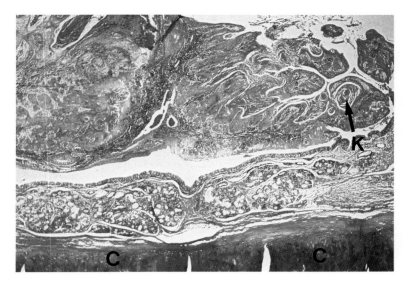

Fig. 11.3 Carcinoma of the larynx (LP)

Squamous cell carcinomas form the vast majority of malignant tumours of the larynx, most commonly originating in the vocal cords (intrinsic), but also occasionally arising in epiglottis, aryepiglottic folds and pyriform fossae (extrinsic carcinoma of larynx). Squamous carcinomas of the larynx are usually well differentiated and exhibit keratin pearl formation.

This micrograph shows a squamous carcinoma arising from a vocal cord; note the presence of keratin pearls **K**. The section also includes part of the normal laryngeal wall including laryngeal cartilage **C**.

The airways and lungs

The trachea and bronchi may become acutely inflamed as a result of infections by viruses or pyogenic bacteria to cause *acute tracheobronchitis* (Fig. 11.4). Bacterial infections of airways are frequently complicated by extension of inflammation into the surrounding lung parenchyma to cause a pattern of lung infection known as *bronchopneumonia* (Fig. 11.5), a common cause of illness and death in the debilitated and elderly. Another common pattern of bacterial lung infection is *lobar pneumonia* which involves a whole segment or lobe; usually a more virulent bacterium such as the pneumococcus is involved and fit young people may be almost as susceptible as the elderly and debilitated. Lobar pneumonia illustrates many important principles of acute inflammation and the phenomenon of resolution, and is discussed in Chapter 2 (Figs. 2.4 and 2.9). In contrast, tuberculosis and sarcoidosis are classical examples of specific chronic inflammations and are discussed fully in Chapter 3.

Recurrent or persistent suppurative bacterial infections of bronchi may lead to irreversible dilatation of airways with marked thickening and chronic inflammation of the walls, a condition known as *bronchiectasis* (see Fig. 3.3).

Abscess formation in the lungs (Fig. 2.13) is a serious complication of certain pneumonias, particularly *Staphylococcal* and *Klebsiella* pneumonias. Lung abscesses may also result from septic emboli causing infarction of the lung, bronchiectasis, bronchial obstruction by tumour or as a complication of pulmonary tuberculosis.

The term *chronic obstructive airways disease* refers to conditions characterised by chronic or recurrent obstruction of air flow and includes chronic bronchitis and emphysema. Recurrent episodes of acute bronchitis or persistent non-infective irritation of bronchial mucosa (e.g. due to cigarette smoking) may produce *chronic bronchitis* (Fig. 11.7), which is frequently associated with persistent dilatation of air spaces and destruction of their walls, a condition known as *emphysema* (Fig. 11.6).

Asthma (Fig. 11.8) is a disorder of the airways characterised by reversible bronchoconstriction often provoked by allergens in susceptible individuals but also triggered by physical agents or infection.

The massive capillary bed of the lungs makes them vulnerable to a variety of haemodynamic and other vascular disorders. Left ventricular failure results in engorgement of pulmonary capillaries and fluid transudation into the alveolar spaces causing *pulmonary congestion* and *oedema* (Fig. 11.9). Two other common vascular disorders of great clinical importance are *pulmonary embolism* and *pulmonary infarction* illustrated in Figures 8.4 and 9.4 respectively.

An important end-stage of many types of parenchymal lung disease, particularly those involving chronic persistent inflammatory processes, is *interstitial fibrosis*. This results in severe impairment of respiratory function and leads to alterations in the physiology of pulmonary vasculature with resultant pulmonary hypertension.

The lungs are a common site of primary malignant tumours which are of three main types: *squamous cell carcinoma* (Fig. 11.12) and *oat cell carcinoma* (Fig. 11.13), which occur most frequently in the main bronchi and their major branches, and *adenocarcinoma* (Fig. 11.14), which tends to arise more peripherally. In contrast, benign tumours of the lung and bronchi are rare. The lung is an extremely common site of metastatic tumour deposits, usually blood-borne from distant organs (see Fig. 6.7b).

Finally the pleura is the site of several important pathological processes. Acute inflammation of the pleura *(pleurisy)* is a frequent accompaniment of lung infections and infarcts, and is characterised by a marked fibrinous exudate typical of serosal surfaces (Fig. 2.7). Rarely, a primary malignant tumour arises in the pleural serosa; this tumour, known as *mesothelioma* (Fig. 11.15), is almost exclusively confined to people with a history of exposure to asbestos.

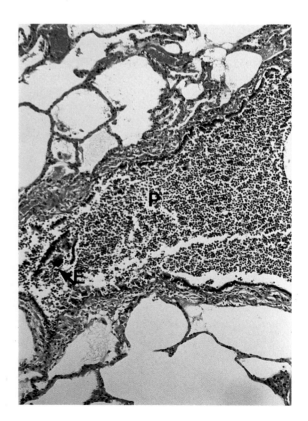

Fig. 11.4 Acute purulent bronchitis (MP)

Bacterial infections of the upper respiratory tract (often following a transient viral infection) tend to spread down the respiratory tract where they may produce an acute purulent *tracheobronchitis* and *bronchiolitis*. The mucosa of the airways becomes acutely inflamed and congested, and the smaller lobular bronchi and bronchioles become filled with purulent exudate **P** composed of fluid and numerous neutrophils; strips of necrotic epithelium **E** are often shed into the pus. The inflammatory process inhibits ciliary activity but promotes secretion of mucus which, with the dead and dying pus cells, pools in the airways and is coughed up as yellow-green sputum. In the early stages, the lung parenchyma is usually unaffected but the alveolar spaces adjacent to the affected bronchioles often become filled with oedema fluid. In susceptible patients, this may then proceed to the development of bronchopneumonia which is illustrated in Figure 11.5.

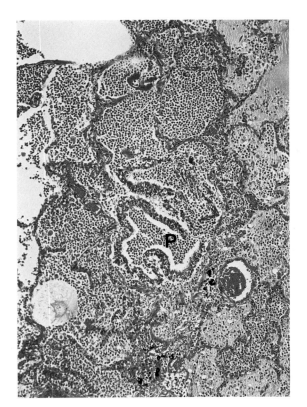

Fig. 11.5 Bronchopneumonia (MP)

Extension of bacterial infection from bronchioles into the surrounding lung parenchyma leads to a patchy pattern of purulent pneumonic consolidation known as *bronchopneumonia*; this is in marked contrast to the involvement from the outset of a whole lobe or lobule as occurs in *lobar pneumonia* (see Fig. 2.4).

Each peribronchial focus of pneumonic consolidation has within it a small bronchus or bronchiole exhibiting the features of acute purulent bronchitis **P**, as demonstrated in Figure 11.4. As each focus of bronchopneumonia expands, it tends to merge with adjacent foci until the consolidation becomes confluent.

Bronchopneumonia is a threat to the very young, elderly or those debilitated by pre-existing illness such as congestive cardiac failure or carcinomatosis, and is a very common terminal event. No single organism is responsible, but *Streptococcus pneumoniae* and *Haemophilus influenzae* are the most frequent.

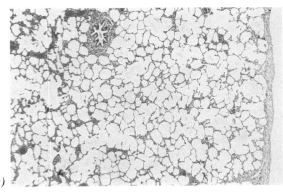

(a)

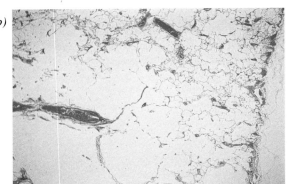

(b)

Fig. 11.6 Pulmonary emphysema
(a) normal lung (LP)
(b) emphysematous lung (LP)

Emphysema is a condition characterised by permanent enlargement of the respiratory spaces distal to the terminal bronchioles in the lung, accompanied by destruction of their walls. Comparison of emphysematous and normal lungs (shown here at the same magnification) demonstrates the marked increase in alveolar volume and consequent marked reduction in area of alveolar wall available for gaseous exchange in emphysema. This problem is compounded by the loss of elastic 'guy rope' support which alveolar walls normally provide to the airways; thus, in emphysema, the airways tend to collapse during expiration. Emphysema is often associated with recurrent or chronic infection of the airways (chronic bronchitis) and some degree of reversible airways obstruction due to bronchospasm.

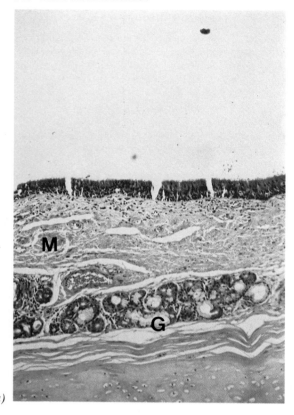

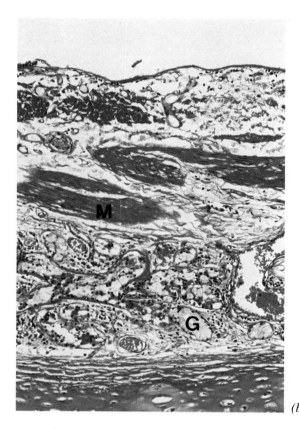

(a)
(b)

Fig. 11.7 Chronic bronchitis
(a) normal bronchial wall (MP)
(b) bronchial wall in chronic bronchitis (MP)

The term chronic bronchitis is used clinically to describe the situation where excess sputum is produced by a patient on most days for at least three months of the year for at least two consecutive years.

Although well defined as a clinical term, pathological changes in chronic bronchitis are variable and relatively non-specific. Chronic irritation of the bronchial mucosa, either by tobacco smoke, atmospheric pollution or by repeated episodes of infection, induces chronic inflammatory and hyperplastic changes resulting in marked thickening of the bronchial wall. This feature is the main abnormality in cases of chronic bronchitis, being well illustrated in micrograph (b) when compared to the normal bronchial wall shown in micrograph (a) at the same magnification.

Three factors contribute to the increased thickness of the bronchial wall: infiltration of the submucosa by chronic inflammatory cells, marked hypertrophy of mucosal smooth muscle **M** and marked hyperplasia of the mucous glands **G** with the production of copious mucus.

In addition, the surface epithelium undergoes hyperplasia or even squamous metaplasia (see Fig. 5.5). The consequent loss of ciliary activity then compounds the problem of excessive mucus production by destroying the 'mucociliary escalator' and provides an ideal environment for superimposed bacterial infection.

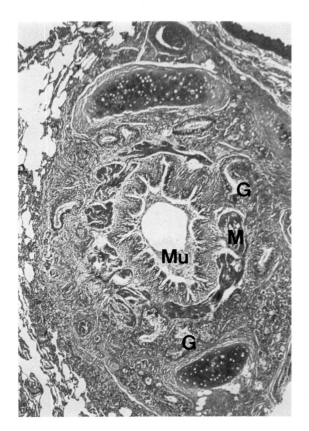

Fig. 11.8 Chronic asthma (MP)

Asthma is a common respiratory disorder characterised by instability of the smooth muscle of bronchiolar walls leading to paroxysmal bronchoconstriction. This results in diminution of airway diameter causing marked resistance to air flow, particularly on expiration. Clinically there is shortness of breath, wheezing and cough. There are several aetiological and trigger factors for bronchospasm including IgE-mediated immune reactions to allergens, bacterial or viral infections, exertion, changes in air temperature, and non-allergic sensitivity to specific environmental agents (often through occupational exposure). In severe asthma, reduction in bronchial diameter has three components: bronchospasm, mucosal oedema and luminal occlusion by excessive mucus production.

Single acute asthmatic attacks resolve with therapy leaving no apparent structural disorder; however, in chronic asthmatics, as in this example, the bronchial walls become thickened due to hypertrophy of smooth muscle **M**, hyperplasia of submucosal mucous glands **G**, protracted oedema of supporting connective tissues and marked infiltration by eosinophils. The bronchial lumen becomes obstructed by mucus **Mu** containing numerous eosinophils.

Eosinophils characteristically accumulate in a variety of allergic states and may be involved in deactivation of some of the chemical mediators.

Fig. 11.9 Pulmonary oedema (LP)

Any condition in which the left ventricle or atrium fails to empty adequately increases pressure in the affected chamber which is transmitted back to the pulmonary venous system and pulmonary capillaries. The pulmonary capilkaries become *congested* and dilated with erythrocytes and the increased hydrostatic pressure results in *transudation* of plasma fluid into the alveolar spaces causing *pulmonary oedema*.

As progressive cardiac failure is a terminal event in many diseases, pulmonary congestion and oedema are common post-mortem findings. This condition also provides an ideal environment for the growth of pathogens of relatively low virulence, so superimposed bronchopneumonia is a common sequel (see Fig. 11.5). Chronic pulmonary congestion, e.g. due to mitral stenosis, may result in numerous small intra-alveolar haemorrhages followed by red cell lysis; phagocytosis of released iron pigments, mainly haemosiderin, leads to the gross appearance known as *brown induration*.

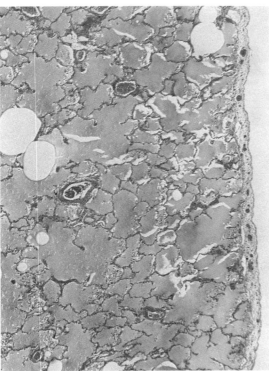

Pneumoconioses and dust-related diseases of the lungs

The commonest forms of pneumoconiosis follow inhalation of *mineral dusts* (e.g. silica and asbestos), usually over a long period of industrial exposure, leading to fibrotic reactions in the lung. Inhalation of *organic dusts* (e.g. fungal spores and plant dusts) may also cause pulmonary disease, usually by the development of chronic allergic responses termed *extrinsic allergic alveolitis.* The end result of these diseases is the development of *interstitial fibrosis* in the lungs. Pulmonary fibrosis of this type results in thickening of the barrier between blood and air causing reduced gas transfer. As the disease progresses, these may cause pulmonary hypertension and respiratory failure.

Fig. 11.10   Silicosis (MP) *(illustration opposite)*

Silicosis is the form of pneumoconiosis which tends to occur in miners and others with industrial exposure to silica dusts. Initially, the inhaled silica particles are phagocytosed by macrophages which accumulate in clumps, very occasionally forming granuloma-like masses. The presence of silica-laden macrophages excites a vigorous focal fibrotic reaction resulting in the formation of nodules of collagenous tissue. The centre of each focus becomes progressively hyaline and acellular, and is surrounded by a variable zone of more cellular fibrous tissue, exhibiting a relatively sparse chronic inflammatory cell infiltrate in which black carbon-laden macrophages abound. Usual histological methods do not reveal the presence of silica which can, however, be demonstrated as refractile particles by polarised light microscopy.

As the process continues, the fibrotic nodules may coalesce, resulting in widespread pulmonary fibrosis.

Silicosis is the most common of the pneumoconioses; other examples are asbestosis (see Fig. 11.11), and berylliosis, in which the inhaled particles excite a giant cell granulomatous reaction similar to that seen in sarcoidosis (see Fig. 3.19).

All the clinically significant inorganic dust diseases of the lung lead to progressive fibrosis, with ventilatory failure and diminished gaseous exchange. Disruption of the pulmonary microvasculature may lead to pulmonary hypertension.

Fig. 11.11   Asbestosis (HP) *(illustration opposite)*

Asbestos, a complex silicate, occurs in the form of long needle-like fibres which when inhaled into the lung parenchyma become coated with proteinaceous material to form segmented *asbestos bodies.* The presence of asbestos fibres excites a macrophage and giant cell response which ultimately leads to fibrosis in a similar manner to that of silicosis described in Figure 11.10. The major fibrotic lesions occur initially in the subpleural zone of the lower lobes.

This micrograph shows an alveolar space containing alveolar macrophages **M** and typical asbestos bodies **A**; the brownish colour of the asbestos bodies derives from the incorporation of haemosiderin in the proteinaceous coat.

Apart from its deleterious effect on pulmonary function, exposure to asbestos predisposes to neoplastic change. Mesotheliomas of the pleura and less often the peritoneum (see Fig. 11.15) may follow exposure to an uncommon form of asbestos known as 'blue asbestos', whilst common asbestos exposure greatly increases the risk of bronchogenic carcinomas, especially in cigarette smokers.

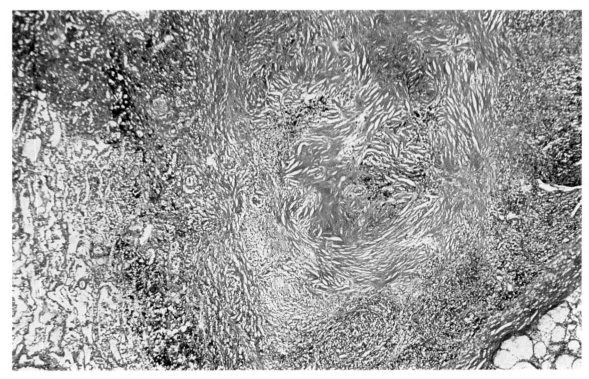

Fig. 11.10 Silicosis *(caption opposite)*

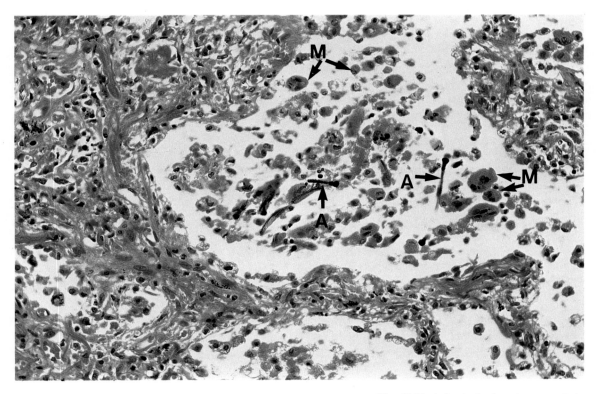

Fig. 11.11 Asbestosis *(caption opposite)*

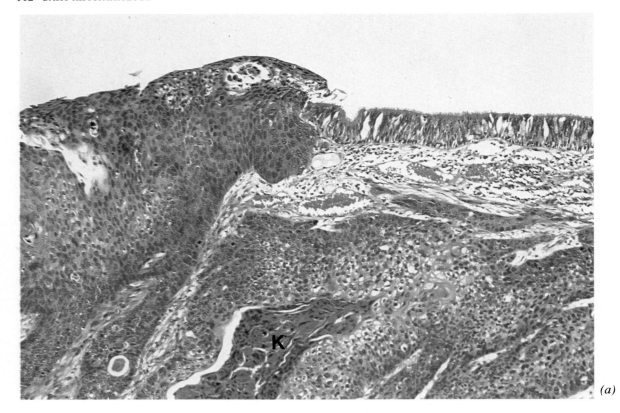

(a)

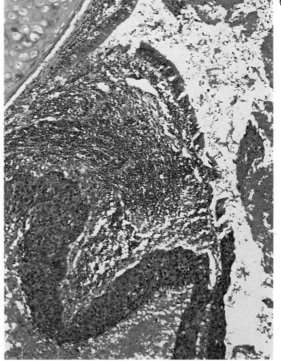

(b)

Fig. 11.12 Squamous cell carcinoma of bronchus
(a) well differentiated (HP)
(b) poorly differentiated (HP)

Squamous cell carcinoma, the commonest primary malignancy of the lung, usually arises in the main bronchi or their larger branches close to the lung hilum and often in an area of epithelium which has previously undergone focal squamous metaplasia, e.g. as a result of cigarette smoking. Such tumours invade the local parenchyma and tend to obstruct the involved airway ,as well as spreading via local lymphatics to regional lymph nodes.

These tumours have the typical features of squamous cell carcinoma but tend to vary widely in degree of differentiation. At one extreme is the well-differentiated keratinising type as in micrograph (a), where a basic stratified squamous pattern is evident and there is formation of keratin **K** in some areas. Towards the other end of the spectrum are tumours such as that shown in micrograph (b), in which squamous characteristics such as intercellular bridges are only visible at high magnification (see Fig. 6.11b). Some tumours are so poorly differentiated that squamous features cannot be seen by light microscopy, and they are often then classified as *large cell undifferentiated carcinoma*.

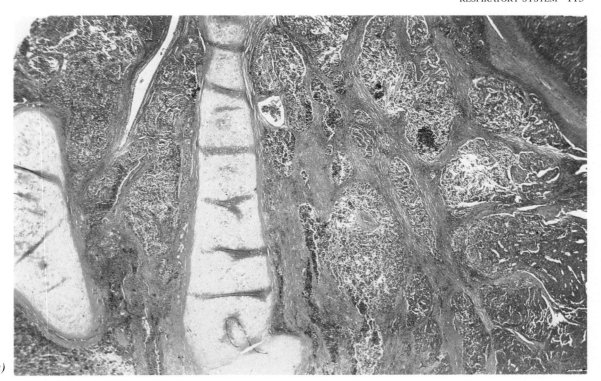

(a)

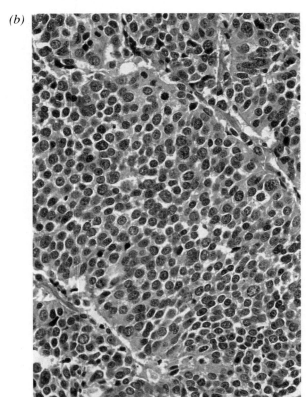

(b)

Fig. 11.13 Oat cell carcinoma
(a) LP **(b)** HP

In addition to squamous carcinoma, the proximal bronchi may also give rise to another important carcinoma known as *oat cell carcinoma*. As seen at high magnification in micrograph (b), the name derives from the supposed resemblance of the small, tightly packed, darkly stained, ovoid tumour cells to oat grains; from these histological features and rampant clinical course, some authorities prefer to apply the term *small cell undifferentiated carcinoma*. These tumours rapidly and extensively invade the bronchial wall and surrounding parenchyma as seen in micrograph (a), and may compress and invade nearby pulmonary veins. Early lymphatic and blood-borne spread is a feature of these tumours: oat cell tumours have the worst prognosis of all bronchogenic carcinomas.

The origin of oat cell tumours is thought to be from pulmonary neuroendocrine cells normally scattered within the bronchial mucosa. Apart from their local and metastatic effects, these tumours may also secrete peptide hormones such, as ADH and ACTH, giving rise to various tumour-related endocrine syndromes (*ectopic hormone secretion*).

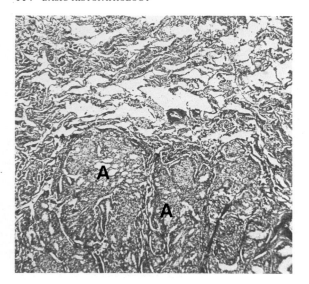

Fig. 11.14 Adenocarcinoma of the lung (LP)

Adenocarcinomas are a third common type of primary lung tumour and tend to arise more peripherally in small bronchi and bronchioles; they have a particular predilection for old areas of scar tissue, e.g. healed tuberculosis. The main histological feature of this type of tumour is the formation of the tumour cells into a glandular acinar pattern **A**, the acini often being filled with mucus. Very poorly differentiated variants of adenocarcinoma constitute another type of *large cell undifferentiated carcinoma* (see also Fig. 11.12); here also, only electron microscopy can demonstrate the glandular origin of such tumours. The cytological features of adenocarcinomas are shown in Figure 6.13. Adenocarcinoma of the lung is not as tightly linked with cigarette smoking as other lung carcinomas.

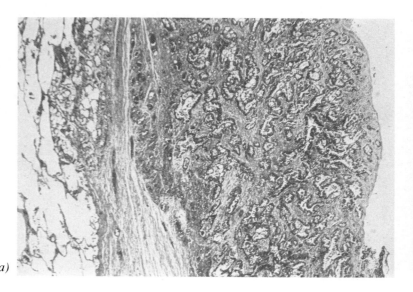

(a)

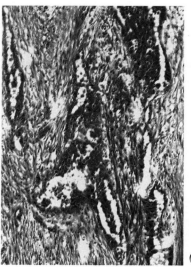

(b)

Fig. 11.15 Mesothelioma of pleura (a) LP (b) HP

The pleura is frequently involved in secondary spread of bronchial and breast carcinoma and primary tumours of the pleura are rare. Nevertheless, these tumours, known as *mesotheliomas* because of their origin from mesothelial cells, are of great interest since they are related to exposure to asbestos dust, although often exposure is trivial and in the distant past. Even more rarely, mesotheliomas of the peritoneum occur, also with a history of exposure to asbestos.

Pleural mesotheliomas present as a dense sheet of tumour extending over the pleural surface as in micrograph (a), often encasing the lung in a hard white shell; the tumour extends only a little distance into the lung parenchyma and metastatic spread is uncommon.

At low magnification, the tumour can be seen to have both a glandular epithelial component and a fibrous stromal component. At high magnification as in (b), both epithelial and spindle-celled stromal components exhibit the pleomorphism characteristic of malignancy. Most mesotheliomas contain both spindle cell and glandular components but occasionally one pattern predominates.

12. Alimentary system

Oral tissues

The mouth and associated structures may be involved in a wide variety of disease states which may be loosely divided into three categories. First, many systemic diseases, particularly dermatological conditions, exhibit oral manifestations (e.g. lichen planus, syphilis). Second, all oral tissues may be subject to acute or chronic inflammatory states, the most common being *dental caries* and its sequelae *periapical abscess formation* and *peridontal disease* (i.e. inflammation of the gums). Of more general histopathological interest is inflammation of the salivary glands leading to *chronic sialadenitis* (Fig. 12.2). Third, many benign and malignant tumours may arise in the oral tissues, the most common being squamous cell carcinomas of the lips, oral mucosa and tongue (see Fig. 12.1). Salivary tumours, both benign (see Figs. 12.3 and 12.4) and malignant (see Fig. 12.5), are relatively common.

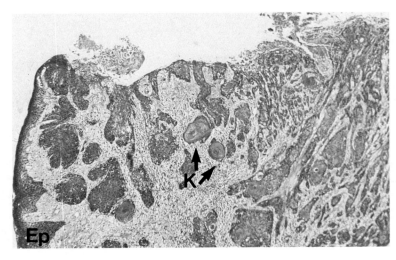

Fig. 12.1 Carcinoma of the tongue (LP)

Malignant tumours of the mucosa of the lips, tongue, cheeks and gums are almost invariably squamous cell carcinomas; they tend to be well differentiated and rarely metastasise beyond regional lymph nodes.

This micrograph illustrates a squamous carcinoma involving the tongue. The tumour has arisen from adjacent normal stratified squamous epithelium **Ep**, and has deeply infiltrated the tongue. It exhibits keratin pearl formation **K**. The cytology is shown in Figure 6.11(a).

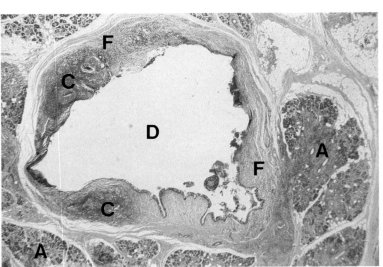

Fig. 12.2 Chronic sialadenitis (LP)

Prolonged obstruction of a large salivary gland duct by a calculus *(sialolith)* results in chronic inflammation and acinar atrophy in the gland termed *chronic sialadenitis*.

This micrograph is from the submandibular gland, the gland most frequently involved. The salivary duct **D** is dilated, with periductal fibrosis **F** and infiltration by masses of chronic inflammatory cells **C**. The surrounding secretory acini **A** have undergone marked atrophy and the expanded interstitial spaces have become filled by fibrous and adipose tissue.

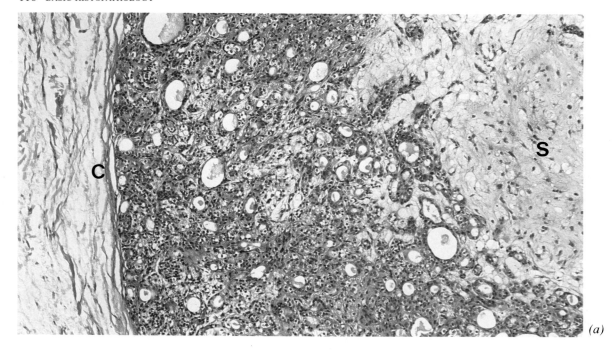

(a)

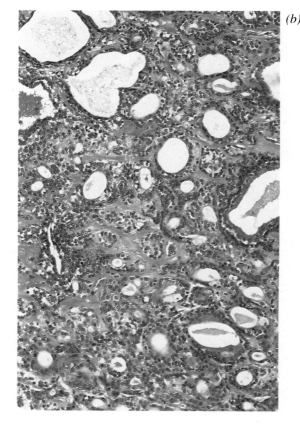

(b)

Fig. 12.3 Benign pleomorphic salivary adenoma
(a) typical pleomorphic form (MP)
(b) monomorphic variant (HP)

The most common salivary gland tumour is the *pleomorphic adenoma*, formerly known as *mixed salivary tumour*; the latter term was acquired from the histological appearance of columns and islands of benign epithelial tumour tissue separated by loose myxomatous connective tissue stroma in which areas resembling immature cartilage may be found.

Pleomorphic adenomas occur most commonly in the parotid gland and are often irregular in shape and poorly circumscribed; in the parotid gland this leads to difficulty in achieving total excision (bearing in mind the facial nerve) and local recurrence is common.

Micrograph (a) demonstrates the typical features of benign pleomorphic adenomas, namely a strongly staining neoplastic glandular element and a pale blue-stained, loose connective tissue stroma **S**, somewhat resembling cartilage. Note that the tumour is circumscribed by a thin fibrous capsule **C**.

Much less commonly, salivary adenomas are entirely composed of the glandular epithelial component and contain none of the myxomatous stromal component which often dominates the picture in the typical pleomorphic salivary adenoma; this variant is described as a *monomorphic salivary adenoma* and an example is shown in micrograph (b).

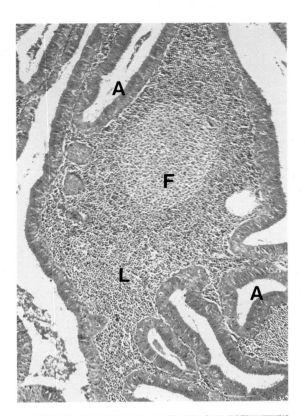

Fig. 12.4 Adenolymphoma (MP)

This unusual benign tumour occurs almost exclusively in and around the parotid gland; it commonly arises in middle-aged and older men.

The tumour is composed of large glandular acini **A** embedded in dense lymphoid tissue **L** in which typical lymphoid follicles **F** are sometimes seen. The glandular element consists of tall columnar epithelium rather resembling that of large salivary ducts.

The histogenesis of this tumour is not understood but the glandular element may represent hamartomatous salivary duct tissue within lymph nodes in and around the parotid gland. Adenolymphomas are also known by the eponymous name, *Warthin's tumour.*

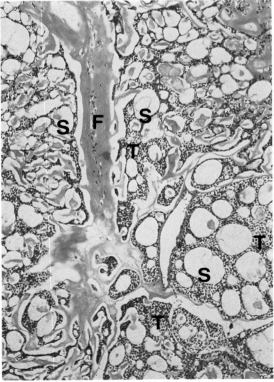

Fig. 12.5 Adenocystic carcinoma (MP)

The most common malignant tumour of salivary tissue is the *adenocystic carcinoma,* formerly known by the unsatisfactory and inaccurate term *cylindroma.* Histologically, it has a characteristic cribriform (sieve-like) appearance due to the presence of small spaces **S** in an otherwise solid mass of tightly packed tumour cells **T**. The tumour cells are arranged in clumps and cords separated by a fibrous stroma **F** which may exhibit a marked degree of hyalinisation.

As well as occurring in the major salivary glands, adenocystic carcinomas commonly arise in the minor or accessory salivary glands of the palate. These tumours are locally invasive and prone to recurrence following surgical excision. Spread to regional lymph nodes is frequent and wide systemic spread is common.

Oesophagus

The lower oesophagus frequently becomes inflamed as a result of gastric acid reflux, producing either oesophagitis or sometimes chronic peptic ulceration analogous to that seen in the stomach and duodenum (see Figs. 3.1 and 12.7). In response to reflux of acid-pepsin, the squamous mucosa of the lower oesophagus may undergo metaplastic transformation into a form of glandular epithelium similar to that seen in the stomach. This metaplastic condition is eponymously termed *Barrett's oesophagus*.

The most common oesophageal neoplasm is squamous cell carcinoma (Fig. 12.6), although adenocarcinomas may arise in metaplastic glandular epithelium at the lower end of the oesophagus. The lower oesophagus may also be involved by local spread of adenocarcinoma of the upper stomach.

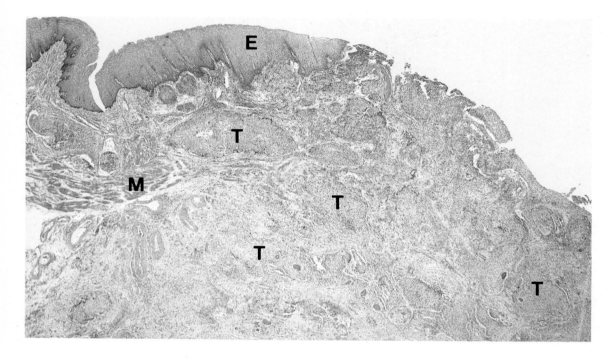

Fig. 12.6 Squamous carcinoma of oesophagus (LP)

The oesophagus is lined by stratified squamous epithelium and the majority of malignant oesophageal tumours are typical squamous carcinomas with occasional keratin pearl formation (cytological details are shown in Fig. 6.11); most are only moderately well differentiated.

Obstructive symptoms do not usually occur until the lesions are well advanced, with extensive local invasion of surrounding mediastinal tissues and metastases, particularly to regional lymph nodes and the liver; prognosis is thus usually very poor. In this example, note the origin of the tumour from normal stratified squamous epithelium **E** and infiltration of the muscular wall **M** by blue-staining islands of tumour **T**.

Adenocarcinomas (see Fig. 6.13) form a small proportion of oesophageal malignancies and usually arise from metaplastic gastric mucosa; their clinical course is similar to that of squamous carcinomas.

Stomach

Gastritis

Inflammation of the stomach is termed *gastritis* and may be divided into acute and chronic forms:

- **Acute gastritis** may be associated with the use of aspirin and other anti-inflammatory drugs, excessive alcohol, and severe stress.

- **Chronic gastritis** is associated with both autoimmune causation and less well-defined environmental factors. It is manifest by inflammatory changes as well as glandular atrophy in the gastric mucosa. *Helicobacter pylori* is a recently recognised spiral-shaped bacteria which can colonise the gastric mucosa and is associated with chronic gastritis as well as gastric ulceration.

Peptic ulceration

The histological details of chronic peptic ulceration in the stomach have already been described in Chapter 3 (Fig. 3.1) as an example of non-specific chronic inflammation. Acid-induced necrosis of the gastric wall, the acute inflammatory response to that necrosis, organisation of the acute inflammatory exudate to form granulation tissue, and fibrous repair to form a fibrous scar all occur concurrently. The outcome of this dynamic process depends on which is the dominant element; the damaging stimulus (in this case, gastric acid) or the attempts of the body to heal the damage (organisation and fibrous repair). There are three main complications of chronic peptic ulceration: perforation, haemorrhage and obstruction. These are illustrated in Figure 12.7.

- **Perforation** - if tissue destruction proceeds at a pace which outstrips the attempts to confine or repair it, the process may extend rapidly through the full thickness of the wall of the bowel, leading to perforation.

- **Haemorrhage** - tissue necrosis, although not involving the full thickness of the intestine wall, extends deeply enough to involve the wall of a large artery. This is most common in long-standing chronic gastric ulcers situated on the posterior wall in the region of the left gastro-epiploic artery. This vessel tends to become incorporated in the fibrous scar on the serosal aspect of a chronic gastric ulcer, and its wall may then be eroded in a subsequent episode of tissue necrosis during an acute exacerbation of the ulceration. This may produce torrential haemorrhage leading to haematemesis, melaena and death.

- **Obstruction** - persistent attempts at repair leads to progressive formation of dense fibrous scar tissue which undergoes shrinkage (cicatrisation) and ultimately causes distortion and thickening of the wall of the viscus, commonly at the lower end of the oesophagus or in the pyloric region of the stomach. The narrowing may be so great as to cause stricture formation with partial or even complete obstruction of the lumen. When the ulcerative process is still active, this obstruction may be compounded by the inflammatory oedema of the mucosa surrounding the ulcer.

Neoplasia

Malignant tumours of the stomach are common and are almost invariably adenocarcinomas; examples are shown in Figure 12.8. Benign tumours of the stomach are relatively uncommon, most being derived from connective tissues, e.g. leiomyomas.

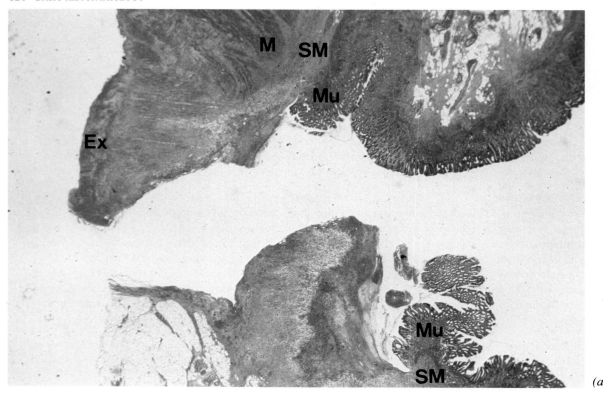

(a)

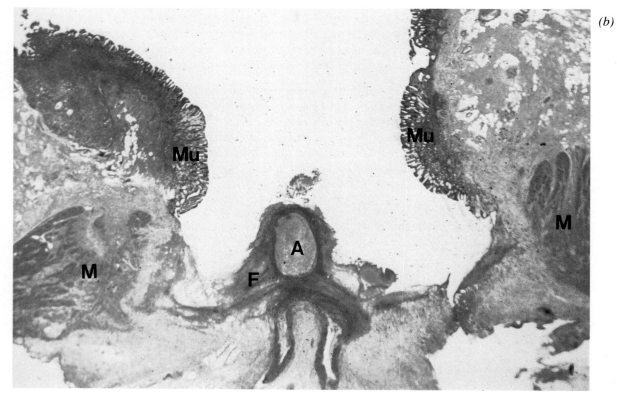

(b)

Fig. 12.7 Complications of peptic ulceration *(caption opposite)*

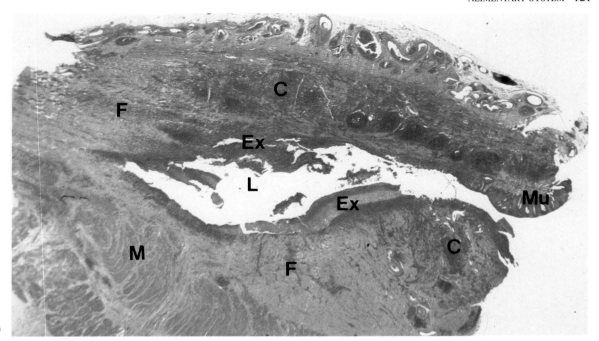

(c)

Fig. 12.7   Complications of peptic ulceration
(a) perforated gastric ulcer (LP) *(illustration opposite)*
(b) bleeding gastric ulcer (LP) *(illustration opposite)*
(c) peptic stricture of oesophagus (LP)

Perforation of peptic ulcers is a common complication and results in liberation of gastric contents into the peritoneal cavity with resulting acute peritonitis. In the perforated gastric ulcer shown in micrograph (a), note that tissue necrosis has extended through the full thickness of the wall, with complete destruction of the mucosa **Mu**, submucosa **SM** and muscle layers **M**. Discharge of gastric contents into the peritoneal cavity has excited an acute inflammatory exudate **Ex** on the serosal surface of the stomach. The margins of the perforated ulcer are lined by necrotic tissue, beneath which is a zone of acute inflammation similar to that found in the floor of a more chronic ulcer (see Fig. 3.1b), but there is no evidence of fibrous granulation tissue or fibrous scar since the destructive process has been too acute. Perforations such as this occur most commonly in peptic ulcers in the first part of the duodenum, but also occur in the stomach as in this example.

Haemorrhage from erosion of a large artery in the base of an ulcer is common in chronic gastric ulcers. Micrograph (b) illustrates such a chronic gastric ulcer; note the eroded artery **A** trapped in the fibrous scar tissue **F** forming the floor of the ulcer. Part of the wall of the artery is undergoing necrosis as a result of the acid attack and massive haemorrhage will follow.

Stricture formation may result from contraction of fibrous tissue formed in response to chronic peptic ulceration. Micrograph (c) shows a longitudinal section of a long-standing peptic ulcer of the lower oesophagus which demonstrates such a process. Note how the lumen **L** is narrowed by fibrous scarring **F**; the mucosa is extensively ulcerated and replaced by inflammatory exudate **Ex** and there is considerable chronic inflammation **C** in the wall. The presenting feature of this type of stricture is usually difficulty in swallowing *(dysphagia)*.

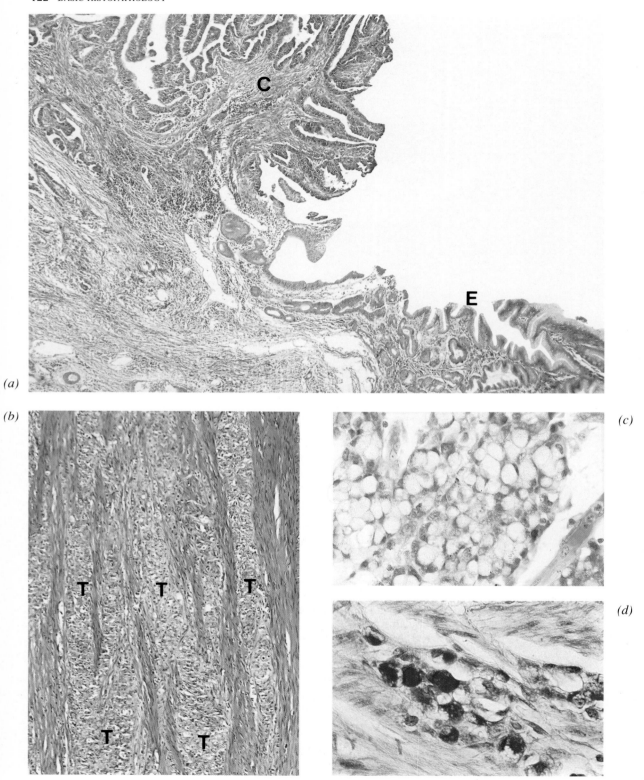

(a)

(b)

(c)

(d)

Fig. 12.8   Carcinoma of the stomach *(caption opposite)*

Fig. 12.8   Carcinoma of the stomach   *(illustrations opposite)*
(a) well-differentiated, polypoid adenocarcinoma (LP)   **(b) poorly differentiated adenocarcinoma** (MP)
(c) signet ring cells (HP)   **(d) signet ring cells** (P.A.S. staining method; HP)

Gastric carcinoma may assume a wide variety of gross morphological forms such as malignant ulcer, fungating polypoid tumour and diffuse infiltration of the wall *(linitis plastica)*. Nevertheless, the histological form is invariably that of adenocarcinoma (Fig. 6.13).

In the majority of cases, gastric adenocarcinoma is only moderately well differentiated although the whole spectrum of differentiation through to marked anaplasia can be encountered. In general, the tumours which take the form of a fungating polypoid tumour are moderately well differentiated; in the example shown in micrograph (a), a polypoid moderately differentiated carcinoma **C** arises from normal epithelium **E** and the neoplastic epithelium invades the underlying lamina propria.

In contrast, in linitis plastica, as illustrated in micrograph (b), sheets of blue-stained cells **T** infiltrate in narrow cords and strands between the red-stained bundles of muscle fibres. Glandular spaces cannot be seen as this type of tumour is almost invariably very poorly differentiated. Micrograph (c) shows some of the cells from this tumour, termed *signet ring cells,* at high magnification. The cells are ovoid in shape with the darkly staining nucleus pushed to one pole of the cell by a large non-staining mucin vacuole which occupies most of the cytoplasm (see also Fig. 6.13). The vacuoles can be demonstrated by special staining methods such as P.A.S., illustrated in micrograph (d), in which mucin droplets (mucopolysaccharide) stain magenta.

Small intestine and appendix

Primary inflammatory disorders of the small intestine are relatively uncommon with the exception of *coeliac disease* (see Fig. 12.9), and *Crohn's disease* (see Fig. 12.12). Primary tumours of the small intestine and appendix are very rare with the exception of *carcinoid tumours* (see Fig. 12.10). *Appendicitis* (see Fig. 12.11) is an extremely common disorder and is a classical example of acute inflammation.

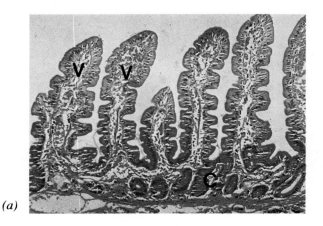

(a)

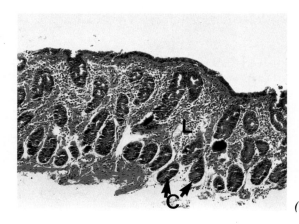

(b)

Fig. 12.9   Coeliac disease (gluten enteropathy)
(a) normal jejunal mucosa (MP)   **(b) atrophic jejunal mucosa** (MP)

Hypersensitivity to gluten (a constituent of wheat, oats and rye flour) gives rise to *coeliac disease* or *gluten enteropathy,* a condition in which the villi of the small bowel mucosa undergo complete or almost complete atrophy leaving a flat mucosal surface with greatly diminished absorptive capacity. Clinically this results in a malabsorption syndrome characterised by weight loss and *steatorrhoea* (diarrhoea containing unabsorbed lipid).

Diagnosis is usually confirmed by jejunal biopsy. Micrograph (a) shows normal mucosa with villi **V** and small crypts **C**. In coeliac disease shown in micrograph (b), there is infiltration of the mucosa by lymphoid inflammatory cells **L**, loss of villi, and hyperplasia (elongation) of crypts **C**. The result is a flat small bowel mucosa. Change to a gluten-free diet results in eventual restoration of the normal villous pattern.

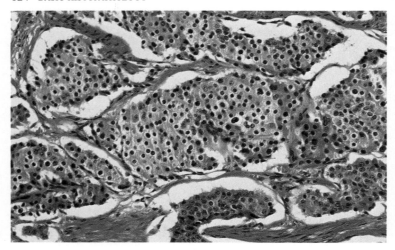
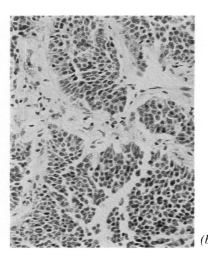

(a) *(b)*

Fig. 12.10   Carcinoid tumour of appendix
(a) H&E (HP)   (b) alkaline diazo staining method (HP)

The most common tumour of the appendix is the carcinoid tumour which is often discovered incidentally in appendices removed for appendicitis; this is also the commonest primary tumour of the small intestine. Carcinoid tumours arise from mucosal neuroendocrine APUD cells.

As seen in micrograph (a), the tumour cells are arranged in clumps or cords and are polygonal or cuboidal in shape with regular rounded nuclei. A characteristic feature is brightly-pink granular cytoplasm reflecting the

content of neuroendocrine granules. Carcinoid tumours may invade through the intestinal wall and metastasise to the liver.

Special stains such as the alkaline diazo method shown in micrograph (b) demonstrate neuroendocrine granules (brick-red by this technique) in the cytoplasm of carcinoid cells; this characteristic is common to many cells with neuroendocrine function. In carcinoid tumours, the most important secretory product is 5-hydroxytryptamine.

Fig. 12.11   Acute appendicitis   *(illustrations opposite)*
(a) early acute appendicitis (MP)
(c) late appendicitis with peritonitis (LP)
(b) later acute appendicitis (MP)
(d) gangrenous appendicitis (MP)

Acute inflammation of the appendix is one of the most common surgical emergencies. The earliest change, shown in micrograph (a), is ulceration of the mucosa **U** with overlying acute fibrinopurulent inflammatory exudate **Ex** and a purulent exudate **P** entering the lumen. At this stage, the patient may experience vague central abdominal pain.

As the condition progresses, the inflammation spreads throughout all layers of the wall of the appendix and the mucosal ulceration becomes more extensive as illustrated in micrograph (b); few of the original mucosal glands **G** now remain intact and large numbers of neutrophils have infiltrated through the submucosa **SM** and muscle layer **M** to the serosa **S**, where at one point a fibrinous exudate **F** is beginning to form on the peritoneal surface. This peritonitis, involving the parietal peritoneum in the right iliac fossa, is responsible for the classical clinical features of acute appendicitis.

The peritoneal exudate often spreads to cover most of the serosal surface of the appendix and the mesoappendix

even though the point at which the inflammation spreads through the appendix wall may remain well localised. This stage has been reached in micrograph (c); the peritoneal surface is covered by a thick fibrinopurulent exudate **Ex** extending onto the fatty mesoappendix, even though the appendix wall is not markedly inflamed at the level at which the histological section was taken. Note, however, that there is some purple-staining pus in the lumen of the appendix.

Severe continuing inflammation of the appendix wall often leads to extensive necrosis of the muscle layer *(gangrenous appendicitis)* which predisposes to perforation of the appendix with more widespread peritonitis. This feature can be seen in micrograph (d); the red-staining muscle layer **M** is identifiable up to a point where it has undergone necrosis **N**. Perforation of the appendix is imminent and will almost certainly take place at this point; the pus **P** which fills the lumen will then be discharged into the peritoneal cavity.

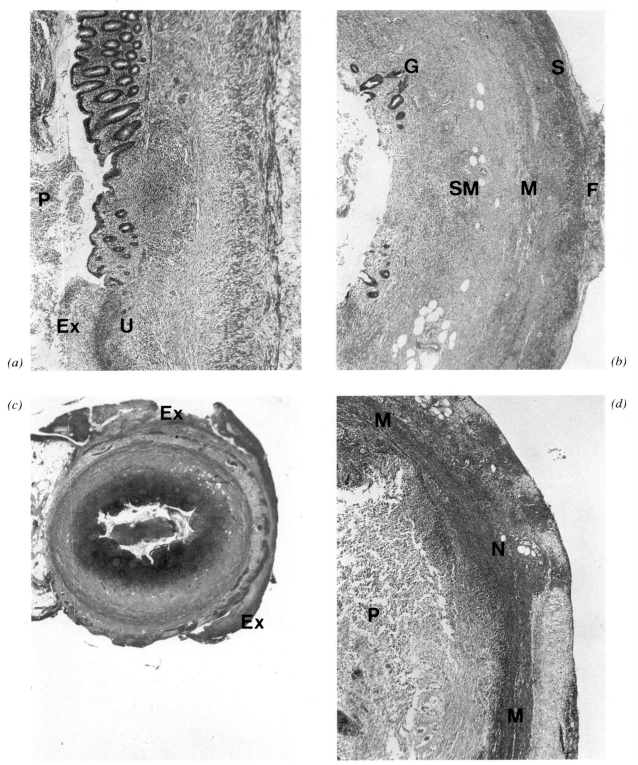

(a)

(b)

(c)

(d)

Fig. 12.11   Acute appendicitis *(caption opposite)*

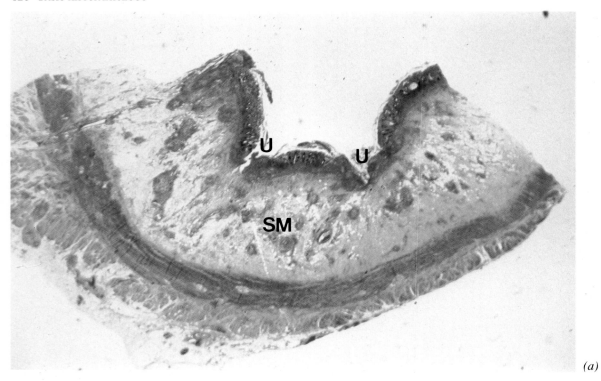

(a)

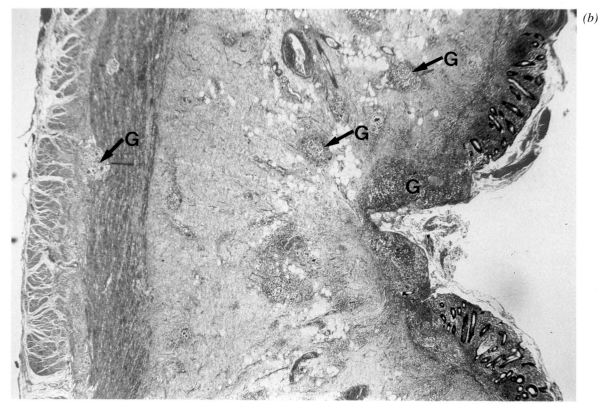

(b)

Fig. 12.12 Crohn's disease *(caption opposite)*

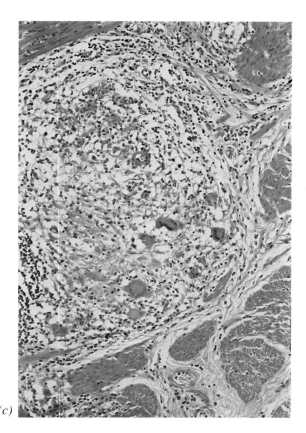

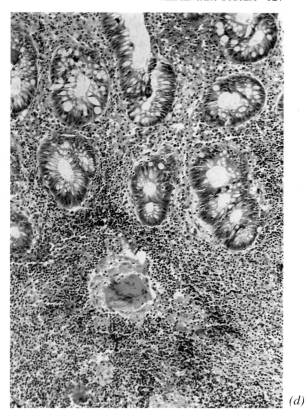

(c)   *(d)*

Fig. 12.12   Crohn's disease *(illustrations (a) and (b) opposite)*
(a) ileal lesion (LP)   **(b) fissured ulcer** (MP)
(c) Crohn's granuloma (HP)   **(d) rectal biopsy** (HP)

Crohn's disease is a chronic inflammatory disease of unknown aetiology which mainly involves the small intestine, especially the terminal ileum, but may also often affect the large bowel and anus. In the latter sites it may be confused clinically with ulcerative colitis and anal fissures and fistulae respectively. In the small intestine it is characteristically patchy in distribution, affecting short segments with lengths of normal bowel in between *(skip lesions)*.

As shown in micrograph (a), the affected segments of small intestine show gross thickening of the wall, mainly due to marked oedema and inflammation of the submucosa **SM**. This oedema produces the typical *'cobblestone'* macroscopic appearance of the mucosa in which domed areas of swollen mucosa and submucosa are criss-crossed by linear depressions caused by narrow *fissured ulcers* **U**. A typical fissured ulcer can be seen more clearly in micrograph (b), which also demonstrates two other features of Crohn's disease, namely, that the

chronic inflammatory changes are *transmural* (i.e. affect all layers from mucosa to serosa), and that *histiocytic granulomas* **G**, often containing giant cells, may be found in all layers. A granuloma between the muscle layers is illustrated at higher magnification in micrograph (c). Although granulomas in Crohn's disease contain histiocytes and multinucleate giant cells as well as lymphocytes, they are often loosely aggregated when compared to those seen in TB or sarcoidosis. Giant cell granulomata such as these may also be found in lymph nodes draining the affected segment of bowel. Micrograph (d) shows a similar, but smaller, giant cell granuloma in the chronically inflamed mucosa obtained by rectal biopsy in a case of suspected chronic ulcerative colitis; its presence resulted in Crohn's disease being diagnosed.

The result of this long-standing chronic inflammation is widespread fibrosis which may cause bowel obstruction; the deep fissured ulceration predisposes to the formation of fistulae, a common complication of Crohn's disease.

Large intestine

The colon and rectum are subject to various viral, bacterial and parasitic infections which are short lived and readily diagnosed by microbiological methods; an important exception is *amoebic colitis* which is often diagnosed only after histological examination of biopsy specimens. Of great importance is the chronic relapsing inflammatory disease of the large intestine known as *ulcerative colitis* (see Fig. 12.13).

Raised intraluminal pressure in the colon, probably due to low residue diet, commonly leads to saccular herniation of mucosa through the muscle layers of the bowel wall; the diverticula so formed may become infected giving rise to *diverticulitis* (see Fig. 12.16) which may have serious sequelae.

The large intestine may undergo infarction either as a result of mesenteric artery occlusion by thrombus or embolus, or more commonly by venous infarction following hernial strangulation or volvulus as shown in Figure 9.6.

The most common benign tumours of the large bowel are *adenomas* of the glandular epithelium. Most adenomas present as smooth-surfaced ovoid nodules arising from a short stalk *(polyps)*, however, a minority develop as frond-like *(villous)* outgrowths arising from a broad base. Benign colonic adenomas of all types usually present with rectal bleeding, and importantly, all have the potential for malignant transformation. The main types are illustrated in Figure 12.14.

Malignant tumours of the colon and rectum are very common, and almost all are adenocarcinomas (see Fig. 12.15); most appear histologically moderately differentiated with a clearly defined glandular pattern. The anal canal, being lined by squamous epithelium, is occasionally the site of a squamous carcinoma (see Fig. 6.11), although local invasion of the anal canal by an adenocarcinoma of the lower rectum also occurs.

Fig. 12.13   Ulcerative colitis   *(illustrations opposite)*
(a) active disease with pseudopolyp formation (LP)   **(b) quiescent phase** (HP)
(c) reactivated chronic disease (HP)

Ulcerative colitis is a chronic relapsing inflammatory disease of unknown cause affecting the large bowel. The disease always involves the rectosigmoid region but often extends to involve the whole colon; it is sometimes accompanied by systemic features such as anaemia, arthritis and uveitis.

In active disease, there is acute inflammation of the mucosa with neutrophils accumulating in the lamina propria and in the lumina of the colonic glands to form *crypt abscesses*; ulceration of the mucosa occurs, but the ulcers are superficial rather than fissured as in Crohn's disease (see Figs. 12.12a & b).

In severe cases, ulceration may develop extensively throughout the length of the colonic mucosa; an example is shown in micrograph (a). Note that the ulcerative process has destroyed much of the mucosa and submucosa in this field, leaving an isolated island of non-ulcerated mucosa which is swollen by acute and chronic inflammatory changes; some of the colonic glands **G** remain. Non-ulcerated areas such as this project above the surrounding ulcerated areas to produce so-called *inflammatory pseudopolyps*. Despite the severity and extent of the inflammation and ulceration, the changes are mainly confined to the submucosa and mucosa, and the muscularis **M** is not involved; inflammatory changes are rarely transmural, a useful distinguishing feature from Crohn's disease (cf. Figs. 12.12 a & b). In micrograph (a),

a peritoneal exudate is present but this resulted from peritonitis due to surgical instrumentation causing perforation; this does not represent true transmural inflammation.

During quiescent periods between acute exacerbations, the mucosa damaged by earlier severe inflammation or ulceration shows mixed features of chronic inflammation and attempts at restitution. Micrograph (b) shows a mucosal biopsy taken during a quiescent phase. The lamina propria **LP** is infiltrated by lymphocytes and plasma cells; the colonic glands show marked reduction in the numbers of mucin-secreting goblet cells and there are mild dysplastic changes with some cellular pleomorphism and increase in nuclear/cytoplasmic ratio.

Micrograph (c) illustrates the features indicative of residual or renewed acute inflammatory activity, namely the presence of crypt abscesses **A** in the glands, dilatation of superficial capillaries **C** in the lamina propria often with polymorph margination, and neutrophilic infiltration amongst the chronic inflammatory cells.

Repeated episodes of inflammation, ulceration and epithelial regeneration lead to dysplastic change in the constantly irritated surface and glandular epithelium; this factor may contribute to the high incidence of colonic adenocarcinoma arising in patients with a long history of ulcerative colitis.

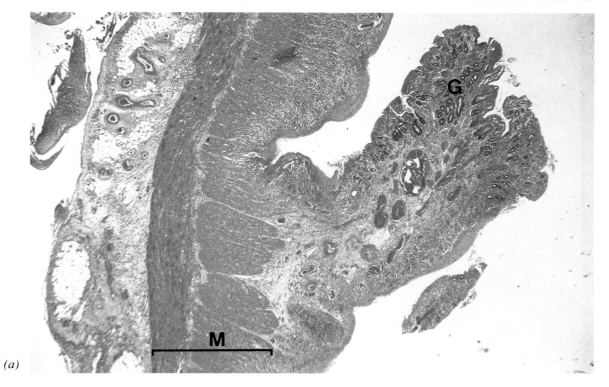

(a)

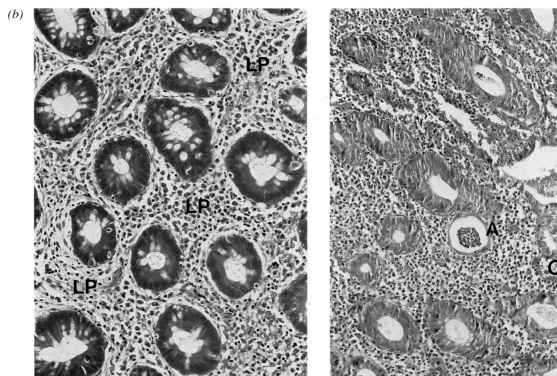

(b)

(c)

Fig. 12.13 Ulcerative colitis *(caption opposite)*

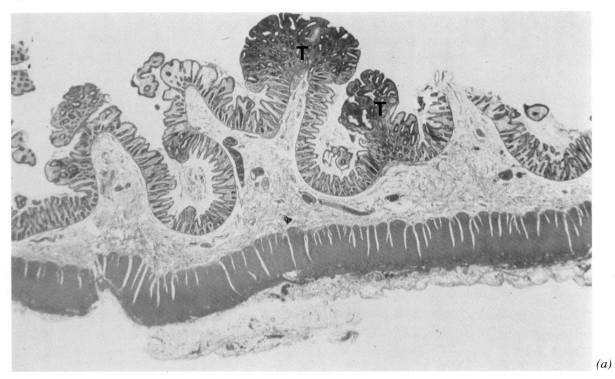

(a)

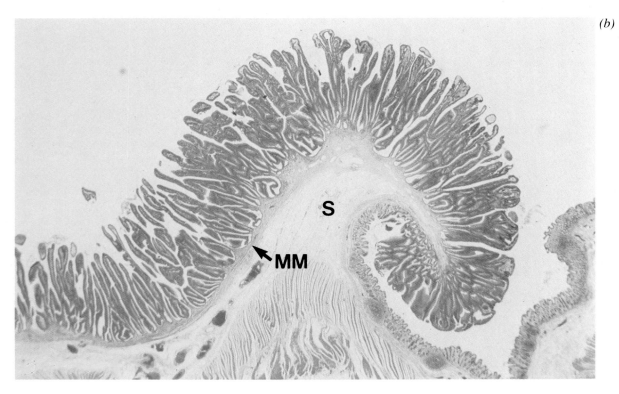

(b)

Fig. 12.14 Colonic polyps *(caption opposite)*

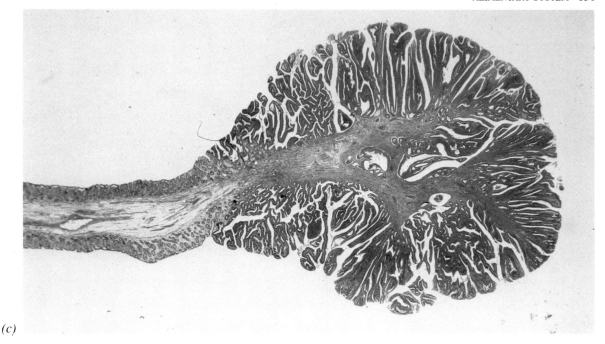

(c)

Fig. 12.14   Colonic polyps   *(illustrations (a) and (b) opposite)*
(a) tubular adenomas: polyposis coli (LP)   **(b) villous adenoma** (LP)
(c) tubulovillous adenoma (LP)

Colonic polyps are usually benign adenomas of the epithelium of the colonic mucosa. There are three main histological patterns, *tubular adenoma, villous adenoma (papilloma)* and *tubulovillous adenoma.*

Tubular adenomas are almost always pedunculated polypoid lesions, the adenoma proper being connected to the mucosa by a narrow stalk of normal tissue. The adenoma consists of dysplastic colonic epithelium arranged in straight tubular glands, the cells being dark staining because they lack the usually abundant cytoplasmic mucin and have a high nucleus/cytoplasm ratio. When seen with the naked eye, these tumours have a smooth or slightly bosselated appearance. Tubular adenomas may be either solitary or multiple. In one heritable condition, known as *familial polyposis coli,* numerous tubular adenomas develop throughout the colon and there is a strong predisposition to the transformation of original benign lesions into adenocarcinoma.

Micrograph (a) shows two tubular adenomas **T** in a segment of colon from a patient with polyposis coli. Note the darkly stained adenomatous masses connected to the underlying mucosa by stalks which merely represent extensions of the normal mucosa and submucosa. The cytological detail of glands in a colonic adenoma are shown in Figure 6.2 (b).

Villous adenoma (or *papilloma*) is a sessile, rather than pedunculated lesion, arising from a broad base; it is composed of narrow, frond-like outgrowths of epithelial cells arranged on a delicate connective tissue stroma, giving a papillary appearance both histologically and with the naked eye. A typical sessile villous adenoma is illustrated in micrograph (b); in this case, the lesion is completely benign and shows no evidence of invasion across muscularis mucosae **MM** into submucosa **S**. Further cytological detail of this tumour is shown in Figures 6.5 (a) and (b).

Many long-standing tubular adenomas acquire a partially villous histological pattern, particularly at the surface, although the general configuration of the lesion (pedunculated and non-sessile) resembles that of a pure tubular adenoma. Such adenomas are called *tubulovillous adenomas*. In the example shown in micrograph (c), note that the stalk is covered by normal colonic-type mucosa which contrasts markedly with the densely staining dysplastic epithelium of the adenoma.

All the above types of colonic polyps have the potential for malignant change with the development of invasive adenocarcinoma. This is more frequently in the villous adenoma than the other types.

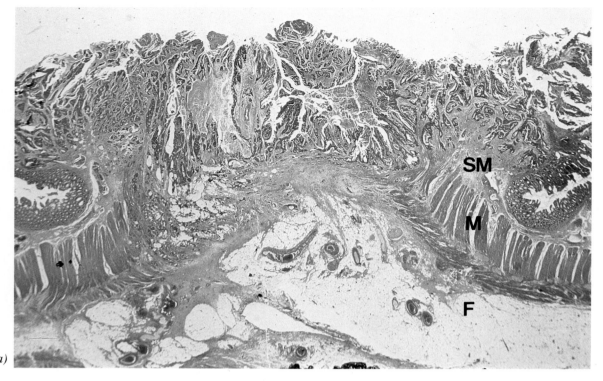

(a)

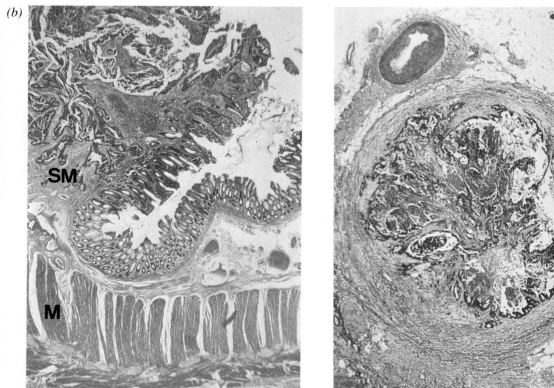

(b)

(c)

Fig. 12.15 Adenocarcinoma of the colon *(caption opposite)*

Fig. 12.15 Adenocarcinoma of the colon *(illustrations opposite)*
(a) invasive tumour (LP)   **(b) edge of lesion in (a)** (MP)
(c) invasion of vein (MP)

Adenocarcinoma is the most common and important malignant tumour of the large bowel and arises most frequently in the descending and sigmoid colon as well as the rectum. There are three common macroscopic patterns of growth; tumours may be raised with central ulceration and elevated margins, extensive lesions may involve the whole circumference of the bowel forming an annular stricture, or lesions may develop as a protruberant cauliflower-like mass most commonly seen in the caecum and proximal colon.

Micrograph (a) shows an ulcerated adenocarcinoma of the rectum; the tumour has infiltrated deeply through the submucosa **SM**, muscularis **M**, and out into the paracolic fat **F**. This tumour is moderately well differentiated as evidenced by the well-defined glandular pattern.

Micrograph (b) shows the raised everted edge of this tumour at higher magnification; note the abrupt transition between normal rectal mucosa and the abnormal malignant epithelium. In this area, the tumour has infiltrated into the submucosa **SM**, but not into the muscularis **M**.

The prognosis of colonic and rectal carcinomas depends on a number of factors, the most important being tumour stage as assessed by the depth of invasion of the bowel wall, the presence of distant metastases and evidence of tumour invasion into veins. Micrograph (c) shows a vein in the serosa of the colon; it is filled with colonic adenocarcinoma which is growing along it as a solid cord.

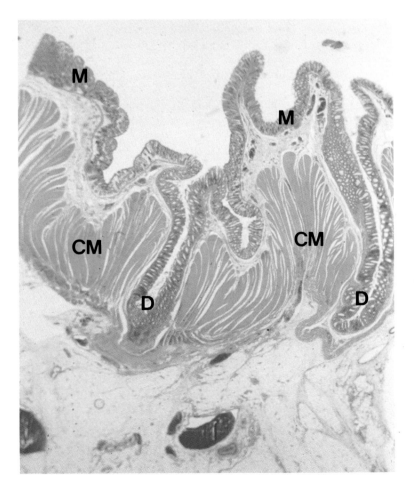

Fig. 12.16 Diverticular disease
(LP)

Diverticular disease is a common condition in the elderly; it may involve any part of the colon, although the sigmoid colon is the most frequently and most severely affected part.

The normal muscular wall of the colon consists of an inner circular layer and a discontinuous outer longitudinal layer represented by the taeniae coli. Diverticula **D** are formed by herniation of pouches of colonic mucosa **M** through unsupported areas of the circular muscle between the taenia coli. This possibly results from abnormally high intraluminal pressure associated with low residue diets. A characteristic histological feature is marked hypertrophy of the circular muscle layer **CM**. The diverticula **D** bulge towards the outer surface and often contain faecal material. Acute inflammation, *diverticulitis,* may develop following obstruction of the narrow neck of the diverticulum. Complications include rectal haemorrhage, perforation, peritonitis, paracolic abscess formation and fistula formation with other viscera such as bladder and vagina.

13. Hepatobiliary system and pancreas

Acute inflammation of the liver

Hepatocytes, with their high degree of metabolic activity, are readily disturbed by toxins, especially drugs or alcohol, and demonstrate the histological cellular responses known as cloudy swelling, fatty change and necrosis as described in Chapter 1. Since the connective tissue component of liver is normally inconspicuous apart from in the portal tracts, acute inflammation of the liver is not characterised by the usual vascular and exudative changes seen in other tissues where connective tissue is a more significant constituent. Instead, acute inflammation of the liver parenchyma is usually marked by focal accumulations of inflammatory cells usually in relation to the site of necrotic hepatocytes. The exception to this is in the formation of *hepatic abscesses* which usually develop either as a result of bacterial infections from the biliary tract or from a septic focus in the abdomen drained by the portal venous system to the liver.

Acute hepatitis is a general term for inflammation of the liver parenchyma which can then be further classified according to aetiology. The four most important groups of conditions causing acute hepatitis are:

- **Viral hepatitis** - caused by viruses which are trophic to the liver giving the histological appearance shown in Figure 13.3. *Hepatitis A and E viruses* are enterically transmitted and cause a benign form of acute hepatitis *(infectious hepatitis)*. *Hepatitis B and C viruses* are transmitted parenterally and cause acute hepatitis *(serum hepatitis)* but also commonly lead to chronic forms of liver disease such as chronic hepatitis. *Hepatitis D virus* superinfects patients with hepatitis B infection.
- **Toxins** - alcohol is the most common hepatic toxin, and liver biopsy may be used to confirm the diagnosis or establish its severity (Fig. 13.2).
- **Drugs** - hepatitis may be caused by the anaesthetic gas halothane, particularly after repeated exposures. Isoniazid, a drug commonly used in the treatment of tuberculosis, results in acute hepatitis in a small proportion of cases
- **Systemic infections** - infections such as *Leptospira* and *Toxoplasma* usually involve the liver secondarily as part of disseminated disease. Other systemic infections may cause multiple minute infective lesions as in bacterial septicaemia and miliary tuberculosis.

Although not classed as hepatitis, other parasites give rise to specific inflammations of the liver, e.g. around cysts in *hydatid disease* and the granulomata in portal areas in *schistosomiasis*. Chronic granulomatous lesions *(gummata)* also occur in tertiary syphilis (see Fig. 3.20a).

Chronic inflammation of the liver

Apart from the forms of acute hepatitis described above, some patients develop clinical and biochemical manifestations of chronic inflammation of the liver. When this situation continues without improvement for 6 months or more, the condition is described as *chronic hepatitis;* this term, however, excludes chronic inflammation of the liver caused by alcohol, bacterial agents and biliary obstruction. There are many causes of chronic hepatitis but the commonest are persistent viral infection, certain drugs, and a large group where there is no obvious causative agent and in which abnormal immunological phenomena play an important role.

In clinical terms, chronic hepatitis exhibits a spectrum of activity from self-limiting and relatively transient to severe and progressive. There are two main histological patterns at opposite ends of this spectrum:

- **Chronic persistent hepatitis** - a prolonged relapsing but self-limiting form of hepatitis with no evidence of active destruction of liver cells (Fig. 13.4)
- **Chronic aggressive hepatitis** - an insidiously progressive form of hepatitis with evidence of liver cell destruction which may cause cirrhosis and liver failure (Fig. 13.5).

Primary biliary cirrhosis is a chronic autoimmune inflammatory disease characterised by destruction of intrahepatic bile ducts with associated inflammatory changes (Fig. 13.6).

Cirrhosis

Cirrhosis is a general term applied to the end result of a variety of chronic liver disorders having the common features of diffuse persistent destruction of hepatocytes, regeneration of hepatocytes to form nodules and the development of fibrosis. The end result is impairment of liver function and gross distortion of liver architecture leading to portal hypertension. Various different types of cirrhosis are illustrated and discussed in Figure 13.8.

Other important liver disorders

- **Right sided cardiac failure** involves the liver when raised pressure is transmitted to the central veins resulting in congestion of sinusoids with blood. Hepatocytes in the centrilobular zones frequently then undergo atrophy.
- **Inborn errors of metabolism**, in most cases probably reflecting single gene defects, result in the abnormal accumulation of various metabolites within hepatocytes. These are known as *storage diseases* and include glycogen storage diseases, mucopolysaccharidoses, lipidoses, haemochromatosis and Wilson's disease. Liver biopsy may be useful in the diagnosis of such disorders and, as an example, haemochromatosis is illustrated in Fig. 13.7.
- **Amyloidosis** (see Fig. 4.5) involves extracellular accumulation of abnormal protein in the liver.
- **Malignant disease** frequently involves the liver, most commonly as secondary spread, especially from primary lesions in gut, breast and lung (see Fig. 6.7a); less frequently the liver becomes diffusely infiltrated in lymphoreticular malignancies such as Hodgkin's disease and other lymphomas.
- **Primary malignancy** of the liver, *hepatocellular carcinoma* (see Fig. 13.9), is uncommon and most often arises in pre-existing cirrhosis.

Fig. 13.1   Clinical features of hepatobiliary diseases and their pathophysiology

Sign/symptom	Clinical feature	Mechanism
Jaundice	Yellow colouration of tissues due to bile	Failure of metabolism or excretion of bile pigments
Bleeding	Easy bruising and prolonged clotting time of blood	Failure of synthesis of clotting factors
Oedema	Swelling of dependent parts due to extracellular accumulation of water	Failure of synthesis of albumen resulting in reduced plasma oncotic pressure
Ascites	Fluid in peritoneal cavity	Low serum albumen and portal hypertension
Gynaecomastia	Enlarged male breast	Failure to detoxify endogenous oestrogens
Encephalopathy	Altered consciousness; lack of co-ordination; may lead to coma	Failure to detoxify ammonia and excitatory amino acids which result from protein breakdown
Haematemesis and melaena	Vomiting blood and passing blood per rectum	Bleeding from oesophageal varices due to portal hypertension

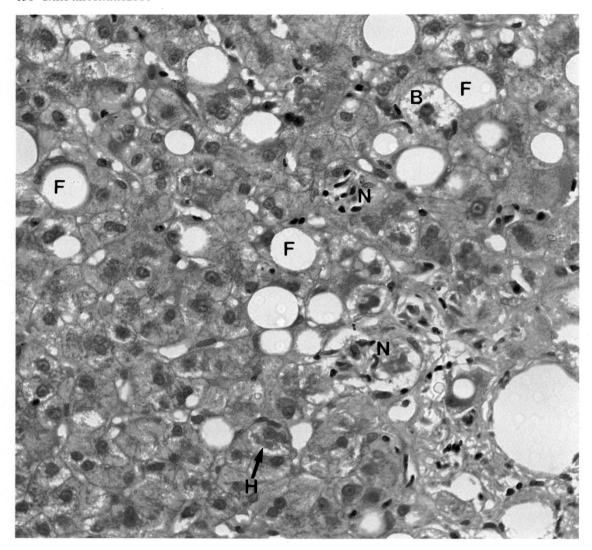

Fig. 13.2 Alcoholic hepatitis (HP)

Alcohol is a potent hepatotoxin when taken in large quantities and liver changes occur even after isolated bouts of heavy drinking.

Early evidence of metabolic injury to the hepatocytes is the appearance of fatty change **F** manifest by the accumulation of lipid in the form of large cytoplasmic vacuoles within some hepatocytes, usually displacing the nucleus to one side (see also Fig. 1.5). With more severe metabolic disruption, the hepatocytes undergo hydropic degeneration (see Fig. 1.4) and become swollen and vacuolated, an appearance described as *ballooning degeneration* **B**; in some cases, the metabolic disruption may be irrecoverable and some hepatocytes undergo necrosis. The location of necrotic hepatocytes **N** is marked by foci of neutrophils and lymphocytes. Some hepatocytes accumulate an eosinophilic material, derived from cytoskeletal cytokeratin intermediate filaments, termed *Mallory's hyaline* **H**; this material forms irregular cytoplasmic globules, usually near the nucleus, and stains a glassy pink colour, slightly darker than the normal cytoplasm. The hepatocytes around the centrilobular veins appear to be most vulnerable to alcohol toxicity and in some individuals delicate fibrosis may be seen around the central veins.

With prolonged alcohol abuse there is progressive fibrosis due to hepatocyte necrosis and regeneration of liver cells which can develop into alcoholic cirrhosis, illustrated in Figure 13.18.

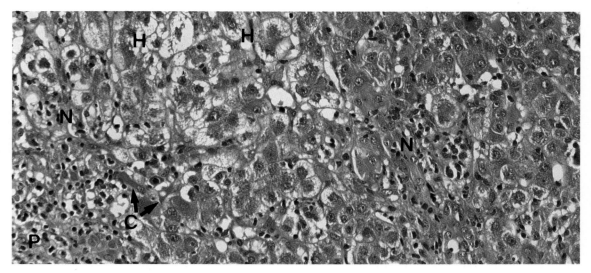

Fig. 13.3 Acute viral hepatitis (HP)

The viral agents of acute hepatitis all produce a similar histological picture.

There is widespread swelling and ballooning of hepatocytes due to hydropic degeneration **H** and this progresses to focal or spotty necrosis throughout the lobule; the areas of necrosis are identified by aggregates of neutrophils **N** or round eosinophilic (pink-stained) bodies called *Councilman bodies* **C**, representing the cytoplasm of necrotic liver cells. The Kuppfer cells are very active and within portal tracts **P** there are increased numbers of chronic inflammatory cells.

In time, regeneration of the dead hepatocytes occurs. In hepatitis A and E (infective type) the changes usually completely resolve but in hepatitis B and C (serum type) activity may persist or progress to chronic active hepatitis (Fig. 13.5).

Rare cases of viral hepatitis occur in which there is massive liver necrosis instead of the focal type seen here. This is particularly seen with hepatitis E in pregnancy and such fulminant cases are usually fatal.

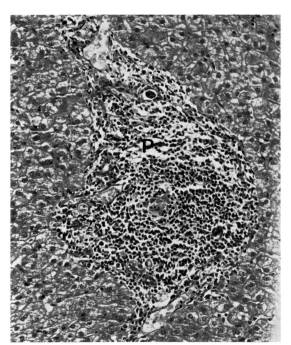

Fig. 13.4 Chronic persistent hepatitis (HP)

This form of chronic hepatitis is encountered after a previous episode of acute viral hepatitis. Clinically, it is noted that biochemical tests of liver function fail to return to normal and biopsy is performed to assess the degree of liver damage. Histologically, there is expansion of the portal tract **P** by mononuclear chronic inflammatory cells, mainly lymphocytes but with some plasma cells. Note that the inflammation is sharply limited to the connective tissue of the portal tract, in contrast to chronic aggressive hepatitis (see Fig. 13.5), where the inflammation spills out into the liver parenchyma. No necrosis of liver cells is seen in chronic persistent hepatitis.

This form of chronic hepatitis has a good prognosis and the histological changes remain stable or improve over a period of time. This biopsy was from a patient who had an episode of acute hepatitis due to hepatitis B virus; liver function tests were still mildly abnormal 8 months after the illness prompting the biopsy.

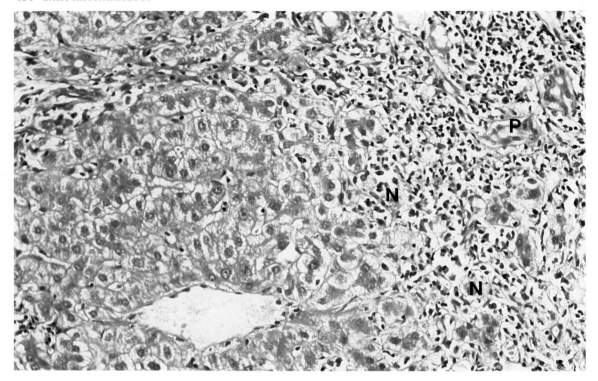

Fig. 13.5 Chronic aggressive hepatitis (HP)

This disease is a form of chronic hepatitis characterised by continued active inflammation and hepatocyte damage commonly resulting in progressive fibrosis. The disease may progress to cirrhosis and liver failure if untreated.

There are several causes of this histological picture including persistent hepatitis B infection; other patients have high titres of auto-antibodies, particularly against smooth muscle, and an auto-immune aetiology has been postulated in such cases. Certain drugs may also cause this pattern of reaction.

Histologically, chronic aggressive hepatitis has three main features: chronic inflammation, hepatocyte necrosis and fibrosis. These are illustrated in the micrograph above.

Marked chronic inflammatory infiltration occurs in the portal tracts which become expanded by lymphocytes and plasma cells. The layer of liver cells immediately adjacent to the portal tracts, known to pathologists as the *limiting plate*, undergoes necrosis **N** with lymphocytes and plasma cells spilling out of the portal tracts **P** into the liver parenchyma; this necrosis of cells in the limiting plate is patchy and is termed *piecemeal necrosis*. The hepatocyte necrosis around the portal areas leads to fibrosis which may link the portal tracts with fibrous bridges. With further liver damage the condition progresses to cirrhosis as shown in Figure 13.8(d).

This histopathological appearance is known by the term *chronic aggressive hepatitis* and corresponds to the clinical condition described as *chronic active hepatitis*.

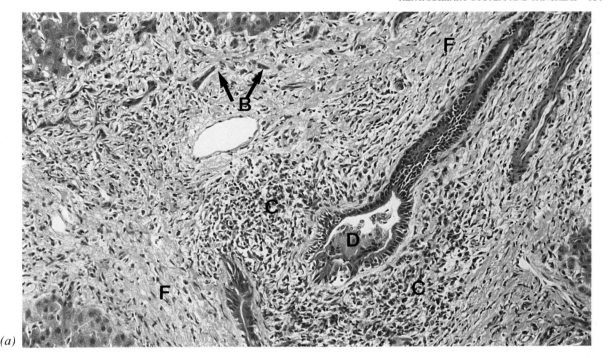

(a)

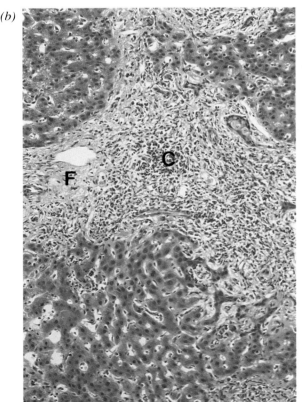

(b)

Fig. 13.6 Primary biliary cirrhosis
(a) early lesion (HP) **(b) later lesion** (HP)

Primary biliary cirrhosis is a chronic inflammatory disease of the liver in which destructive inflammatory changes are centred primarily on bile ducts; hepatocytes are, however, also affected.

The earliest changes are seen in the epithelium of the larger bile ducts **D** as shown in micrograph (a). There is vacuolation of the epithelial cells and infiltration of the wall and surrounding tissues by chronic inflammatory cells. A characteristic feature at this stage, though not shown here, is the formation of *histiocytic granulomata* in relation to damaged bile ducts. Portal tracts then become progressively expanded by chronic inflammatory cells **C**.

As seen in micrograph (b), the inflammatory cells progressively extend from the portal tracts into the liver parenchyma, with piecemeal necrosis occurring along the limiting plate in a manner similar to chronic aggressive hepatitis (see Fig. 13.5). As liver cells are destroyed, the portal tracts also become expanded by fibrosis **F**. Large bile ducts are no longer visible, having been destroyed.

At the periphery of the portal tracts there is proliferation of small bile ducts **B** which do not appear to be canalised; this feature is best seen in micrograph (a).

If primary biliary cirrhosis proceeds unchecked, true cirrhosis develops (see Fig. 13.8); note that this disease is referred to as primary biliary cirrhosis even in the early stages when there is no evidence of cirrhotic changes.

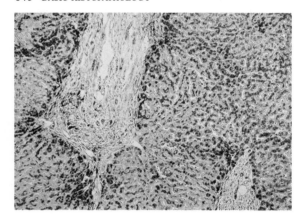

Fig. 13.7   Haemochromatosis (Perls stain; MP)

Haemochromatosis is a condition characterised by excessive deposition of iron in the tissues. It is due to an inherited defect of iron transport such that excessive iron is absorbed from a normal diet. Pathologically excessive iron is deposited in many tissues especially the myocardium, the liver, the adrenal glands and the pancreas.

Hepatic involvement causes cirrhosis. As seen in this micrograph, liver cells accumulate enormous amounts of iron which are stained blue by Perls stain. Excessive iron may also be stored in the liver due to dietary excess or frequent blood transfusion. This is termed *secondary haemosiderosis*.

Fig. 13.8   Cirrhosis   *(illustrations opposite)*
(a) alcoholic cirrhosis (MP)
(c) cryptogenic cirrhosis (van Gieson stain; MP)

(b) cryptogenic cirrhosis (MP)
(d) cirrhosis due to chronic active hepatitis (MP)

Cirrhosis is the end result of continued damage to liver cells from a great many causes. It is characterised by fibrous septa which cut across the liver lobules and the formation of nodules of regenerating liver cells. Portal tracts become interconnected by broad bands of fibrous tissue with distortion of the normal liver architecture.

There are two main effects of this altered liver architecture and cellular damage: reduced liver cell function with consequences listed in Figure 13.1, and disturbance of blood flow through the liver from portal vein to hepatic vein.

The effect of vascular obstruction within the liver is an increase in portal venous pressure termed *portal hypertension*. Anastomoses open up between the portal circulation and the systemic venous system resulting in large dilated veins called *varices*. The most important site of varices is in the lower oesophagus but they can occur elsewhere. These dilated thin-walled varices are liable to rupture and this is a common fatal event in patients with cirrhosis.

The classification of cirrhosis is based on the disease which caused the underlying liver damage. The most important causes are chronic alcohol abuse, chronic aggressive hepatitis and biliary cirrhosis (primary and secondary to obstruction). In a large percentage of cases no underlying disease can be found; this is known as *cryptogenic cirrhosis*.

The diagnosis of cirrhosis is confirmed by liver biopsy, usually using a wide-bore needle. Histological examination is directed towards identifying the nature of any underlying disease process as well as establishing evidence of cirrhosis.

In micrograph (a), the features of cirrhosis are broad fibrous bands **F** connecting portal areas **P**, and intervening nodules of liver cells **L** showing marked fatty change; this

is an example of alcoholic cirrhosis.

Micrograph (b) shows a typical cirrhotic pattern, with bands of fibrous tissue **F** disrupting the lobular architecture; there is no inflammation, fatty change or specific features. If there are also no clinical pointers to the aetiology, this is classified as cryptogenic cirrhosis. Micrograph (c) is from the same case, this time stained by a method which emphasises the fibrosis (stained red).

Cirrhosis following chronic aggressive hepatitis is illustrated in micrograph (d). The portal tracts **P** contain large numbers of chronic inflammatory cells and in some areas these inflammatory cells spill over the limiting plate into nodules of hepatocytes. There are also focal areas of inflammation **I** in the liver parenchyma. The portal tracts show evidence of fibrosis and fibrous bands **F** containing chronic inflammatory cells have formed bridges between adjacent portal areas. These features are all characteristically seen in chronic aggressive hepatitis (see Fig. 13.5).

Treatment of cirrhosis is aimed at controlling the underlying liver disease which is the cause of the progressive fibrosis. Repeated liver biopsy can be used to monitor the progress of the disease.

Older classifications of cirrhosis grouped the diseases according to the size of the regeneration nodules seen at post-mortem or laparotomy. In *macronodular cirrhosis* large nodules up to several centimetres in diameter are present. *Micronodular cirrhosis* is characterised by uniform small nodules of regeneration up to one centimetre in diameter. While useful to describe macroscopic features, this classification does not help in assessing disease type or progress.

In *active cirrhosis* there is evidence of continuing damage to liver cells, whereas in *inactive cirrhosis* there is no evidence of continuing liver damage.

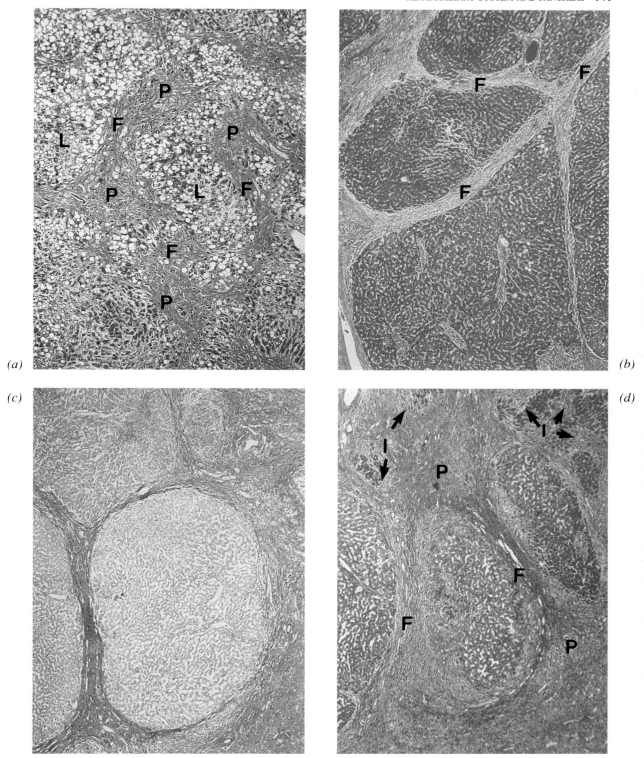

(a)

(b)

(c)

(d)

Fig. 13.8 Cirrhosis *(caption opposite)*

Fig. 13.9   Hepatocellular carcinoma (HP)

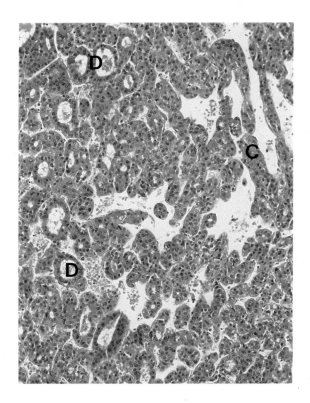

Primary carcinoma of the liver is a relatively uncommon condition compared to secondary malignant deposits. On a world-wide basis the incidence of hepatocellular carcinoma is closely related to the prevalence of hepatitis B virus infection. In some parts of Africa it accounts for up to 40% of all cancers, however, in Europe and USA it only accounts for around 2%. Cirrhosis from any cause also predisposes to the development of hepatocellular carcinoma.

The tumour may form a single massive nodule, multiple small nodules, or exhibit a diffuse infiltrating pattern. In this example, the tumour cells resemble normal hepatocytes; in some places they are arranged in cords **C,** in others in a duct-like pattern **D**. In well-differentiated tumours, bile may be present in the tumour cells.

Alphafetoprotein is secreted by a large proportion of hepatocellular carcinomas and is a useful diagnostic marker.

These tumours are associated with rapid clinical progression with average survival from diagnosis being around six months.

Disorders of the biliary system

Gall bladder disease is a common surgical problem in developed countries and is often associated with stone formation and chronic obstruction of the cystic duct leading to *chronic cholecystitis* (see Fig. 13.11). Tumours of the biliary system are relatively rare and usually take the form of highly malignant adenocarcinomas (see Fig. 13.10).

Fig. 13.10   Cholangiocarcinoma (HP)

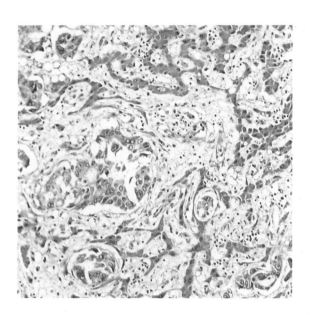

Cholangiocarcinoma arises from bile duct epithelium and may be extrahepatic (in the extrahepatic bile ducts) or intrahepatic in location. Histologically, a dense fibrous stroma is a conspicuous feature. The malignant epithelium forms small gland-like structures and the cells are often very pleomorphic.

Bile duct tumours may spread along intrahepatic portal tracts or may form large nodular growths in the liver; obstructive jaundice is a common mode of presentation. Cholangiocarcinomas also arise in the gall bladder, usually in the very elderly; invading locally they present later and have an even worse prognosis.

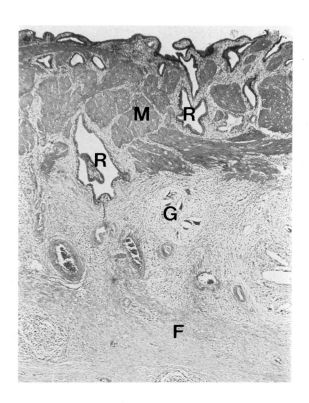

Fig. 13.11   Chronic cholecystitis (LP)

Many gall bladders containing stones are removed surgically because of abdominal pain. On histological examination, there is evidence of low grade chronic inflammation with marked muscle hypertrophy **M** and an infiltrate of lymphocytes and plasma cells in the submucosal layer. Irregular gland-like mucosal pockets extend deep into the thickened muscle layer and are known as *Rokitansky-Aschoff sinuses* **R**.

Outside the muscle layer, aggregates of histiocytes form around inspissated bile forming *bile granulomata* **G**. There is fibrosis **F** and mild chronic inflammation beneath the serosa.

If bile becomes inspissated and concentrated within the gall bladder, it may cause an acute chemical cholecystitis with a more neutrophilic inflammatory component.

Pancreatic disorders

Inflammation of the pancreas *(pancreatitis)* may present in acute or chronic form. Acute pancreatitis has a high mortality partly due to the release of pancreatic enzymes into surrounding tissues causing severe local tissue destruction and is discussed in Figure 13.12. Chronic pancreatitis is frequently associated with intractable pain and in some cases causes chronic pancreatic insufficiency.

Malignant disease of the pancreas is now appearing with increasing frequency; these adenocarcinomas (see Fig. 13.13) are highly malignant and metastases are almost always present by the time of diagnosis.

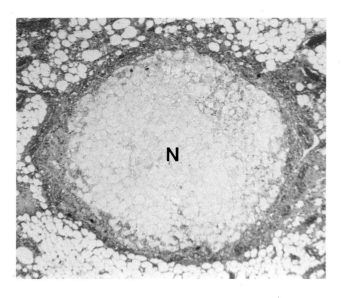

Fig. 13.12   Fat necrosis in acute pancreatitis (MP)

Acute pancreatitis is a condition in which there is destruction of the pancreatic gland due to liberation of pancreatic enzymes. Severe cases result in a massive chemical peritonitis causing severe abdominal pain and shock. The two most important predisposing conditions are *alcoholism* and *biliary tract disease* (usually stones).

Histologically, there is extensive haemorrhagic necrosis of pancreas and surrounding tissues. Release of pancreatic enzymes gives rise to a characteristic feature termed *fat necrosis*. With the naked eye, numerous chalky-white spots are seen in peripancreatic and omental fat. Histologically, they represent foci of necrotic adipose tissue **N**, surrounded by a darker staining rim of inflammatory cells.

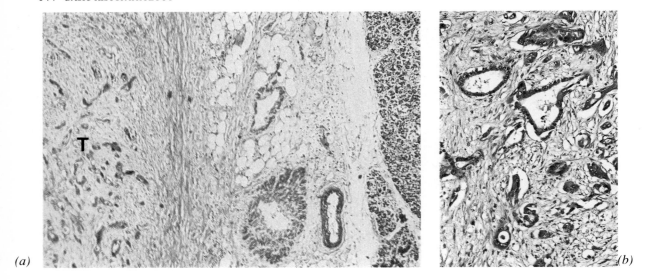

(a) *(b)*

Fig. 13.13 Adenocarcinoma of the pancreas
(a) LP   **(b)** HP

These tumours virtually all arise from the pancreatic
ductal epithelium and are of great importance because of
their insidious manner of growth, often remaining
undetected until a very advanced stage.

The majority of tumours arise in the head of the gland
where they tend to obstruct the bile duct thus presenting
early with painless jaundice.

Macroscopically, the tumours are hard and white.
Micrograph (a) shows tumour **T** with normal pancreas on
the right. Note the characteristic tortuous, irregular glands
in a dense fibrous stroma. At higher magnification in
micrograph (b), the tumour is seen to have a ductular
pattern, with marked variation in size and shape of
neoplastic gland-like spaces.

14. Urinary system

Introduction

The urinary system comprises the kidneys, pelvicalyceal systems, ureters, bladder and urethra (collectively called the urinary tract). The kidney is responsible for the excretion of waste products from body metabolic processes, the waste products being excreted in the form of an aqueous solution called urine. The urine passes from the kidney into the pelvicalyceal systems and thence via the ureter to the bladder which acts as a reservoir. Urine is held in the bladder by a series of muscular sphincters until sufficient volume has accumulated, when opening of the sphincters and contraction of smooth muscle in the bladder wall allows the urine to be voided to the exterior through the urethra (micturition).

Congenital disorders of the urinary system

There are a number of important congenital disorders of the urinary system. These are summarised in Figure 14.1.

Fig. 14.1 Congenital abnormalities of the urinary system

Kidneys	
Renal agenesis	Commonly part of other malformations. Incompatible with life when bilateral
Renal dysplasia	Abnormal metanephric development. Kidneys multicystic with mesenchymal elements such as cartilage present. May be unilateral or partial
Polycystic kidney (autosomal dominant)	Usually presents in adult life with hypertension, renal failure and/or haematuria
Polycystic kidney (autosomal recessive)	Presents in newborn children with renal failure
Ectopic kidney	Commonly pelvic. Result of abnormal metanephric development
Horse-shoe kidney	Kidneys are fused across the midline into one organ. Common abnormality (1/1000 adults). Usually an incidental finding
Ureters	
Double and bifid ureter	Commonly associated with duplication of renal pelves. May be asymptomatic but can cause urinary obstruction through abnormal drainage or kinking
Bladder	
Extrophy	Bladder communicates with surface of the anterior abdominal wall as an open sac due to failure of embryological closure

The kidney

The main functions of the kidneys are the excretion of nitrogenous by-products of body metabolism and the maintenance of water and electrolyte homeostasis. The structural unit responsible for these functions, the *nephron,* has two components, the *glomerulus* and the *renal tubule.* The glomerulus consists of a highly specialised capillary network from which water, electrolyte ions and nitrogenous waste products are filtered into the lumen of the renal tubule. The ultrafiltrate then passes along the tubular system where selective reabsorption of water and electrolytes occurs leaving unwanted water and electrolytes, together with nitrogenous waste materials such as urea and creatinine, to pass out of the kidneys as urine.

From a functional viewpoint, the activity of the glomerulus depends virtually entirely on the integrity of its structure whereas in contrast, the activity of the renal tubule is mostly determined by the metabolic activity of the lining epithelial cells. Glomerular function tends to be disrupted by pathological phenomena which alter (often in a subtle way) glomerular structure, whereas disorders of renal tubular function are more often brought about by a metabolic insult to the tubular cells such as hypoxia, or exposure to circulating toxins. Importantly, both glomerulus and tubule are utterly dependent for their normal function on adequate perfusion of the kidney by circulating blood and if this is disrupted there are serious consequences to both nephron components. Once disease has affected one part of the nephron then it is not uncommon for secondary abnormalities to develop in the other because of the intimate structural and functional relationships which exist in the kidney. The kidneys have a considerable degree of functional reserve but when disease processes damage sufficient numbers of nephrons to exceed the homeostatic ability of the remaining nephrons, renal failure ensues.

Renal impairment syndromes

For simplicity, renal disorders can be divided into two main types: *total,* in which all functions of the nephron are impaired, or *partial* (selective), in which only certain functions are disturbed.

The syndromes of total renal impairment are known clinically as *chronic* and *acute renal failure.* Partial renal dysfunction is the hallmark of the clinical conditions known as the *nephritic syndrome,* the *nephrotic syndrome* and the *mixed nephritic-nephrotic syndrome,* together with minor or precursor stages.

Total renal failure syndromes

- **Chronic renal failure**: progressive retention of nitrogenous metabolites (uraemia) due to insufficient glomerular filtration. Concomitant failure of tubular function produces widespread abnormalities in biochemical homeostasis, including salt and water retention, metabolic acidosis, and other electrolyte imbalances particularly hyperkalaemia. Many renal lesions can produce the chronic renal failure syndrome but all have as their common basis the *slowly progressive, irreversible destruction of almost all nephron units,* both glomerular and tubular components. The primary lesion may be disease of the vessels (e.g. hypertension or vasculitis), disease of glomeruli (e.g. glomerulonephritis), or disease of tubules. Chronic renal failure may also result from destruction of the whole nephron secondary to severe bacterial infection or urinary outflow obstruction. A kidney in which all nephrons have been irreversibly damaged is macroscopically small and shrivelled and is known as an *end-stage kidney* (see Fig. 14.2).
- **Acute renal failure:** abrupt cessation of activity of the nephrons, usually manifest initially as a marked fall in urine production *(oliguria)* which may even be total *(anuria).* Disturbances of fluid and electrolyte balance soon follow, particularly a rise in the serum potassium level and metabolic acidosis; if nephron failure persists, features of nitrogen retention develop. Again, many different types of lesion can produce acute renal failure, but all have as their common basis the *acute cessation of nephron activity.* The initiating lesion may primarily involve the blood supply, as in hypovolaemic shock, causing hypoxic injury or necrosis of tubular epithelial cells (see Fig. 1.4), the glomerulus, as in some forms of glomerulonephritis, or the tubules as in papillary necrosis (see Fig. 14.3). The important difference from chronic renal failure is that the acute syndrome is sometimes reversible and normal nephron function may be restored if the pathological stimulus is removed either spontaneously or as a result of treatment.

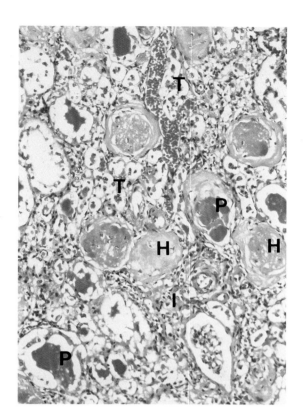

Fig. 14.2   End-stage kidney (MP)

Many progressive renal diseases of greatly differing pathogenesis are followed by progressive nephron destruction paralleled clinically by insidious deterioration of renal function culminating in death due to chronic renal failure. At necropsy, the kidneys are usually found to be small and hard with symmetrical atrophic thinning of the cortex and poor demarcation of cortex from medulla. This condition is known as *end-stage kidney*, and both in gross and histological appearance there is often little clue to the original renal pathology.

In the cortex, there is widespread replacement of glomerular tufts by avascular, acellular hyaline material **H** *(hyalinisation)*. The cortical tubules **T** also become shrunken and atrophic and the relatively expanded interstitial spaces **I** undergo fibrosis; some atrophic tubules may become cystically dilated with *casts* of inspissated proteinaceous material **P** which is highly eosinophilic (pink staining). The shrunken cortex is sometimes marked by scars, formerly attributed to chronic infection; this is now believed to contribute to only a small proportion of cases and most of the scars are probably ischaemic in origin.

Fig. 14.3   Renal papillary necrosis (LP)

This low power photomicrograph shows the condition known as *papillary necrosis* or *necrotising papillitis*.

The tip of the papilla **P** undergoes necrosis of a coagulative type, with preservation of ghost-like outlines of the papillary tubules and collecting ducts. In the early stages there is a neutrophil inflammatory response at the junction **J** between normal and necrotic papilla but this largely disappears at a later stage when the necrotic papilla separates and is shed.

This condition, which is probably ischaemic in nature, often occurs in association with acute infection of the urinary parenchyma and pelvicalyceal system, particularly when accompanied by an obstructive lesion in the lower urinary tract. It may also be seen with or without overt infection in *diabetic nephropathy* and in *analgesic nephropathy.* If there is sudden loss of many papillae, the patient may develop acute renal failure.

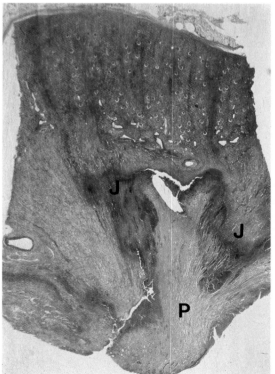

Partial renal failure syndromes

• **Acute nephritic syndrome** (formerly inaccurately called acute glomerulonephritis) - characterised by *haematuria* and *oliguria, oedema* (often periorbital) and a *rise in blood pressure* and *blood urea concentration* (usually transient). It generally results from primary glomerular lesions (often immunological in origin) which cause *obstruction to the glomerular capillary lumina* by proliferation of cellular elements. When glomerular blood flow is reduced, glomerular filtration also falls causing the oliguria, rise in blood pressure and retention of nitrogenous metabolites. Swollen and damaged glomerular capillary endothelial cells are usually responsible for the obstruction of the glomerular capillary lumina and this permits leakage of red blood cells and some protein into the urine.

• **Nephrotic syndrome** - characterised by *severe proteinuria* which leads to a fall in serum protein concentration *(hypoalbuminaemia)* and consequent marked *oedema* of peripheral tissues. Many types of renal lesion can produce heavy proteinuria and the nephrotic syndrome, but most have as their basis a *disturbance of glomerular capillary basement membrane function* permitting the leakage of plasma proteins across the filtration barrier and into the urine. In most cases of nephrotic syndrome, there is some detectable structural abnormality of the glomerular basement membrane, either alone, or as part of a disease process affecting other glomerular components such as the mesangium or endothelial cells. Such structural abnormalities commonly arise from deposition of immune complexes as in *membranous nephropathy* (see Fig. 14.6) and lupus nephritis, infiltration by amyloid (see Fig. 4.3), and non-specific thickening as in diabetes mellitus (see Fig. 14.12). The commonest cause of the nephrotic syndrome in children is *minimal change nephropathy*, so named because the glomeruli appear normal by light microscopy. Electron microscopy shows loss of the normal structural relationship between podocyte foot processes and the glomerular basement membrane and it is possible to demonstrate loss of normal glomerular polyanionic charge (normally involved in preventing protein leakage).

• **Mixed nephritic-nephrotic syndrome** - exhibits some of the features of both syndromes. It is mainly seen in association with glomerular lesions with both a proliferative (capillary lumen-obstructing) and membranous (protein-leaking) component. The most common lesion of this type is *mesangiocapillary glomerulonephritis,* also known as *membranoproliferative glomerulonephritis,* illustrated in Figure 14.9.

Proteinuria and renal haematuria

Persistent proteinuria, resulting from excessive loss of plasma protein in the glomerular filtrate, is an important indicator of early glomerular damage and merits further investigation of renal function. Persistent proteinuria may precede the onset of the true nephrotic syndrome by many years.

   Haematuria of renal origin is an important indicator of early glomerular damage, particularly in some forms of focal segmental glomerulonephritis such as *IgA mesangial disease.*

Role of renal biopsy

The introduction of safe and reliable techniques of percutaneous needle biopsy of the kidney has greatly increased knowledge about the natural history of renal diseases, particularly in elucidating the underlying lesion in partial renal failure syndromes, acute renal failure and unexplained proteinuria or haematuria. It is of limited value in chronic renal failure when the kidney is shrunken and histological changes non-specific, e.g. end-stage kidney (Fig. 14.2).

   Maximum information is obtained from a needle biopsy of renal tissue using the following methods:

• light microscopy applying stains to define the basement membrane

• electron microscopy to show the presence and precise location of immune complexes

• immunohistochemical techniques to identify and localise immunoglobulins and complement factors.

Glomerulonephritis

Primary lesions of the glomerulus are often referred to by the loose term *'glomerulonephritis'*, a word incapable of accurate definition. Its use persists in the classification and nomenclature of primary active proliferative and destructive lesions of the glomerulus (see Figs. 14.6 to 14.10); the term *'chronic glomerulonephritis'*, formerly used in an imprecise way to describe what is now called end-stage kidney, has fortunately been largely discontinued.

In response to damaging stimuli, the glomerulus appears to react in one or more of the following ways:

- swelling or proliferation of the normally flat endothelial cells lining the glomerular capillaries

- proliferation of the epithelial cells investing the outer surface of the glomerular capillary tuft (the podocytes) and the cells lining Bowman's capsule

- thickening of the glomerular basement membranes

- proliferation of the cells of the mesangium and excessive production of acellular mesangial material.

Irreversible glomerular damage, whatever the cause, is usually followed by progressive replacement of the vascular glomerular tuft by mesangial material, leading to the condition of *glomerular hyalinisation,* also illustrated in Figures 14.2 and 14.11(a). Many of the subtleties of these glomerular disorders are difficult to visualise in standard H&E-stained paraffin sections and require specially prepared thin sections stained by special techniques to highlight different structural components, or ultrastructural examination.

(a)

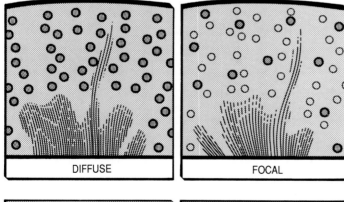

(b)

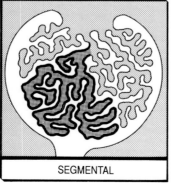

Fig. 14.4 Nomenclature of patterns of glomerulonephritis
(a) diffuse or focal
(b) global or segmental

Primary glomerular lesions can be categorised according to the extent of glomerular involvement: *diffuse* - affecting all glomeruli in the kidney, and *focal* - affecting only some glomeruli. This is illustrated in diagram (a).

Glomerulonephritis can be further categorised according to the degree of involvement of each individual glomerulus; *global* - affecting the entire glomerular tuft, *segmental* - affecting only some segments of each glomerular tuft. This is illustrated in diagram (b).

Thus a particular type of glomerulonephritis may be described as diffuse global (e.g. acute proliferative glomerulonephritis, Fig. 14.7) , focal segmental (e.g. Henoch-Schönlein nephritis, Fig. 14.9), or any combination.

Outcome of glomerular disorders

The renal disorders in which the major abnormality includes the glomerulus may subside spontaneously or with treatment. However, if they progress, glomerular blood flow is obstructed, glomerular filtration ceases and the tubules associated with affected glomeruli become involved; thus many nephrons may cease to function. When sufficient nephrons have been affected, the clinical features of the disease will evolve from a partial renal failure syndrome, i.e. nephritic, nephrotic or mixed syndrome, into a total impairment syndrome, i.e. chronic renal failure.

By way of illustration, a patient with the nephrotic syndrome due to diabetic glomerular disease may slowly develop the features of chronic renal failure as individual nephrons are progressively converted into functionless units by glomerular hyalinisation and tubular atrophy. In contrast, a patient who initially presents with the acute nephritic syndrome due to a rapidly progressive crescentic glomerulonephritis (see Fig. 14.8) may quickly progress to the syndrome of acute renal failure as the glomeruli are rapidly destroyed by the disease process. Some of the more important clinical and pathological features of the various patterns of renal impairment are summarised in Figure 14.5.

Disorders of the renal tubule

The tubular components of the nephron may be primarily damaged as a result of hypovolaemic shock, by inorganic and organic toxins, or as the result of infection. In hypovolaemic states and intoxication, tubular epithelial cells may exhibit marked cytoplasmic degenerative changes or frank necrosis leading to the pathological term *acute tubular necrosis* and producing the clinical syndrome of acute renal failure. Tubular epithelial cells have considerable powers of recovery and regeneration, and acute renal failure may be reversible under such circumstances if the patient can be sustained in the interim by dialysis and other supporting measures. An example of renal tubular abnormality is shown in Figure 1.4.

Fig. 14.5 Renal impairment syndromes: summary of general principles

Syndrome	Main features	Pathophysiology
Acute renal failure	Oliguria, hyperkalaemia, acidosis, uraemia (rapid rise)	Abrupt cessation of all nephron activity (often reversible), e.g. all tubules damaged (Fig. 1.4), or all glomeruli damaged (Fig. 14.8)
Chronic renal failure	Uraemia (slow rise), chronic electrolyte disturbances (acidosis, hyperkalaemia)	Slowly progressive cessation of nephron function due to irreversible nephron destruction, leads to end-stage kidney (Fig. 14.12)
Nephritic syndrome	Haematuria, oedema, transient uraemia, hypertension	Obstruction to blood flow through glomerular capillaries, usually due to blockage by proliferating endothelial cells, leading to decreased glomerular filtration, increased blood urea and hypertension (Fig. 14.6)
Nephrotic syndrome	Proteinuria, hypoalbumenaemia, oedema	Structural abnormality of the glomerular capillary basement membrane leading to protein leakage into the urine (Figs. 14.6, 14.12, 4.3)
Mixed nephritic/ nephrotic syndrome	Nephrotic syndrome with some nephritic features, usually haematuria	Combined abnormality of capillary lumina and basement membranes (Fig. 14.10)

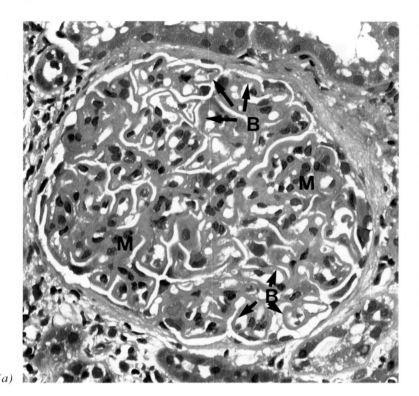

(a)

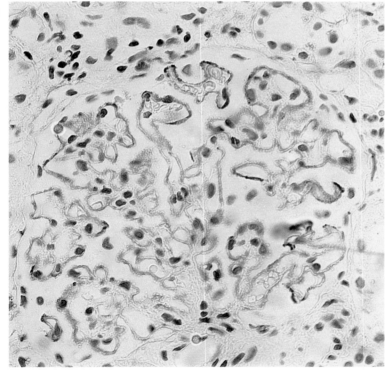

(b)

Fig. 14.6 Membranous nephropathy
(a) **H&E** (HP)
(b) **Immunoperoxidase method** (HP)

In *membranous nephropathy*, the filtration properties of the glomerular basement membrane are disrupted, allowing leakage of plasma proteins, especially albumin, into the urine; the condition usually presents clinically as the *nephrotic syndrome*.

In this condition the glomerular basement membranes are diffusely and fairly uniformly thickened, often reaching 5 or 6 times normal thickness. With the H&E stain, the basement membranes **B** appear thick, eosinophilic and sometimes slightly refractile. There is no associated endothelial or epithelial (podocyte) proliferation although there may be a slight increase in mesangial material **M** in severe and long-standing cases. Much of the basement membrane thickening appears to be due to the presence of immune complexes which can be demonstrated by electron microscopy, or, as in micrograph (b), by immuno-histochemical methods; in micrograph (b) the brown stain represents immunoglobulin (in this case IgG) incorporated in the glomerular basement membranes.

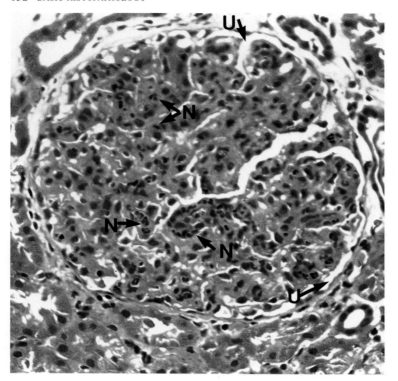

Fig. 14.7 Acute proliferative ('endocapillary') glomerulonephritis (HP)

This form of glomerulonephritis most commonly occurs in children and often follows a streptococcal infection, usually of the throat. As seen in this micrograph the cellularity of the glomerulus is increased due to proliferation of endothelial cells which have virtually obliterated the capillary lumina; increased numbers of neutrophils **N** are present in the glomerular tufts. The urinary space **U** remains clear since there has been no proliferation of podocytes.

The obstruction of glomerular capillary lumina diminishes glomerular filtration and causes leakage of erythrocytes, hence this condition usually presents with haematuria, transient hypertension and oedema, i.e. the acute nephritic syndrome.

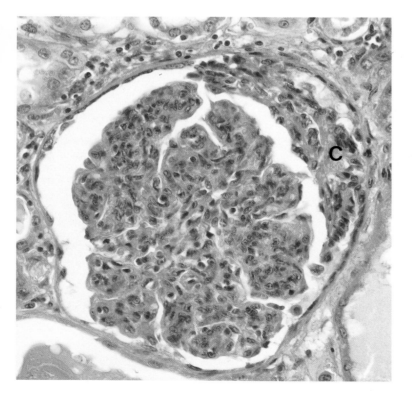

Fig. 14.8 Acute crescentic glomerulonephritis (HP)

Sometimes the changes illustrated and described in Fig. 14.7 are accompanied by proliferation of podocytes and the epithelial cells lining Bowman's capsule. Uneven proliferation of Bowman's capsule epithelial cells around only part of the circumference of Bowman's capsule produces a so-called *crescent* **C**. Continued proliferation of the crescent may obliterate the glomerular tuft, leading to irreversible glomerular destruction and subsequent nephron atrophy, with rapidly progressive renal impairment and total renal failure.

The formation of crescents may develop in a variety of different proliferative glomerular diseases.

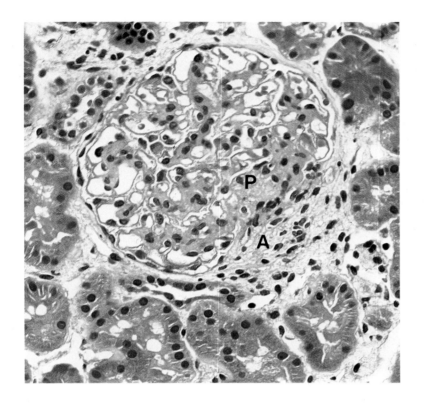

Fig. 14.9   Focal segmental glomerulonephritis (HP)

In the types of glomerulonephritis discussed in Figures 14.7 and 14.8, the pathological changes were global and diffuse. In contrast, there are a number of glomerular disorders, such as *Henoch-Schönlein purpura* (shown here) and *IgA mesangial disease,* in which endothelial and epithelial proliferation is segmental and focal. (see Fig. 14.4).

Note the segmental area of proliferation **P** in the glomerular tuft, largely the result of increase in size and number of mesangial cells and (at the later stage shown here) increase in acellular mesangial material; there is also proliferation and swelling of endothelial cells and irregular basement membrane thickening. Note the normality of the remaining segments of the glomerular tuft. Sometimes the abnormal segments of the tuft come to adhere to Bowman's capsule to form a *tuft adhesion* **A** as in this example.

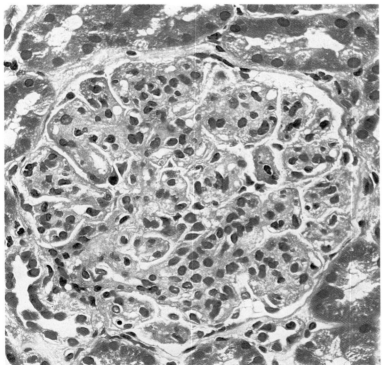

Fig. 14.10   Mesangiocapillary (membranoproliferative) glomerulonephritis (HP)

In this condition, all segments of all glomeruli undergo both mesangial and endothelial cell proliferation as well as marked widespread basement membrane thickening. The latter is due to a combination of extensive immune complex deposition and interpositioning of mesangial material between basement membrane laminae. Unfortunately, neither of these basement membrane features are discernible in H&E-stained paraffin sections, and special stains or electron microscopy are necessary to demonstrate them adequately. More easily seen, as in this micrograph, is the expansion of each segment of the tuft producing an exaggerated lobular appearance. The combination of basement membrane abnormality and cellular proliferation usually results in the nephrotic syndrome, often with some superadded features of the nephritic syndrome (e.g. haematuria).

Systemic causes of renal disease

The kidney is commonly involved in systemic disease, particularly where the disease affects the blood vessels. The most commonly occurring systemic disorders to produce abnormalities in the kidney are *diabetes mellitus* and *arterial hypertension.*

In diabetes mellitus, renal disease may occur in several ways. Diabetics have an increased predisposition to the development of renal infections (see Fig. 14.13) and papillary necrosis (see Fig. 14.3), as well as a tendency to severe large vessel atherosclerosis increasing the risk of renal ischaemia. Diabetes also particularly affects small renal arterioles and glomerular capillaries in the kidney producing *diabetic glomerulosclerosis.*

The kidney is especially vulnerable to the effects of arterial hypertension as seen in Figures 10.6 and 10.7, and irreversible damage to nephrons may result either acutely from accelerated hypertension or progressively over a period of years in essential benign hypertension; both these forms of *hypertensive nephrosclerosis* are illustrated in Figure 14.11.

The kidney may also be involved, along with other organs, in *systemic amyloidosis* (see Ch. 4). A variety of other diseases associated with vascular abnormalities may damage the kidney and these include *polyarteritis nodosa* and other *primary arteritis disorders, embolic disease* and *connective tissue disorders* such as *SLE* and *scleroderma.*

Fig. 14.11   Hypertensive nephrosclerosis *(illustrations opposite)*
(a) benign hypertensive nephrosclerosis (HP)
(b) malignant hypertensive nephrosclerosis (HP)

The vessel changes in systemic hypertension have been discussed and illustrated in some detail in Figures 10.6 and 10.7. The kidney is particularly vulnerable to the damaging effects of these vessel changes and renal failure is an important complication of untreated hypertension.

The pathological changes in the kidney depend on the severity and rate of progress of the hypertension. In *benign (essential) hypertension,* where the hypertension is of gradual onset and progression, reaching only moderately elevated diastolic pressure, the large and medium-sized renal arteries show marked thickening of their walls by a combination of medial hypertrophy, elastic lamina reduplication and fibrous intimal thickening (Fig. 10.6a); arterioles show hyaline thickening of their walls (Fig. 10.6b). These changes reduce the calibre of all renal afferent vessels and the resulting chronic ischaemia leads to progressive *sclerosis* (hyalinisation) of the glomerulus and subsequent disuse atrophy of the tubular component of the nephron.

Micrograph (a) shows a clump of glomeruli, two of which have become converted into hyaline amorphous pink-staining masses **H** as a result of chronic ischaemia due to hyalinisation of the walls of their afferent arterioles **Aa**; the other glomeruli are as yet unaffected.

Slowly progressive loss of functioning nephrons may eventually lead to chronic renal failure and the morphological state known as end-stage kidney.

In contrast, in *malignant (accelerated) hypertension,* where the rise in blood pressure is rapid and severe, the arterial and arteriolar changes are different. Large and medium-sized arteries may show only concentric thickening of the intima by loose, rather myxomatous, fibroblastic tissue (see Fig. 10.7a), and there is no elastic lamina reduplication or significant medial hypertrophy. Small arteries may show marked concentric fibroblastic intimal thickening so that the lumen is often virtually obliterated. Arterioles frequently show patchy acute necrosis of their walls with the accumulation of amorphous, brightly eosinophilic proteinaceous material *(fibrinoid)* in the damaged walls (Fig. 10.7b). This change is known as *fibrinoid necrosis* and as seen in the micrograph (b) often affects the afferent arterioles **Aa** at the glomerular hila and may extend into the glomerular tuft to affect some segments **S** of the glomerular capillary network. These small vessel changes are acute in onset and may produce an abrupt reduction in blood supply to the nephrons, often producing glomerular micro-infarction and tubular epithelial necrosis. The effect is to produce a catastrophic reduction in glomerular filtration, and the patient may develop acute oliguric or anuric renal failure. Not infrequently, the patient with long-standing benign hypertension may suddenly develop an accelerated phase, and the histological changes in the kidney may be those of mixed benign and malignant nephrosclerosis.

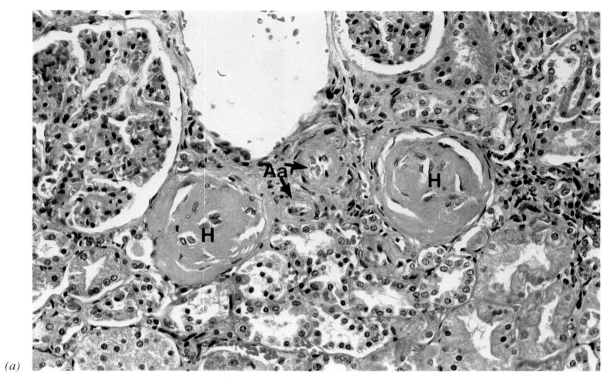

(a)

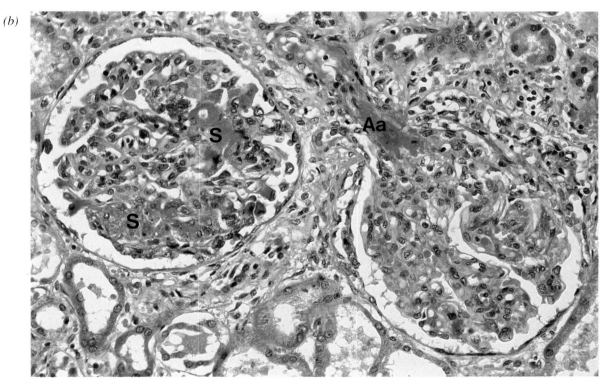

(b)

Fig. 14.11   **Hypertensive nephrosclerosis** *(caption opposite)*

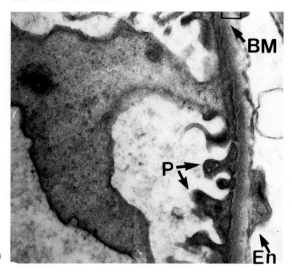

Fig. 14.12 Diabetic glomerulosclerosis *(illustrations (c) and (d) opposite)*
(a) normal glomerular basement membrane (EM)   **(b) diabetic basement membrane** (EM)
(c) nodular diabetic glomerulosclerosis (HP)   **(d) diffuse diabetic glomerulosclerosis** (HP)

In addition to a predisposition to urinary tract infections, papillary necrosis, and renal effects of arteriosclerotic vascular disease, diabetes may cause glomerular damage. Characteristic changes occur in the glomeruli *(diabetic glomerulosclerosis)*, and in the walls of afferent and efferent arterioles. Among the early glomerular changes is a uniform and homogeneous thickening of the glomerular capillary basement membrane, best seen by electron microscopy; this feature is illustrated in micrograph (b), with the normal shown for comparison in micrograph (a). In both electron micrographs, note the glomerular capillary basement membrane **BM** invested by thin endothelial cell cytoplasm **En** on the inner aspect, and by epithelial cell (podocyte) foot processes **P** externally. In diabetes, the basement membrane may be up to 4 or 5 times normal thickness.

In more advanced glomerular involvement, the basement membrane thickening is associated with an increase in mesangial cells and matrix. The mesangial matrix increase is often segmental and localised to produce characteristic acellular nodules, often with compressed mesangial cell nuclei pushed to their periphery; these nodules are called *Kimmelstiel-Wilson nodules*. This pattern of diabetic glomerular involvement is shown in micrograph (c), and is called *nodular diabetic glomerulosclerosis*; note the Kimmelstiel-Wilson nodules **K.**

In another pattern, the mesangial cell and material increase is diffuse and global, not segmental and nodular, producing the change called *diffuse diabetic glomerulosclerosis,* illustrated in micrograph (d). Both patterns may occur in the same kidney, and nodule formation may be superimposed upon the diffuse change

within the same glomerulus. In both patterns, there is escape of plasma protein across the thickened but leaky glomerular capillary wall into the urinary space; occasionally, inspissated protein may be deposited on the outer surface of the glomerular tuft *(fibrin caps)* or on the inner surface of Bowman's capsule *(capsular drops)*. A fibrin cap **Fc** is demonstrated in micrograph (d), associated with diffuse diabetic glomerulosclerosis. These features are also seen in chronically ischaemic glomeruli and are not specific to diabetic glomerular disease.

A frequent feature of diabetic renal disease is hyalinisation of afferent and efferent arteriole walls, a further manifestation of the predisposition of the diabetic kidney to vascular disease ranging from large renal artery atherosclerosis to capillary wall basement membrane thickening. This arteriolar hyalinisation **H**, well shown in association with nodular diabetic glomerulosclerosis in micrograph (c), may also extend into the vascular hilum of the glomerulus.

The combination of arterial atherosclerosis and arteriolar hyalinisation progressively reduces the blood flow to the glomeruli; thus chronic ischaemic changes, such as hyalinisation of glomeruli and periglomerular fibrosis, are common associated findings in diabetic renal disease.

The initial glomerular basement membrane changes result in proteinuria and even the nephrotic syndrome, but with progressive diabetic glomerulosclerosis and chronic ischaemic nephron atrophy, the features of chronic renal failure may supervene.

Acute pyelonephritis or renal papillary necrosis (see Figs. 14.13 and 14.3) may precipitate acute renal failure.

(c)

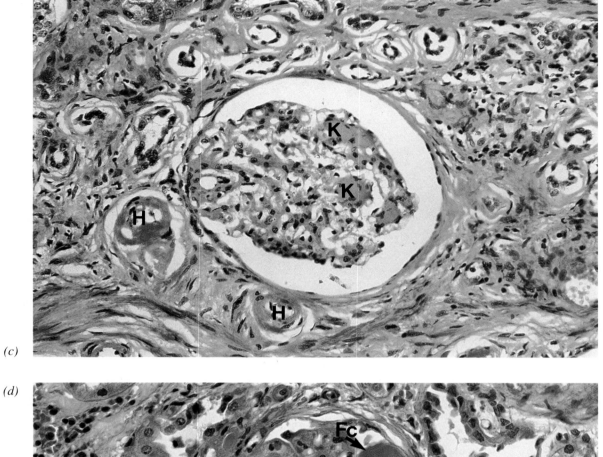

(d)

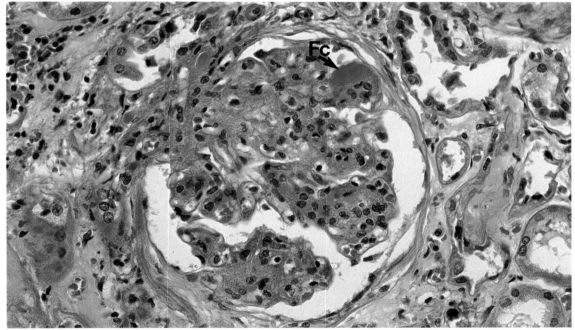

Fig. 14.12 Diabetic glomerulosclerosis *(caption opposite)*

Infections of the kidney

Pyogenic infections of the renal parenchyma *(pyelonephritis)* are usually caused by Gram-negative bacilli which are normally commensals in the lower intestinal tract; they gain access to the kidney either by ascending infection from the lower urinary tract or by blood stream spread. Acute pyogenic pyelonephritis is illustrated in Figure 14.10. Tuberculous pyelonephritis may also arise by similar routes of spread and is shown in Figure 3.13.

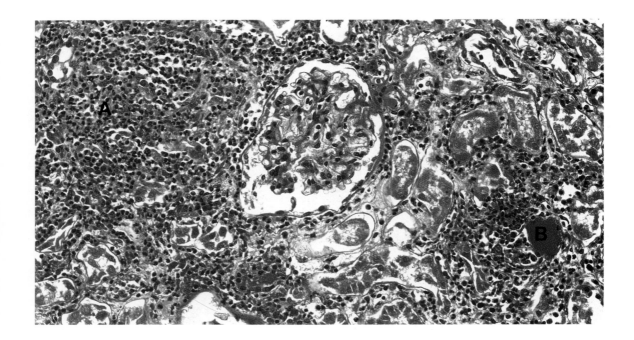

Fig. 14.13 Acute pyelonephritis (HP)

Acute suppurative bacterial infections of the kidney usually follow ascending infection from the lower urinary tract, particularly when there is obstruction to urinary outflow such as in benign prostatic hyperplasia or pressure from the fetus in pregnancy; in such cases, coliform organisms (such as *Escherichia coli* and *Proteus* species) are the most frequent infecting agent. Infection may also arise in the kidney by the haematogenous route during episodes of bacteraemia.

In established *acute pyelonephritis* there may be extensive infiltration of the kidney by neutrophil polymorphs, often with abscess formation. In the micrograph, note the infiltration of the kidney by small dark-staining neutrophils, abscess formation **A**, and a clump of purple-staining bacteria **B**.

Acute pyelonephritis may be complicated by the development of *papillary necrosis* (Fig. 14.3) or pus accumulation in a dilated, obstructed pelvicalyceal system *(pyonephrosis)*. In untreated cases, the small multiple abscesses may merge to produce larger abscesses which may discharge into the pelvicalyceal system to produce pyonephrosis, or through the capsule into perinephric fat to produce a *perinephric abscess.*

Patients with urinary reflux or obstruction are prone to develop recurrent pyelonephritis; repeated attacks lead to scarring on healing and after many episodes the kidney becomes coarsely scarred (chronic pyelonephritis).

Tumours of the kidney

The most common tumour of the kidney in adults is the *renal adenocarcinoma* derived from the tubular epithelial cells; it is illustrated in Figure 14.14 and one of its important methods of spread, by venous invasion, is shown in Figure 6.6. The kidney is the site of an important malignant tumour of children, *nephroblastoma* (or *Wilms' tumour),* an example of a so-called embryonal tumour (Fig. 14.15).

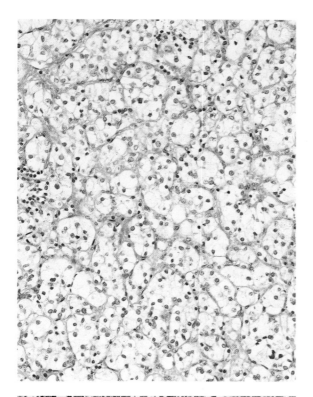

Fig. 14.14   Renal tubular carcinoma (HP)

The most common malignant tumour of the kidney is the *renal adenocarcinoma* derived from renal tubular epithelium. The tumour cells are large and polygonal in shape and, as in this example, often have characteristically clear cytoplasm, the result of cytoplasmic glycogen and lipid accumulation. In other histological variants, the tumour cell cytoplasm is granular and pink staining, more closely resembling the tubular epithelium from which these tumours are derived. Renal tubular carcinoma tends to breach the walls of intrarenal venous tributaries and to grow as solid cords along the lumen of the renal vein towards and into the inferior vena cava (see Fig. 6.6). From here venous emboli spread tumour deposits to the lung producing typical 'cannon-ball secondaries'. Renal adenocarcinoma also has a particular propensity for metastasis to bone and brain.

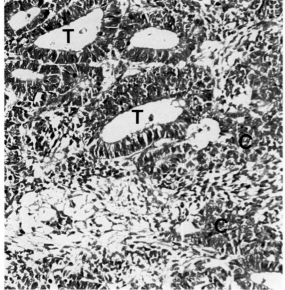

Fig. 14.15   Nephroblastoma (HP)

The kidney is the site of one of the most common of the embryonal tumours, the *nephroblastoma* or *Wilms' tumour.* This tumour of infants and children is believed to originate from embryonic renal blastema, and, although largely composed of primitive and undifferentiated cells **C**, usually shows a tendency in some areas to form tubular structures **T** resembling primitive renal tubules; occasionally, structures resembling immature glomeruli are found. There are many histological variants of this tumour, some of which contain primitive tissue cells such as skeletal muscle cells (rhabdomyoblasts).

The lower urinary tract

The most important disorders of the lower urinary tract are infection and neoplasia. Infections are common, but usually remain confined to the bladder *(cystitis);* ascending spread up into the ureters and pelvicalyceal systems may result in involvement of the parenchyma of the kidney *(acute pyelonephritis)* shown in Figure 14.13. Persistent or repeated infection in the urinary tract predisposes to the development of urinary stones, particularly in the bladder and pelvicalyceal systems.

Infections of the urethra (urethritis) are commonly associated with sexually transmitted diseases with the organisms *Gonococcus* and *Chlamydia.*

The pelvicalyceal system, ureters and bladder are lined by a specialised transitional epithelium, the *urothelium.* Tumours of the urothelium *(transitional cell carcinoma)* are common and of particular interest because of the possible role of chemical carcinogens such as aniline dyes in their pathogenesis (see Figs. 6.12 and 14.16)

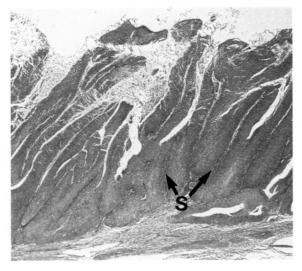

(a)

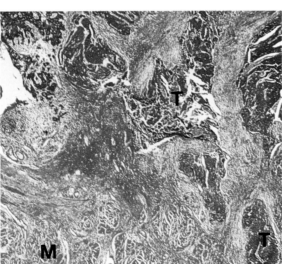

(b)

Fig. 14.16 Transitional cell carcinoma
(a) well differentiated (LP)
(b) poorly differentiated (LP)

Tumours of the urothelium are common and all are regarded as malignant despite the fact that many are well differentiated histologically and show no evidence of invasion when first detected.

As in the pelvicalyceal tumour shown in micrograph (a), well-differentiated tumours commonly arise as frond-like papillary outgrowths from the urothelial surface and have a slender connective tissue stroma **S** supporting the layers of neoplastic cells.

In less well-differentiated tumours, some semblance of this papillary pattern is retained, but it is lost in the most poorly differentiated tumours, usually in the bladder. The less well-differentiated tumours often appear as sessile ulcerated plaques and, as shown in micrograph (b), the tumour **T** extends deeply through the bladder submucosa and muscular wall **M**.

Urothelial tumours are frequently multifocal in origin, and there is a strong link between their development and exposure to certain industrial chemicals such as aniline dyes. Cigarette smoking has also been causally linked with the development of urothelial tumours.

The prognosis of urothelial tumours depends on their location, the histological pattern, the degree of cytological differentiation, and the extent of local invasion when the tumour is first detected. The cytology of transitional cell tumours is shown in more detail in Figure 6.12.

Occasionally, squamous carcinomas may develop in the bladder from metaplastic epithelium associated with chronic inflammation by a stone or parasitic infection *(Schistosomiasis)*. Rarely, adenocarcinoma arises from embryological urachal remnants.

15. Lymphoid and haemopoietic systems

Functions of lymphoreticular system

The lymphoreticular system is composed of various organs and tissues which facilitate the interaction of lymphocytes with cells of monocyte-macrophage lineage in the generation of immune responses. The main tissues of the system are the thymus, spleen, lymph nodes, bone marrow and mucosal-associated lymphoid tissue (MALT) such as tonsils and Peyer's patches of the gut. Virtually every tissue in the body also has a resident population of specialised interstitial dendritic cells of macrophage type which have important roles in presenting new antigens to lymphoid cells.

- Lymphocytes are produced in the bone marrow, their number being selectively expanded mainly in the thymus and lymph nodes in response to specific immunological requirements; many circulate through peripheral tissues via blood and lymphatic vessels in a constant search for antigens (immunological surveillance).

- The monocyte-macrophage system includes the tissue macrophages (histiocytes) found in virtually every tissue which become activated following tissue damage and, together with monocytes recruited from the blood, act as phagocytic cells in the process of organisation. It also includes the specialised dendritic antigen-presenting cells with a role in initiating new immune responses by presenting antigen to T-cells.

The lymphoreticular system is thus composed of both specific tissues as well as dispersed elements in all peripheral tissues.

Reactive disorders of lymph nodes

The lymphoreticular system is remarkably labile and quickly responds to the presence of infective agents or foreign material in the activation of an immune response. There are two main patterns of immune response:

- the *cell-mediated response,* involving the activity of T-lymphocytes which are either directly or indirectly cytotoxic

- the *humoral response,* which involves the activation of B-lymphocytes which transform into antibody-secreting plasma cells; interaction of antibody with antigen leads to destruction of the antigen.

Following tissue damage, particularly infection, local draining lymph nodes become particularly active and enlarged; this is histologically termed *reactive hyperplasia*. This may involve one or more of the principal cellular constituents of the node, depending on the nature of the foreign material encountered:

- in a predominantly humoral response, there is hyperplasia of the cortical follicles mainly composed of B-lymphocytes and large B-cell germinal centres develop *(follicular hyperplasia)*

- in a predominantly cell-mediated response, there is hyperplasia of the paracortical (parafollicular) region of the node, mainly occupied by T-lymphocytes *(parafollicular* or *paracortical hyperplasia)*

- certain stimuli evoke intense phagocytic activity leading to dilatation of subcapsular and medullary sinuses with increased numbers and activity of macrophages and phagocytic sinus-lining cells *(sinus hyperplasia).*

Examples are shown in Figure 15.1. Certain foreign agents stimulate characteristic and unique patterns of reaction in lymph nodes which allow a diagnosis of disease to be made on lymph node biopsy; for example multiple minute histiocytic clusters are seen in nodes in toxoplasmosis. In addition, lymph nodes are classically involved by specific chronic granulomatous inflammations such as tuberculosis, sarcoidosis and syphilis; these are described in Chapter 3.

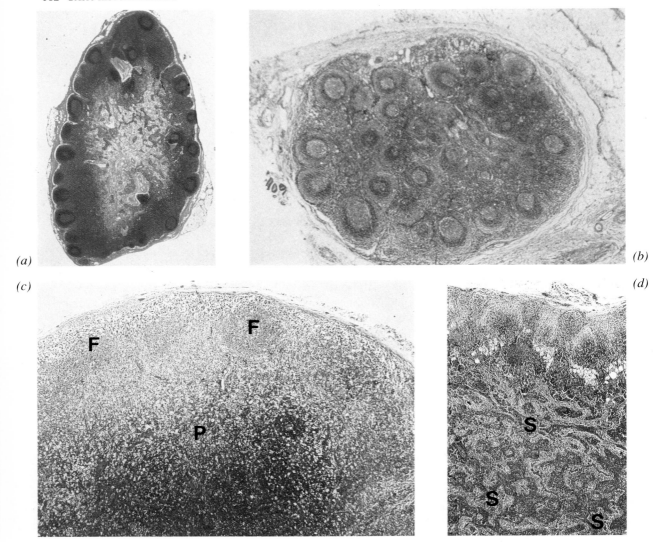

(a)

(b)

(c)

(d)

Fig. 15.1 Reactive hyperplasia of lymph nodes
(a) normal lymph node (LP)   **(b) follicular hyperplasia** (LP)
(c) paracortical hyperplasia (MP)   **(d) sinus hyperplasia** (MP)

Damage or inflammation of any tissue may excite a reactive response in the draining lymph nodes. The three basic patterns of response, follicular hyperplasia, paracortical hyperplasia, and sinus hyperplasia, may be seen separately or in combination according to the nature of the stimulus.

   In follicular hyperplasia, illustrated in micrograph (b), there is an increase in number and size of cortical lymphoid follicles evident on comparison with the normal in micrograph (a). This is a reflection of a B-cell (humoral) response and results in the production and clonal expansion of antibody-secreting B-cells.

   In paracortical (parafollicular) hyperplasia, seen in micrograph (c), there is expansion of the T-cell parafollicular zone of the lymph node **P** with small B-cell follicles **F** pushed to the periphery of the node beneath the capsule. This pattern is common in response to viral infection.

   In sinus hyperplasia, shown in micrograph (d) there is no great increase in the lymphoid component of the node, but the medullary sinuses **S** are extremely prominent by virtue of dilatation, and by hyperplasia of histiocytic cells lining the sinuses. This pattern of reaction is seen in nodes draining tissues from which endogenous particulate matter such as lipid is released, for example a necrotic tumour.

Acquired immune deficiency syndrome (AIDS)

The *human immunodeficency virus type 1 (HIV-1)* is a lymphotropic virus which gains access to cells by way of the CD4 surface protein, normally found on T-helper cells as well as most monocytes and other macrophages. Infection with HIV-1 is associated with several clinical and pathological syndromes. Some patients develop fever, weight loss, diarrhoea and generalised lymphadenopathy in which there is generalised follicular hyperplasia. In patients with the full-blown immunodeficient state of AIDS, lymph nodes commonly show loss of follicles, lymphocyte depletion, vascular proliferation and fibrosis. The main consequences of the immune deficient state seen in AIDS are:

- **opportunistic infections** - *Pneumocystis carinii pneumonia, cytomegalovirus infection, toxoplasmosis, mycobacterial infections* (tuberculosis as well as atypical organisms), *cutaneous fungal infections*

- **neoplasia** - development of *Kaposi's sarcoma* (Fig. 10.13) as well as *non-Hodgkin's lymphomas.*

Malignant disorders of the lymphoid system

Apart from reactive changes in which the lymphoreticular system is mounting an immune response to some foreign agent, the most common disorder encountered in the lymphoreticular system is the development of primary neoplastic proliferation of various lymphocytic cell lines. Such neoplastic proliferations are divided into two broad groups depending on histopathological identification of the type of neoplastic cell.

- **Hodgkin's disease** is characterised by neoplastic proliferation of large lymphoid cells of uncertain origin eponymously termed *Reed-Sternberg cells.*

- **Non-Hodgkin's lymphomas** are derived from neoplastic proliferations of lymphocytes (either T or B) or rarely histiocytic cells.

These diseases usually present by involvement of a group of lymph nodes but then spread to involve multiple lymph node groups, spleen, and bone marrow. Eventually, peripheral sites such as liver, skin or nervous system may also become involved. There are also a small group of non-Hodgkin's lymphomas which arise in lymphoid tissue outside the main lymphoid organs, for example the gut, lung, brain, salivary gland, thyroid, and testis. These conditions and their classification are discussed in detail in Figure 15.3.

The lymphoreticular system is also the seat of a group of disorders termed *histiocytoses* which, although not certainly neoplastic, behave as disseminated infiltrative cellular proliferations. In these conditions, which are usually seen in childhood, there is widespread infiltration of tissues by histiocytic cells with features of *Langerhans cells* (a type of dendritic antigen-presenting cell normally found in its skin and draining nodes). There is a spectrum of severity from localised and benign to disseminated and fatal which may involve skin, viscera, bone marrow, and lymph nodes.

Organs of the lymphoreticular system are also commonly sites of metastatic deposits of tumour, in particular lymph nodes (see Fig. 6.8b).

Hodgkin's disease

Hodgkin's disease is a malignant neoplasm of the lymphoreticular system which usually first becomes manifest by lymph node enlargement but later by splenomegaly, hepatomegaly and bone marrow involvement. The histogenesis of the tumour cell line in Hodgkin's disease is not known; however it is morphologically distinctive and eponymously named the *Reed-Sternberg cell*. Classical Reed-Sternberg cells are large and binucleate with two mirror image nuclei containing large pink-staining nucleoli (said to resemble owls' eyes). Reed-Sternberg cells usually only form a small proportion of the cell population of lymph nodes in Hodgkin's disease, and the neoplastic cells are hidden amongst a sea of reactive lymphoid cells, histiocytic cells and commonly eosinophils. Multinucleate and mononuclear variants of the Reed-Sternberg cell are also seen.

There are four histological sub-groups of Hodgkin's disease which correlate with prognosis and response to treatment:

- **lymphocyte-predominant** – slowly progressive
- **mixed cellularity** – intermediate progression
- **lymphocyte-depleted** – aggressive disease
- **nodular sclerosis** – slowly progressive.

The delineation of each type depends on the number of Reed-Sternberg cells relative to reactive cells in the node (see Fig 15.2). Nodular sclerosis is a separate type being distinguished by a fibroblastic response in the node with the production of bands of collagen.

The prognosis and treatment of Hodgkin's disease are not only related to the histological type but also to the extent of involvement of the lymphoreticular system as a whole. Investigation usually involves biopsy examination of lymph nodes, bone marrow, and liver, with extent of nodal involvement being assessed by CT scan or lymphangiography.

Fig. 15.2 Hodgkin's disease *(illustrations opposite)*
(a) lymphocyte-predominant pattern (HP)
(c) mixed cellularity pattern (HP)
(b) lymphocyte-depleted pattern (HP)
(d) nodular sclerosing pattern (LP)

The sub-type of Hodgkin's disease with the best prognosis is the *lymphocyte-predominant pattern* seen in micrograph (a). In this type, the lymphocytes (which are structurally normal) form extensive sheets within which are scattered relatively few Reed-Sternberg cells. Many of the large pale-staining cells are forms of mononuclear Reed-Sternberg cell. This sub-type is easy to confuse with forms of non-Hodgkin's lymphoma (see later) if the characteristic Reed-Sternberg cells are not identified.

The next most favourable prognosis applies to the most common form, *mixed cellularity Hodgkin's disease* shown in micrograph (b); there is a numerically even distribution of lymphocytes **L** and histiocyte-like cells **H**; occasional eosinophils **E**, neutrophils **N** and fibroblasts **F** are scattered about. Classical Reed-Sternberg cells **RS** are also present.

The type with the worst prognosis is *lymphocyte-depleted Hodgkin's disease* illustrated in micrograph (c) in which there is little evidence of reactive cells. Affected nodes are replaced by sheets of large pleomorphic cells including some classical Reed-Sternberg cells **RS**; lymphocytes **L** and other reactive cells are scanty.

Most commonly, Hodgkin's disease destroys the normal architecture of the lymph node completely, producing a homogeneous appearance in which no trace of the original cortico-medullary demarcation and follicular pattern remains. However, one form of Hodgkin's disease, the *nodular sclerosing pattern* seen in micrograph (d), results in the deposition of broad irregular bands of collagenous fibrous tissue **C** which separates the cellular Hodgkin's tumour mass into islands, imparting a nodular appearance to the cut surface of the node. The nodular sclerosing pattern is associated with a good prognosis if diagnosed at an early stage.

With modern chemotherapy it is now common to achieve complete cure of Hodgkin's disease. Prognosis depends on histological type and clinical stage of disease. There is, however, a tendency for the lymphocyte-predominant type to present with localised disease (excellent prognosis) while the lymphocyte-depleted type presents with disseminated disease (poor prognosis). The prognosis for mixed cellularity disease depends on stage, with localised disease being associated with an excellent prognosis while disseminated disease, particularly involving extra-nodal tissues, is associated with a less favourable outcome.

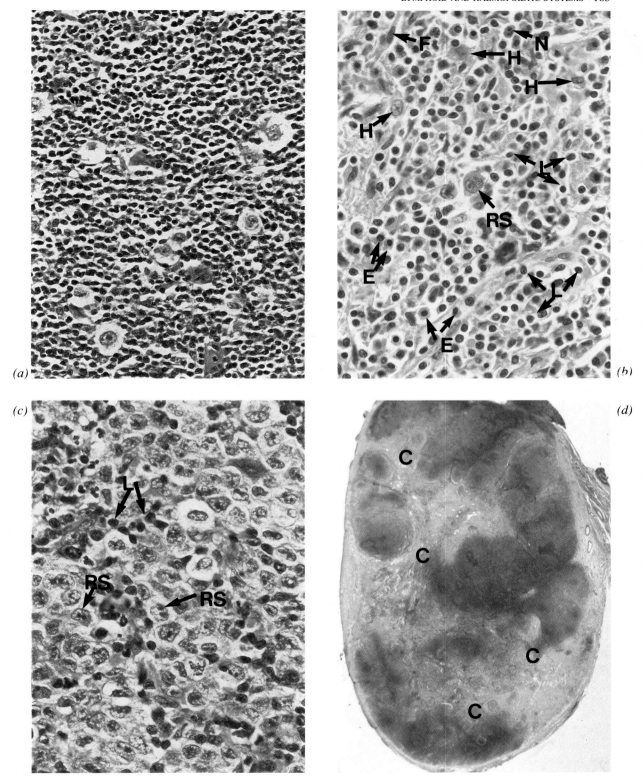

Fig. 15.2 Hodgkin's disease *(caption opposite)*

Non-Hodgkin's lymphomas

The non-Hodgkin's lymphomas are a group of neoplastic proliferations of lymphoid or histiocytic cells. They are collectively known as *lymphomas* and despite the suffix -oma, all are malignant in that they may become widely disseminated. The main features of non-Hodgkin's lymphomas are as follows:

- Clinically the usual presentation is with enlargement of a group of lymph nodes; biopsy is usually performed to establish a diagnosis. As well as conventional histology, immunohistochemistry is used to establish the precise type of cell forming the neoplastic proliferation.

- Early stage disease is localised to one set of nodes and, if untreated, there is spread to other nodal groups, bone marrow, spleen and liver.

- Tumours are derived from either T or B-lymphocytes but only rarely from true histiocytic cells.

- The majority of lymphomas arise in lymph nodes and are B-cell in type.

- Non-Hodgkin's lymphoma may occur in the gut, lung, salivary gland or lacrimal gland and are derived from mucosal associated lymphoid tissues (MALT). These specialised types tend to remain as localised disease without systemic spread.

- T-cell lymphoma may occur in the skin as a disease termed *mycosis fungoides* (see Fig. 20.20).

Classification of non-Hodgkin's lymphomas

There are many different sub-types of non-Hodgkin's lymphoma and as a result there have been a variety of different classifications based on either morphology, immunology or clinical behaviour. It is now evident that the most satisfactory method of classification for clinical purposes is to group disease into good, intermediate and poor prognosis types. The terminology used to describe specific disease types varies between Europe and the USA, however the following general principles apply to most systems.

Cell morphology. Lymphoma cells may be classified according to whether they are small (around the size of a mature lymphocyte) or large (five to six times the size of a small lymphocyte). In general, a high proportion of small cells is associated with less aggressive disease while a high proportion of large cells is associated with aggressive disease.

Growth pattern. Lymphomas may be classified as being either *follicular* or *diffuse*. In the follicular pattern the cells form aggregates which resemble lymphoid follicles but without germinal centres, whereas, in the diffuse pattern, there is diffuse distribution of cells with no evidence of follicular aggregation. In very general terms, for a given cell size, a follicular pattern is associated with a better prognosis than a diffuse pattern.

Lymphocyte maturation. Research on the normal cytology and function of follicular B-lymphoid cells as they undergo transformation from small mature lymphocytes through to plasma cells has revealed characteristic cytological features which are recapitulated in the patterns of differentiation seen in non-Hodgkin's lymphomas. The *Kiel classification,* popularised in Europe, identifies lymphocytic, lymphoblastic, centrocytic, centroblastic, immunoblastic, lymphoplasmacytic and plasma cell variants of lymphoid cells. The *Lukes and Collins classification,* popularised in the USA, applies the terms lymphocytic, lymphoblastic, small and large cleaved cell, small and large non-cleaved cell, and immunoblast to describe the same morphological features.

In clinical practice, the histologist identifies cytological features of neoplastic lymphocytes, including size, shape, content and position of nucleoli, as well as amount and distribution of cytoplasm. On this basis, a type of lymphoma is determined and then its pattern as follicular or diffuse is defined. It is often desirable to determine the cell of origin (B- or T-cell) by immunochemical methods using antibodies which stain specific cell markers. Clinical experience with treatment has allowed different types of non-Hodgkin's lymphoma to be sub-divided into prognostic groups as detailed in Figure 15.3.

Fig. 15.3 Classification of non-Hodgkin's lymphoma

Updated Kiel classification (Europe) 1988		American working formulation
B-cell	**T-cell**	**B- and T-cell types**
Low grade	**Low grade**	**Low grade**
Lymphocytic – chronic lymphocytic and and prolymphocytic leukaemia	Lymphocytic – chronic lymphocytic and prolymphocytic leukaemia	Small lymphocytic
Hairy cell leukaemia		Follicular small cleaved cell
		Follicular mixed large/small cleaved cell
	Small cerebriform cell – mycosis fungoides, Sezary's syndrome	
Lymphoplasmacytic/cytoid	Lymphoepithelioid (Lennert's	**Intermediate grade**
(LP immunocytoma)	lymphoma)	Follicular, large cell
Plasmacytic	Angioimmunoblastic (AILD)	Diffuse small cleaved cell
Centroblastic/centrocytic	T zone	Diffuse mixed small and large cell
–follicular ± diffuse		Diffuse large cell
–diffuse		
Centrocytic	Pleomorphic small cell (HTLV-1 ±)	
High grade	**High grade**	**High grade**
Centroblastic	Pleomorphic, medium and large cell	Large cell immunoblastic
Immunoblastic	Immunoblastic	Lymphoblastic
Large cell anaplastic (Ki-1+)	Large cell anaplastic (Ki-1+)	Small non-cleaved cell
Burkitt lymphoma		
Lymphoblastic	Lymphoblastic	
Rare types	*Rare types*	*Miscellaneous*
		e.g. cutaneous T-cell lymphomas

Note: terms on the same line in different columns from each classification are not meant to be equivalent.

There are several relatively common groups of non-Hodgkin's lymphomas which have distinct clinical and pathological features which are summarised as follows:

- Small-cell lymphomas occur in elderly patients often with widespread disease; they behave as indolent low-grade neoplasms. Bone marrow involvement and an associated leukaemic picture is common.

- Follicular lymphomas with a predominance of small cells occur in older patients and present with generalised lymphadenopathy and frequent marrow involvement. They run a long indolent course and complete remission is difficult to achieve.

- Burkitt's lymphoma is composed of cells intermediate in size between small lymphoid cells and immunoblasts; the disease predominantly affects children, and frequently presents with extranodal tumour especially in the abdomen and jaw.

- Large-cell lymphomas occur particularly in adults, have a high cell proliferation rate and require aggressive chemotherapy to achieve remission.

- Lymphoblastic lymphomas present in childhood and have high cell proliferation rates associated with large masses of tumour requiring aggressive chemotherapy to achieve remission.

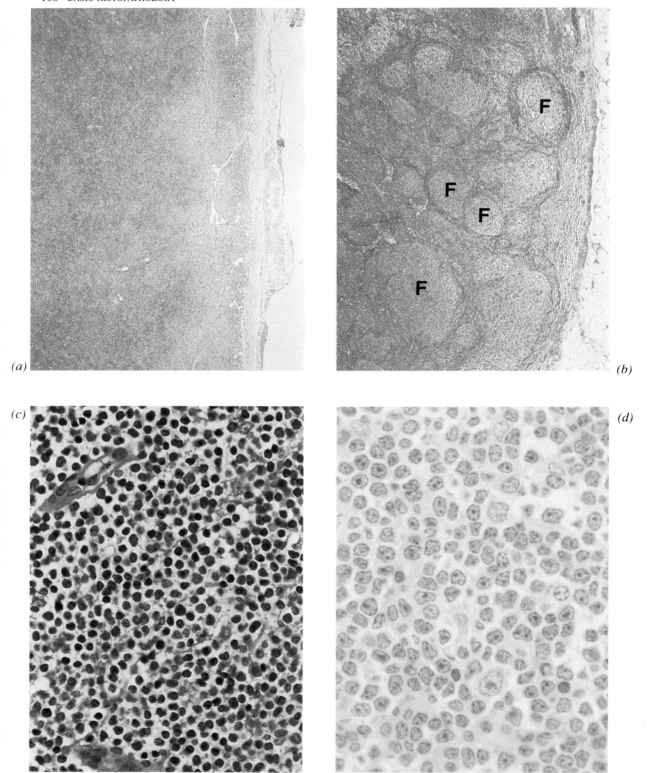

(a)

(b)

(c)

(d)

Fig. 15.4   Non-Hodgkin's lymphoma *(caption opposite)*

Fig. 15.4   Non-Hodgkin's lymphoma *(illustrations opposite)*
(a) diffuse pattern (LP)   **(b) follicular pattern** (LP)
(c) small cell lymphoma (HP)   **(d) large cell lymphoma** (HP)

Lymphocytic lymphomas may be sub-divided by pattern of growth into follicular and diffuse types, and also by size of cell into small and large cell variants. These micrographs show four variants of lymphocytic lymphoma based upon these criteria.

Note in the *diffuse pattern* shown in micrograph (a) how the normal architecture of the node has been completely effaced and replaced by uniform sheets of neoplastic lymphocytes; in contrast, in the *follicular pattern* illustrated in micrograph (b), the neoplastic cells are aggregated into irregular follicles **F**, larger and more variable in size and shape than normal follicles.

Within the follicular and diffuse patterns, there is further sub-division into small and large cell variants which are illustrated at higher magnification in micrographs (c) and (d) respectively. In the *small cell variant*, the tumour cells are like small lymphocytes with round darkly staining nuclei and only an insignificant rim of surrounding cytoplasm. The *large cell variant* exhibits less uniformity of nuclear shape, size and staining intensity, most nuclei being large with an open chromatin pattern and large nucleoli.

Haemopoietic system

The spaces between the bone trabeculae of spongy bone are occupied by *bone marrow* which is the primary site for haemopoiesis. The marrow contains the reservoir of stem cells which give rise to the cellular elements of the blood through a process of differentiation and cell stimulation by specific growth factors.
Bone marrow is traditionally divided into two types according to gross appearance:

- **Red marrow** – this is packed with haemopoietic cells, the precursors of the erythrocytes, neutrophil polymorphs with other granulocytes and platelets. In addition, some lymphocytes are produced in the bone marrow.
- **Yellow marrow** – haemopoietic tissue largely replaced by adipose tissue.

In children, virtually the entire marrow space is occupied by haemopoietic (red) marrow, but as the bones enlarge with maturity much of the red marrow is replaced by adipose tissue until just sufficient haemopoietic tissue remains to supply the body's normal requirement for new blood cells. However, the haemopoietic tissue is able to undergo hyperplasia, with rapid multiplication of one or more of the blood cell precursor lines, to provide additional blood cells if they are required. For example, in the case of infection, the precursors of neutrophil polymorphs (myeloblasts and myelocytes) will proliferate to produce increased numbers of neutrophil polymorphs. Similarly, if there is a sudden requirement for increased numbers of erythrocytes (e.g. after sudden blood loss), then the red cell precursors (erythroblasts) in the marrow will proliferate to increase the supply. These are normal responses to transient changes in demand, and the rate of precursor cell proliferation returns to normal once the immediate demand has been met.

There are, however, some conditions where the requirement for increased numbers of blood cells is constant as a result of disease. This is most commonly the result in some deficiency of the erythrocytes; for example, in haemolytic anaemias the red cells have a shorter life span than normal and are destroyed prematurely, and there is a constant need for rapid production of new red cells. In circumstances such as this, the bone marrow shows erythroblastic hyperplasia, and the red (haemopoietic) marrow occupies more of the marrow space, replacing the adipose tissue of the yellow marrow.

Abnormalities involving red blood cells

Reduction in the functional mass of circulating red blood cells is termed *anaemia* and the effect is to cause a reduction in blood haemoglobin concentration. Anaemia can be caused by many different disorders but the three most common causes are blood loss, increased rate of destruction of red cells *(haemolysis)* and impaired production of red blood cells. Bone marrow biopsy is often of great diagnostic value; for example, in haemolytic anaemia the bone marrow shows a marked increase in red blood cell precursors.

A major cause of defective production of red blood cells is deficiency of dietary factors vital for red cell production. Marrow biopsy is particularly useful in the following situations:

- In *iron deficiency* the bone marrow shows increased red cell precursors but there is absence of iron deposits which can be normally seen with special staining. Circulating red cells are small *(microcytic)* and pale *(hypochromic)*.

- In *vitamin B12 or folic acid deficient states* the bone marrow shows abnormally large red cell precursors *(megaloblasts)*. Circulating red cells are large *(macrocytes)* but the mean amount of haemoglobin per cell is not increased.

Aplastic anaemia is a condition where there is failure of marrow stem cells to form differentiated cell lines. There is a marked reduction in bone marrow cellularity which becomes replaced by fat. There is commonly an associated low neutrophil count *(neutropaenia)* and platelet count *(thrombocytopaenia)*. The common triggering factors are drugs, toxins, irradiation and viral infections, but in 50% of cases there is no known cause.

Abnormalities of white blood cells

The main groups of white blood cells are the lymphocytes, granulocytes, and monocytes. The pathology of lymphocytes has been discussed earlier in relation to diseases of the lymphoreticular system.

An abnormally low white blood cell count *(leukopaenia)* is usually due to reduction in the number of circulating neutrophils *(neutropaenia)*. This is a common sequel to diffuse marrow infiltration by neoplastic disease such as lymphoma and is also common when the bone marrow is suppressed by chemotherapy.

Leukaemias

The *leukaemias* are malignant neoplasms of the various white cell types in circulating blood and their precursors in the bone marrow. *Chronic lymphocytic leukaemia* is a disease of middle-aged and elderly adults in which the bone marrow and circulating blood are flooded by neoplastic proliferation of small lymphocytes similar to those seen in small cell lymphocytic lymphoma (Fig. 15.5). *Acute lymphoblastic leukaemia* is a disease of children in which the marrow becomes overwhelmed by the rapid neoplastic proliferation of immature cells of the lymphoid series which spill over into the circulating blood; the main clinical effects of this disease result from the destruction of normal haemopoietic tissue causing severe anaemia and deficiency of neutrophils and platelets, thus predisposing to overwhelming infection and severe coagulation disorders.

Chronic myelocytic leukaemia and *acute myeloblastic leukaemia,* both usually diseases of adults, are neoplasms of the granulopoietic series; fairly mature neutrophils, metamyelocytes and myelocytes predominate in the chronic form, whilst primitive myeloblasts predominate in the more rapidly fatal acute form (see Figs. 15.6 and 15.7).

Chronic myeloid leukaemia appears to be part of a spectrum of diseases known as *myeloproliferative disorders*. Also included in this group are *polycythaemia rubra vera* and *myelofibrosis*. The former is a neoplastic proliferation of erythrocyte precursors resulting in production of a vast excess of erythrocytes; in the latter the blood-forming areas of bone marrow are replaced by fibrous tissue, leading to defective and inadequate blood formation and compensatory development of haemopoietic tissue in extramedullary sites such as spleen and liver (see Fig. 15.8). The interesting feature of these conditions is that they may transform into chronic myeloid leukaemia which may then undergo *blast transformation* into acute myeloblastic leukaemia. Other forms (including monocytic leukaemia) are relatively rare.

Myeloma and plasma cell tumours

An important bone marrow tumour of white cell origin, although not a form of leukaemia, is *myeloma,* a neoplasm of antibody-producing plasma cells. This may occur as a solitary plasma cell tumour in bone or other tissues *(plasmacytoma),* it may present as multiple osteolytic tumours scattered throughout the skeleton, or as a diffuse infiltration of the bone marrow by plasma cells (Fig. l5.9); the last two are described as *multiple myeloma.*

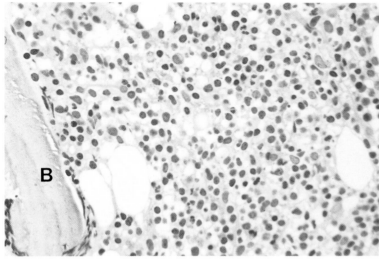

Fig. 15.5 Chronic lymphocytic leukaemia; bone marrow (HP)

In *chronic lymphocytic leukaemia,* the bone marrow in between bone trabeculae **B** becomes infiltrated by small lymphocytes similar to those seen in small cell lymphocytic lymphoma (see Fig. 15.4c) and very large numbers of similar cells appear in the peripheral circulation. Although the occupation of the marrow is extensive, destruction of the normal haemopoietic marrow elements is not as rapid or severe as in acute lymphoblastic leukaemia and the condition runs a less fulminant course.

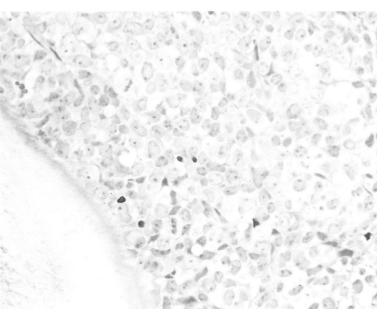

Fig. 15.6 Acute myeloid leukaemia; bone marrow (HP)

Acute myeloid leukaemia is characterised by proliferation of primitive myeloid cells in the bone marrow. There are several sub-groups depending on degree of maturation of the neoplastic cells from primitive myeloblasts, through types with promyelocyte morphology, to types with both myeloid and monocytic morphology. As seen here, the marrow is replaced by large atypical myeloid blast cells with few maturing cells (*cf.* Fig. 15.7).

This type of leukaemia predominates in adults under the age of 60 and presents acutely with anaemia and bleeding secondary to throbocytopaenia. Diagnosis is made on blood and marrow examination.

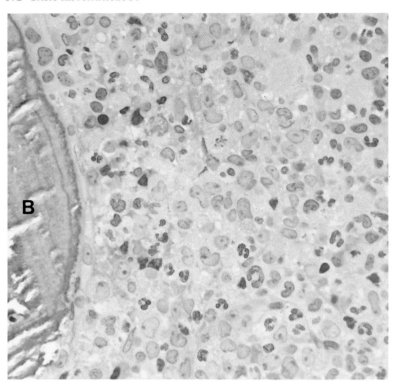

Fig. 15.7 Chronic myeloid leukaemia; bone marrow (HP)

In this disease, there is low grade neoplastic proliferation of neutrophil precursors. Increased numbers of myeloblasts produce greatly increased numbers of myelocytes, metamyelocytes and mature neutrophils, all of which appear in the peripheral blood in greatly increased numbers.

As seen in this micrograph, the marrow cavity in between bone trabeculae **B** is packed with neutrophils and late neutrophil precursors, particularly myelocytes and metamyelocytes; increased numbers of the most primitive precursor, the myeloblast, are also present, but they are a minority population compared to acute myeloid leukaemia (Fig. 15.6). Despite the proliferation of the myeloid series, normal haemopoietic activity continues, but is reduced.

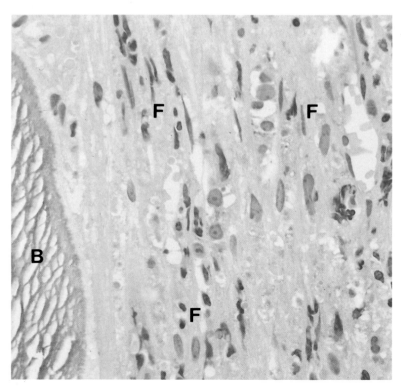

Fig. 15.8 Myelofibrosis (MP)

The replacement of haemopoietic bone marrow by progressive fibrosis in *myelofibrosis* leads to loss of capacity to produce erythrocytes, leucocytes and platelets. In this micrograph, the marrow space in between bone trabeculae **B** is infiltrated by spindle-shaped fibroblastic cells **F**.

This is partly compensated for by *extramedullary haemopoiesis,* when other organs of the lymphoreticular system acquire again their fetal potential for haemopoiesis.

The spleen is the principal organ involved in this compensatory process and becomes greatly enlarged. Histologically the red pulp of the spleen is markedly expanded by the presence of immature erythropoietic and granulopoietic tissues.

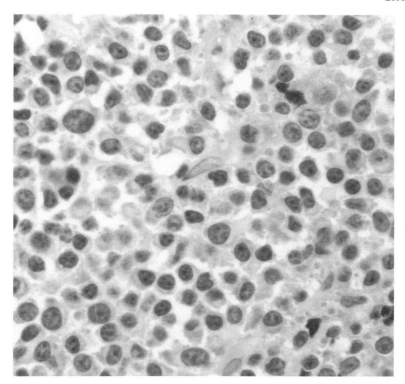

Fig. 15.9   Myeloma (HP)

Myeloma is a tumour of plasma cells which may present with solitary, multifocal or diffuse bone marrow involvement. In this example from a patient with diffuse marrow involvement, the whole marrow space is replaced by plasma cells which, in normal marrow, are only a very minor constituent.

Significant destruction of normal blood-forming marrow usually only occurs at a late stage in the natural history of the disease when bone marrow replacement by neoplastic plasma cells can become very extensive.

Almost all myelomas are derived from a single clone and therefore the tumours produce a vast excess of a single monoclonal antibody which can be easily detected in circulating blood; light chains of the monoclonal antibody may appear in the urine *(Bence-Jones protein)*.

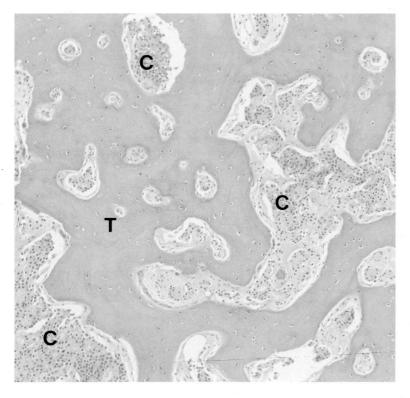

Fig. 15.10   Metastatic tumour in bone marrow (HP)

The bone marrow is a frequent site for deposits of metastatic carcinoma, the common primary tumours being from *prostate, bronchus, breast, thyroid* and *kidney*. Widespread replacement of bone marrow by metastatic tumour causes haematopoiesis in liver and spleen *(extramedullary haematopoiesis)*.

Most metastatic deposits cause bone destruction and, when widespread, can be associated with *hypercalcaemia*. Metastases from carcinoma of the prostate may, however, be associated with bone formation and result in *osteosclerosis*. This is shown in this micrograph where replacement of marrow by carcinoma cells **C** from a carcinoma of the prostate is associated with reactive bone formation forming trabeculae **T**.

16. Female reproductive system

Disorders of the vulva

The vulva is subject to many of the conditions affecting skin elsewhere in the body, including various inflammatory conditions such as dermatitis (see Figs. 20.5 and 20.6), but is also an important site for specific infective lesions which are transmitted sexually, including the chancre of primary syphilis. Many vulval inflammatory lesions lead to intense itching, so the histological features of these conditions are complicated by the effects of trauma from scratching. In elderly post-menopausal women, the vulval mucosa tends to become thickened and white as a result of epithelial atrophy and subepithelial fibrosis, a condition known pathologically as *lichen sclerosus et atrophicus* (see Fig. 16.1). Many pathological lesions may produce the clinical appearance of *leukoplakia,* including chronic inflammatory disease, e.g. neurodermatitis, the early stages of lichen sclerosus, and some forms of vulval *carcinoma in situ;* in the last condition, marked epithelial dysplasia is the classic histological feature (see Fig. 5.6). The most important malignant tumour of the vulva is *squamous carcinoma* (Fig. 16.2).

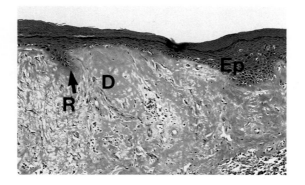

Fig. 16.1 Lichen sclerosus et atrophicus (HP)

This condition of unknown aetiology presents clinically as smooth, whitish plaques around the vulva often with narrowing of the introitus. Histologically there is marked thinning and atrophy of the epidermis **Ep** with virtual disappearance of rete pegs **R** and skin appendages. The epidermal atrophy is associated with hyalinisation of the underlying dermis **D**, seen as homogeneous pink staining. Dermal vessels may show perivascular accumulation of lymphocytes and some plasma cells.

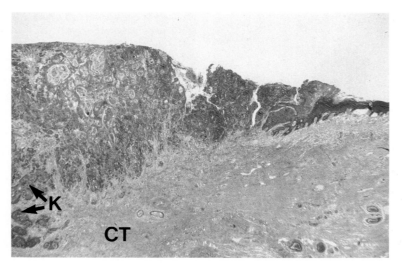

Fig. 16.2 Squamous carcinoma of vulva (MP)

Vulval carcinoma most commonly occurs in the very elderly; it presents as raised indurated areas which eventually undergo central ulceration. These tumours are almost always slow growing, highly differentiated squamous carcinomas and exhibit abundant keratin pearl formation **K** (see also Fig. 6.11). The tumour may originate in the labia majora, labia minora or clitoris, and may spread deeply into underlying connective tissue **CT** and thence via lymphatics to superficial inguinal lymph nodes.

Diseases of the vagina and uterine cervix

The *vagina* is rarely the site of important primary lesions of histopathological interest, although it is frequently the site of infections *(vaginitis)* especially by *Candida*, *Trichomonas* and *Gardnerella vaginalis*. Primary squamous carcinoma and adenocarcinoma of the vagina occur but are very uncommon.   The *cervix* frequently shows chronic inflammatory changes, *chronic cervicitis* (see Fig. 16.3), which may also be associated with polypoid hyperplasia of the endocervical mucosa, sometimes with the formation of a large pedunculated polyp containing distended endocervical glands and stroma (see Fig. 16.4). Clinically, the most important lesions of the cervix are epithelial dysplasia, carcinoma in situ, and squamous carcinoma, all of which originate at the cervical squamocolumnar junction; these related conditions and their pathogenesis are considered in detail in Figures l6.5 to 16.7.

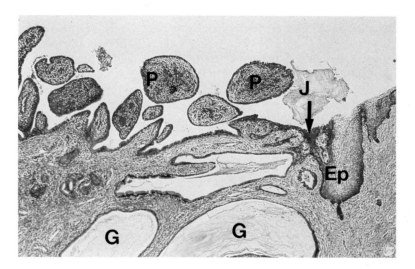

Fig. 16.3   Chronic cervicitis
(MP)

In *chronic cervicitis* the ectocervical squamous epithelium **Ep** is normal except for slight thickening. The major changes are seen in the endocervix immediately above the squamocolumnar junction **J**; here there is micropolyposis, the core of each tiny polyp **P** showing a heavy chronic inflammatory cell infiltrate, mainly lymphocytic. Deeper endocervical glands **G** show cystic dilatation. Long-standing inflammation may lead to squamous metaplasia of the surface endocervical epithelium.

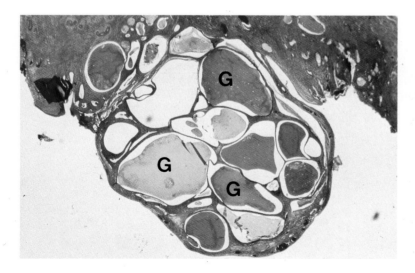

Fig. 16.4   Endocervical polyp
(LP)

This micrograph shows an early benign *endocervical polyp* arising from the endocervical canal. The polyp is composed of cystically dilated glands **G** of varying sizes, each distended by mucin and lined by columnar endocervical mucin-secreting epithelium. As the polyp enlarges it may develop a fibrous stroma between the cystic glands; extrusion through the external os may lead to surface ulceration.

Cervical polyps are an important cause of abnormal vaginal bleeding.

Cervical dysplasia and carcinoma

The vagina and the vaginal aspect of the cervix are covered by stratified squamous epithelium which is well adapted to withstand the normal vaginal environment. The endocervical canal, on the other hand, is lined by a simple columnar, mucin-secreting epithelium; at a microscopic level this is deeply folded so as to form gland-like invaginations into the cervical stroma, the *endocervical glands,* which are responsible for the elaboration of normal cervical mucus.

The junction between stratified squamous and columnar epithelium normally lies at the external os. The volume of the cervical stroma expands under the influence of hormones during each menstrual cycle, at menarche and during pregnancy, and this causes eversion of the vaginal end of the endocervical canal thus exposing some of the simple columnar epithelium to the vaginal environment. This exposed epithelium appears red in relation to the surrounding stratified squamous epithelium and hence became inaccurately known as a *cervical erosion;* more appropriate is the term *cervical ectropion.* Under the influence of the vaginal environment, the ectropic columnar epithelium may undergo squamous metaplasia (see Fig. 5.5) to form stratified squamous epithelium indistinguishable from the lining epithelium native to the vagina. This metaplastic area, described as the *transformation zone,* appears to be unstable and susceptible to dysplastic changes possibly induced by external factors; infection with the genital wart virus, cigarette smoking, and large numbers of sexual partners are associated with a higher incidence of cervical dysplasia and carcinoma; however direct causative roles have not been established. The dysplastic changes may well regress if these uncertain predisposing factors are eliminated, however, it is believed that some undergo irreversible neoplastic change with the development of *carcinoma in situ.* Furthermore, a proportion of untreated cases of carcinoma in situ are thought to transform into frank *invasive squamous carcinoma.*

The development of invasive squamous carcinoma may thus be prevented by intercepting the dysplastic process at some earlier stage and cervical cytology has been developed as a method of screening and monitoring this process in the population of women at risk. Once significant dysplastic changes have been demonstrated cytologically, histological examination of biopsy specimens taken at *colposcopy* is used to define accurately the degree of dysplasia and to plan appropriate treatment.

The *CIN (cervical intraepithelial neoplasia)* classification is a method of grading the degree of abnormality in cervical epithelium. CIN grade I corresponds to mild dysplasia, CIN grade II to moderate dysplasia and CIN grade III includes severe dysplasia and carcinoma in situ. Grade I and grade II lesions may be managed conservatively, but grade III lesions must be eliminated by such methods as laser cautery and local excision *(cone biopsy).* Invasive carcinoma demands radical excision or radiotherapy.

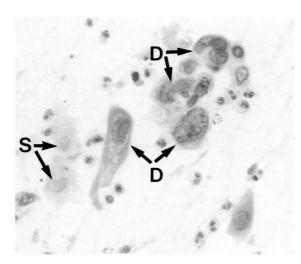

Fig. 16.5 Cervical smear cytology: atypical cells
(PAP stain) (HP)

This micrograph is from a preparation obtained by cervical smear stained by the Papanicolau method (PAP). It exhibits both normal cervical squamous cells **S** and clumps of dysplastic cells **D** which have large dark-stained nuclei, a slightly irregular nuclear contour and a coarse pattern of nuclear chromatin.

Based on the results of such screening, this patient was referred for colposcopic examination and a biopsy was taken of a suspicious area on the cervix that turned white on exposure to acetic acid. The histology is illustrated in Figure 16.6 and shows severe dysplasia, i.e. CIN III.

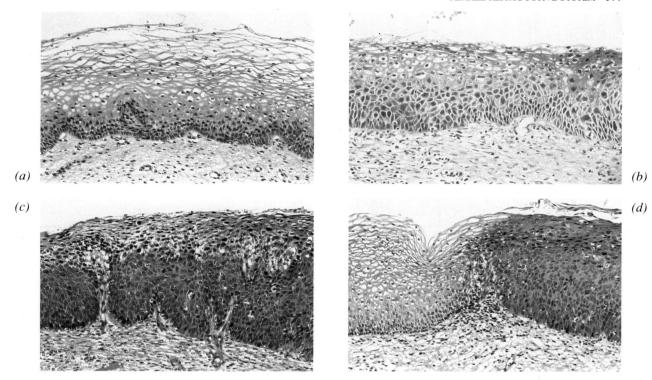

(a)

(b)

(c)

(d)

Fig. 16.6 Cervical dysplasia and carcinoma in situ
(a) normal ectocervix (HP)
(c) severe dysplasia - CIN III (HP)

(b) moderate dysplasia - CIN II (HP)
(d) carcinoma in situ - CIN III (HP)

Micrographs (a) to (d) illustrate the spectrum of cervical epithelial appearances from normal stratified squamous epithelium through to carcinoma in situ.

As seen in micrograph (a), normal ectocervical epithelium has a typical stratified squamous form with all cell division being confined to a single basal layer of small darkly staining cuboidal cells. As the cells undergo maturation, their eosinophilic cytoplasm expands greatly and the cells are pushed upwards into a stratum equivalent to the prickle cell layer of skin. Beyond this, the cells become flattened with further maturation, their nuclei becoming first pyknotic then undergoing karyorrhexis and karyolysis (see Fig. 1.6); the cytoplasm becomes progressively flattened until the cells are finally shed from the surface.

In moderate dysplasia, as shown in micrograph (b), the basal and prickle cell layers occupy about half of the epithelial thickness and exhibit an increased degree of cellular pleomorphism with the nuclei being abnormally large and prominent in the prickle cell layer and mitoses being evident beyond the basal layer; the upper half of the epithelium shows fairly normal maturational changes although nuclei in these layers appear slightly larger than those in the normal. This amounts to moderate dysplasia (CIN grade II).

Micrograph (c) shows more marked dysplasia with the hyperchromatic dysplastic cells extending more than half way towards the surface; although not visible here, mitotic figures were evident far above the basal layer. At the right of the micrograph, dysplastic cells extend almost to the surface with little evidence of normal maturation; this would be classified as CIN grade III.

Micrograph (d) illustrates an abrupt transition from normal stratified squamous epithelium on the left to highly dysplastic epithelium on the right. The pleomorphic dysplastic cells, including mitotic forms, extend right to the surface and there is virtually no evidence of maturation of the surface epithelial cells. These features meet all the cytological criteria for malignant change; nevertheless, the basement membrane remains intact and there is no evidence of invasion of the underlying stroma so this lesion is classified as carcinoma in situ (CIN grade III). The abnormal nucleated surface cells in this lesion were detected in a cervical smear and the clinician then obtained this biopsy for diagnosis.

A critical feature of the dysplastic examples just discussed is that the basement membrane remains sharply defined and intact. With any evidence of microinvasion or more extensive spread into underlying tissues, the lesion is defined as *invasive carcinoma*.

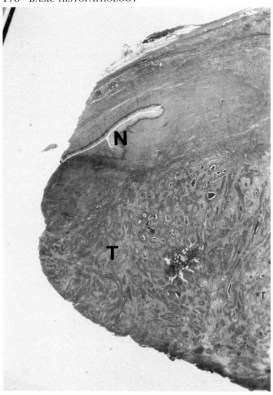

(a)

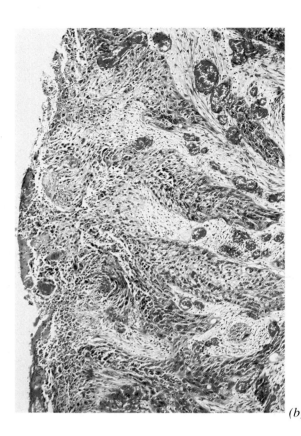

(b)

Fig. 16.7 Invasive squamous carcinoma of the cervix
(a) invasive carcinoma (LP)
(b) poorly differentiated carcinoma (HP)

Extensive lesions which are identified as being CIN III on colposcopic biopsy require cone biopsy to remove the whole area of atypical epithelium; if the dysplastic area does not extend into the endocervical canal this may be amenable to laser or other methods of cautery excision, otherwise cone biopsy is performed; this involves excision of the endocervical canal with surrounding ectocervix.

The earliest forms of invasive carcinoma are seen in a proportion of such excision biopsy specimens as superficial invasion of the cervical stroma. When the lesion is limited in extent it is termed *micro-invasive carcinoma* and relatively conservative surgery such as cone biopsy is adequate to achieve cure.

More extensive and macroscopically obvious carcinoma of the cervix is treated by hysterectomy. Such an invasive squamous carcinoma of the cervix is illustrated at low magnification in micrograph (a). Note that purple-staining tumour **T** has replaced most of the cervical stroma and muscle, although a portion of normal vaginal mucosa **N** remains at the tumour margin. The surface of the tumour is ulcerated and this accounts for the frequent presenting feature of post-coital bleeding.

The surface of this tumour is shown at high magnification in micrograph (b). The lesion consists of islands of darkly staining pleomorphic cells invading the loose cervical stroma; the tumour is poorly differentiated since there is no evidence of pink-staining keratin formation, characteristic of well-differentiated squamous carcinoma (see Fig. 6.11). Such invasive carcinomas of the cervix spread widely into local structures and become disseminated to lymph nodes in the pelvis.

Squamous carcinomas account for about 90% of cervical malignancies, most of the remainder being adenocarcinomas arising in the endocervix.

Disorders of the uterus

The uterine endometrium undergoes monthly cyclical changes under the influence of hormonal stimuli during the period between menarche and menopause, normally only being suspended in pregnancy. Before menarche the endometrial glands and stroma are compact and inactive, a state they return to after the menopause. At menarche, around the menopause, and for the first few cycles after a pregnancy, the endometrium shows a mixture of inactive and normal functional patterns. Under the influence of oral contraceptive drugs and intra-uterine contraceptive devices, the endometrium assumes various other histological patterns.

Excessive or uncoordinated hormonal stimulation of the endometrium may produce diffuse endometrial hyperplasia. Two patterns are recognised, *simple (cystic) hyperplasia* and *atypical hyperplasia;* these are illustrated in Figure 16.9. Localised areas of polypoid hyperplasia forming *endometrial polyps* are common and often contain cystically dilated endometrial glands (see Fig. 16.8). The most common malignant tumour of the endometrium is *endometrial carcinoma,* an adenocarcinoma derived from endometrial glands (see Fig. 16.10).

Endometrial infection is uncommon, but may follow genital tuberculosis or mechanical obstruction to the endocervical canal, e.g. by tumour, often leading to a distension of the endometrial cavity by pus *(pyometra).* Fulminant infection of the uterus by coliform organisms was once a common fatal complication following childbirth *(peurperal fever)* but is now uncommon.

The myometrium is the site of one of the most common benign connective tissue tumours, the *leiomyoma* (see Fig. 16.11 and also Figs. 6.4a and b); in the myometrium these smooth muscle tumours become progressively more collagenous as they enlarge, giving rise to the colloquial term *fibroid.*

The myometrium may also contain islands of ectopic endometrium which may be subject to the usual cycle of proliferative and secretory changes under the influence of ovarian hormones; such changes may give rise to pain and other menstrual disturbances. When involving the uterine muscle, this ectopic endometrium is known as *adenomyosis* (Fig. 16.12); such ectopic endometrial tissue may also be found in various other sites throughout the pelvis when it is described by the more general term *endometriosis* (Fig. 16.15).

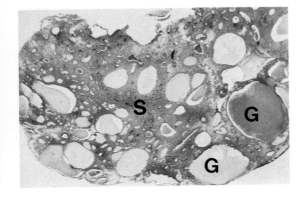

Fig. 16.8   Endometrial polyp (LP)

Endometrial polyps are an important but innocuous cause of abnormal uterine bleeding at or near the menopause; they are pedunculated and often multiple. Most are composed of cystically dilated glands **G** in a typical loose endometrial stroma **S** and covered by a layer of flattened endometrial surface cells. The glands and stroma in some polyps are responsive to ovarian hormones, and thus show evidence of proliferative, secretory or hyperplastic activity accordingly.

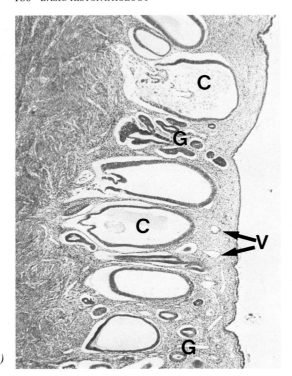

(a)

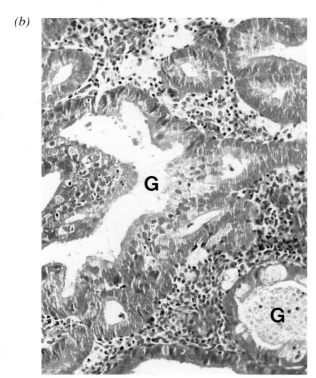

(b)

**Fig. 16.9 Endometrial hyperplasia
(a) simple (cystic) hyperplasia** (MP)
(b) atypical hyperplasia (HP)

Endometrial hyperplasia appears to be a response to excessive or uncoordinated ovarian hormone production and may be either simple or atypical in form.

In *simple (cystic) hyperplasia* as shown in micrograph (a), the endometrial lining becomes thickened as a result of proliferation of the endometrial glandular tissue with the formation of numerous tiny cysts **C** scattered among normal-looking endometrial glands **G**; the cysts result from dilatation of endometrial glands. The intervening stroma frequently contains prominent thin-walled blood vessels **V**; heavy uterine bleeding is the most common presenting symptom.

In *atypical hyperplasia,* shown in micrograph (b) at higher magnification, there is also proliferation of the endometrial glands **G**, however, they show features which indicate possible failure of normal growth regulation. Many are irregular in shape and size, often with papillary infoldings. Adjacent glands are often so closely packed that there appears to be no intervening stroma *(architectural atypia)*. More importantly, many of the glandular epithelial cells show marked *cytological atypia* with nuclear and cytoplasmic pleomorphism and increased mitotic activity. Some foci closely resemble a well-differentiated endometrial adenocarcinoma (see Fig. 16.10).

Both types of hyperplasia may follow excess oestrogen secretion; the specimen in micrograph (b) was associated with the theca cell tumour shown in Figure 16.20.

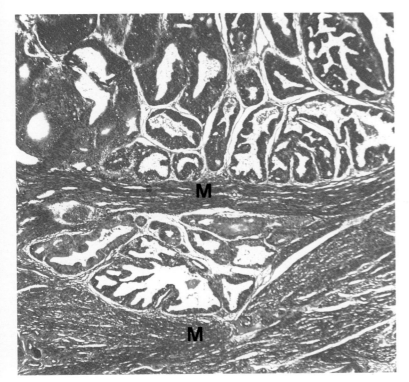

Fig. 16.10 Endometrial adenocarcinoma (MP)

The most common malignancy of the body of the uterus is this malignant tumour of the endometrial glands; it usually occurs in post-menopausal women and is the most important cause of post-menopausal bleeding. Well-differentiated forms bear many histological similarities to the atypical adenomatous hyperplasia shown in Figure 16.9 (b) but malignancy can be recognised by the invasion of the underlying myometrium **M**, as in this micrograph. The tumour also grows into the lumen to distend the uterine cavity. Distorted, irregular, glandular patterns are frequent, and focal squamous metaplasia is seen in some forms. The tumour spreads by local invasion through the myometrium and via lymphatics to iliac and para-aortic lymph nodes.

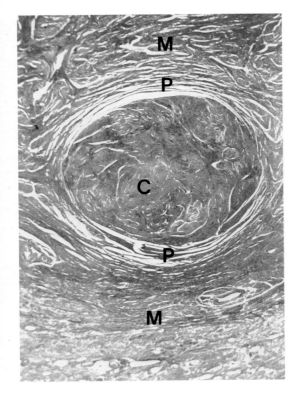

Fig. 16.11 Leiomyoma (fibroid) of myometrium (LP)

This benign tumour of myometrial smooth muscle is a very common cause of abnormal or excessive uterine bleeding and pelvic discomfort. It provides a good illustration of the growth pattern of benign tumours within solid organs and is also illustrated in Figure 6.4. The tumour is composed of fascicles of smooth muscle cells but larger tumours also show foci of fibroblastic collagen formation **C**, particularly towards the centre of the tumour. Gradual expansion of the tumour compresses the surrounding myometrium **M**, leading to atrophy of normal myometrial smooth muscle cells; this leaves only the scanty collagenous stroma which becomes compacted to form a distinct pseudocapsule **P**. Some tumours arise near the endometrial cavity and may protrude into the cavity to produce a polypoid *submucous fibroid*. Secondary changes may also occur, including extensive collagenisation and calcification (especially with increasing age), liquefactive necrosis to form fluid-filled areas of cystic degeneration, and, very rarely, sarcomatous change. To an extent, the growth of these tumours is hormone-dependent, since they almost always shrink and partially regress after the menopause.

Fig. 16.12   Adenomyosis of the uterus (MP)

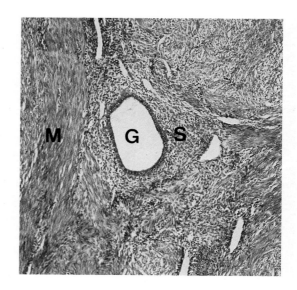

Adenomyosis is the term applied to a condition in which islands of ectopic endometrial glands **G** and stroma **S** are found embedded deep within the myometrium **M**, often at a considerable distance from the normal endometrium. Their presence is often associated with symmetrical increase in myometrial bulk thus enlarging the uterus; occasionally they stimulate a more localised increase in smooth muscle to produce a leiomyoma-like mass containing endometrial islands, a lesion called an *adenomyoma*.

This ectopic endometrium is responsive in the normal manner to ovarian hormones but, being abnormally confined by surrounding tissues, may give rise to pain. Ectopic endometrium may occur elsewhere in the pelvic region when it is known by the term *endometriosis* (see Fig. 16.15).

Diseases of the Fallopian tubes

The Fallopian tubes may become infected by pyogenic bacteria, particularly gonococcus, and the acute inflammation may be complicated by obstruction of the tubal lumen, leading to chronic suppurative inflammation and abscess formation. These conditions, known as *acute salpingitis, chronic salpingitis* and *tubo-ovarian abscess* respectively, are discussed with Figure 16.13. Along with tuberculous infection of the Fallopian tube (see Fig. 3.14), they constitute an important cause of female infertility due to tubal lumen obliteration. Scarring of the tube and other disorders may prevent the free passage of a fertilised ovum into the endometrial cavity and implantation may occur in the oviduct leading to *tubal ectopic pregnancy* (see Fig. 16.14); this usually culminates in massive haemorrhage caused by the placenta eroding through the tubal wall.

Fig. 16.13   Acute salpingitis (MP)

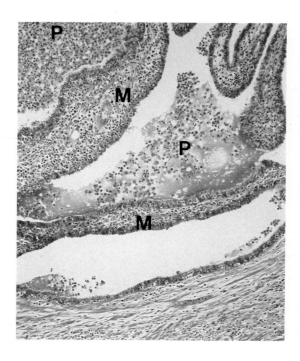

In *acute salpingitis* the tubal mucosa **M** becomes hyperaemic, oedematous, and infiltrated with neutrophil polymorphs and the lumen becomes filled with purulent exudate **P** containing abundant neutrophils. Blockage of the tubal lumen often follows, preventing drainage and leading to distension of the tube by pus *(pyosalpinx)*. Sometimes the inflammation produces adhesions between tube, fimbriae and ovary, and extension of suppuration to these areas may produce multiple locules of pus, the *tubo-ovarian abscess*. Without the intervention of antibiotics, the combination of adhesions and suppuration rarely permits total resolution of the acute inflammation and a state of chronic inflammation generally ensues. This state, known as *chronic salpingitis,* may persist for many years resulting in fibrosis and tubal obstruction and is an important cause of female infertility. Chronic salpingitis may be a component of more widespread chronic inflammation involving ovaries, clinically termed *pelvic inflammatory disease*.

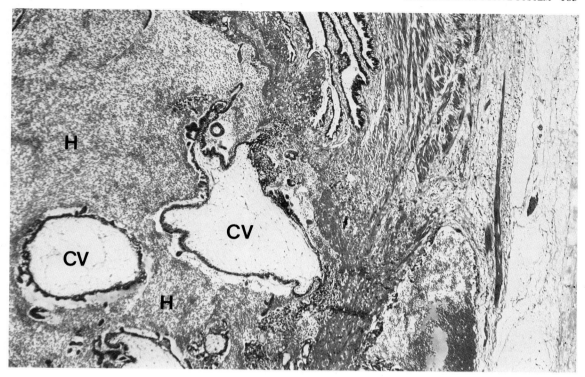

Fig. 16.14   Tubal ectopic pregnancy (MP)

The Fallopian tube is the most frequent location for inappropriate implantation of the fertilised ovum, *ectopic pregnancy.* The tubular lumen becomes filled with developing embryo, placenta and associated membranes, including chorionic villi **CV** and decidual tissue. The tubal wall is often deeply congested and thinned, and stromal cells in the mucosa near the implantation site may shows decidual change. Ectopic pregnancies usually become dramatically apparent by severe haemorrhage **H** into the lumen *(haematosalpinx),* often followed by tracking of blood into the peritoneal cavity; tubal ectopics therefore most often present as acute abdominal emergencies; only very rarely does the pregnancy continue to near normal term.

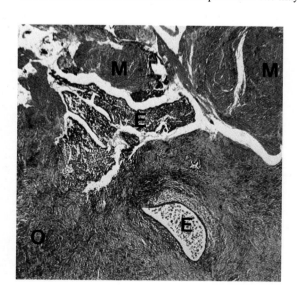

Fig. 16.15   Pelvic endometriosis (MP)

The Fallopian tube, paratubular connective tissues and ovaries are a frequent site for the condition known as *endometriosis,* in which islands of ectopic endometrial glands and stroma are found outside the uterine body.

  This micrograph shows islands of endometriosis **E** in both ovarian stroma **O**, and pink-staining smooth muscle **M** of Fallopian tube wall. Fibrosis secondary to the endometriosis has led to adhesion of the ovary to the tube, forming an ill-defined tubo-ovarian mass. Endometriosis affecting the serosal surfaces may also lead to adhesion between tube, ovary, uterus and loops of bowel. Ectopic endometrium may also occur in the myometrium when it is termed *adenomyosis,* illustrated in Figure 16.12.

Disorders of the ovary

Non-neoplastic cysts

Under the influence of pituitary gonadotrophins, the ovary undergoes cyclical changes providing for the development and release of a mature ovum at the mid-point of each monthly menstrual cycle, and for the production of the ovarian hormones which control the menstrual cycle. During the proliferative phase of the menstrual cycle, a number of follicles enlarge culminating in maturation of one follicle which discharges its single ovum into the Fallopian tube (ovulation); the follicle, until this time also responsible for production of oestrogens, now develops into the corpus luteum responsible for producing progesterone until the beginning of the next menstrual cycle when the follicle atrophies to form the redundant collagenous corpus albicans. This regular sequence of changes is normally only interrupted by the advent of pregnancy, in which case the corpus luteum persists until the end of the first trimester. On occasions however, the sequence is aborted at some stage and small *follicular* or *luteal cysts* may form. Some small cysts may also form by inclusion of islands of surface 'germinal' epithelium of the ovary; these are known as *germinal inclusion cysts*. These three types of cysts are shown in Figure 16.16.

Tumours of the ovary

Tumours may arise from each of the specialised elements which make up the ovary and may be classified into four broad groups:

- **Epithelial origin** - benign and malignant tumours of the surface ovarian epithelium are common and are usually cystic. The most frequent have either a *serous* or *mucinous* content (Figs. 16.17 and 16.18). Epithelial tumours which resemble those seen in the endometrium also develop in the ovary where they are termed *endometrioid carcinoma of the ovary.*

- **Stromal origin** - tumours may develop from *granulosa cells* and *thecal cells* (Fig. 16.20) as well as from spindle cells of the ovarian stroma forming *fibromas*. These stromal tumours may produce oestrogenic hormones and cause endocrine effects such as endometrial hyperplasia (Fig. 16.9).

- **Germ cell origin** - the classification is similar to that for testicular germ cell tumours (Fig. 18.5) and includes *teratoma* (*dermoid cyst*, see Fig. 16.19) and *dysgerminoma* (ovarian equivalent of the seminoma) as well as specialised tumours such as *choriocarcinoma* and *yolk-sac tumour.*

- **Metastatic** - the ovary is a common site for metastatic carcinoma. A well known example is the so-called *Krukenberg tumour* in which there is infiltration of the ovary by mucin-secreting adenocarcinoma of signet ring pattern (see Figs. 6.13 and 12.8) usually derived from stomach or colon, and possibly reaching the ovary by either transcoelomic or lymphatic spread.

Other disorders of the ovary

The ovary may be involved in endometriosis (see Fig. 16.15), as well as being involved by chronic inflammation in the form of tubo-ovarian abscesses caused by primary infection of the Fallopian tube (Fig. 16.13).

Placental tissues

Details of the various structural and functional abnormalities of the placenta, decidua, membranes and umbilical cord are generally outside the scope of this book, however hydatidiform mole (Fig. 16.20) and choriocarcinoma (Fig. 16.22) are included as examples of disorders of placental growth. Ectopic pregnancy is discussed in Figure 16.14.

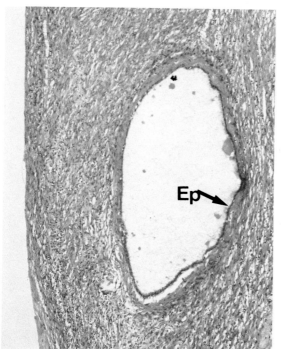

(a)

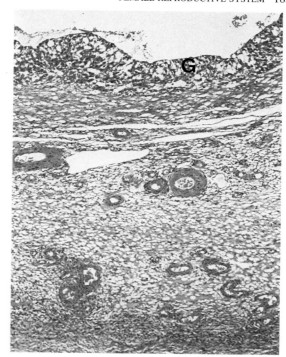

(b)

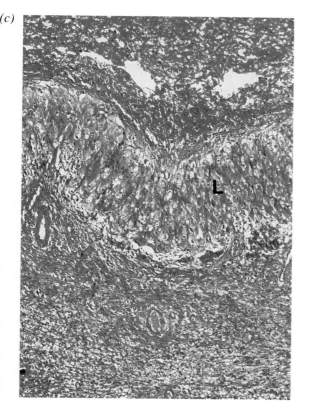

(c)

Fig. 16.16 Non-neoplastic cysts of ovary
(a) germinal inclusion cyst (MP)
(b) follicular cyst (MP)
(c) luteal cyst (MP)

The most common type of ovarian cyst is the so-called
germinal inclusion cyst illustrated in micrograph (a);
these cysts are commonly multiple, small and lined by a
simple cuboidal epithelium **Ep**. They are thought to be
derived from entrapped portions of the ovarian surface
epithelium which is referred to as germinal epithelium.

Follicular cysts are lined internally by granulosa cells
G which usually form a thicker layer than do the
flattened cells lining the germinal inclusion cyst;
continuing enlargement of the follicular cyst leads to
atrophy of the lining cells so that distinction between a
large follicular cyst and a germinal inclusion cyst may be
difficult.

The *luteal cyst* is probably derived from a corpus
luteum which has not undergone the normal transition to
a corpus albicans. The cyst is usually ovoid with a
slightly irregular outline; microscopically it contains
clear or brownish fluid and is lined by a yellow-coloured
layer of variable thickness. Histologically, as shown in
micrograph (c), the yellow layer is composed of plump
luteal cells **L** with lipid-rich cytoplasm.

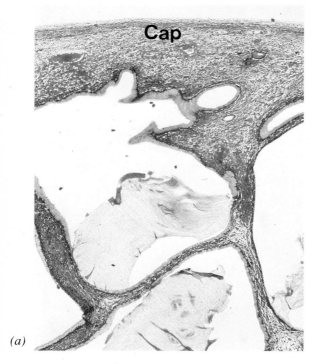

(a)

Cap

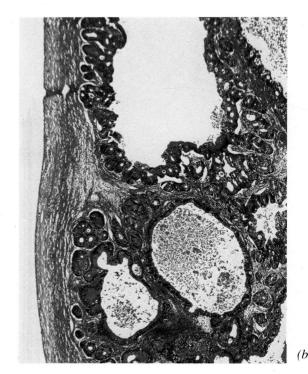

(b)

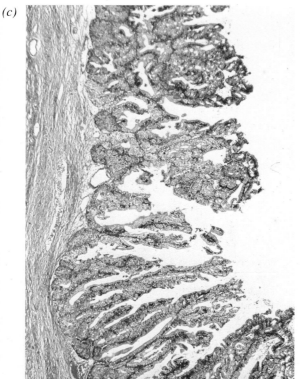

(c)

Fig. 16.17 Mucinous cystic tumours of ovary
(a) benign mucinous cystadenoma (MP)
(b) mucinous cystadenocarcinoma (MP)
(c) mucinous cyst of borderline malignancy (MP)

Mucinous tumours of the ovary may be benign or malignant and are composed of cystic spaces filled with mucin. The *benign cystadenoma*, as shown in micrograph (a), has a characteristically smooth outer surface composed of the ovarian capsule **Cap**. The cystic locules are lined by tall columnar epithelium with uniform basal nuclei and copious mucin-containing cytoplasm at the luminal aspect.

The malignant variant, *mucinous cystadenocarcinoma*, illustrated in micrograph (b), is less common. The tumour is more solid, with smaller cystic spaces. The cells are usually recognisably columnar, but the nucleus occupies much more of the cell, and the remaining cytoplasm usually contains less mucin than its benign counterpart, thereby being less pale staining. Evidence of malignancy is usually demonstrated by invasion of tumour cells through the capsule (not shown in this micrograph).

Some mucinous tumours, apparently benign to the naked eye, show evidence of cytological or architectural atypia without features of invasion; they are regarded as showing *borderline malignancy* and their prognosis is better than for overtly malignant tumours; an example is shown in micrograph (c).

Fig. 16.18 Serous ovarian cystic tumours
(a) serous cystadenoma (MP)
(b) serous papillary cystadenocarcinoma (MP)

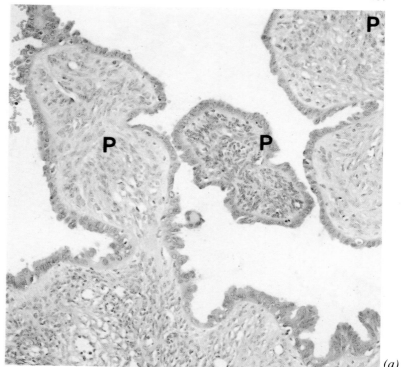

(a)

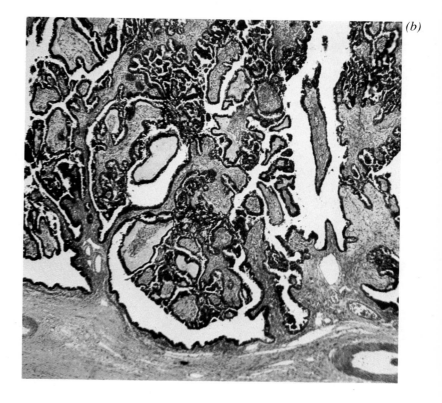

(b)

Like the mucinous cystic tumours, the serous tumours may also develop into very large cystic masses replacing the ovary. In the *benign serous cystadenoma* the cysts are multilocular, though usually less so than the mucinous tumours, and are filled with a clear watery (serous) fluid. The benign cysts are lined by columnar epithelium, often ciliated in places, but the epithelium may be partly flattened in the larger, tense cysts. A characteristic feature of benign serous cystadenomas, as seen in micrograph (a), is the presence of variable numbers of small rounded or papilliferous ingrowths **P** composed of a variably dense stroma covered by tall columnar epithelium.

In the malignant variant, as shown in micrograph (b), the papillary ingrowths are more numerous and papilliferous and tend to fill the cystic cavity.

The benign tumours have a smooth serosal surface, since the epithelial components show no tendency to invade and breach the capsule, whereas the malignant variant eventually invades through the capsule, often producing warty outgrowths on the serosal surface. The overtly malignant variety also shows marked cellular atypia and the cells become heaped up into irregular solid masses.

Some of the papillary growths contain spherical, concentrically laminated, calcified bodies in their stroma; these *psammoma bodies* are typical of papillary tumours of the ovary, although they are also seen in papillary tumours of the thyroid and in meningiomas (see Fig. 22.12). As with the mucinous equivalent, tumours of borderline malignancy occur.

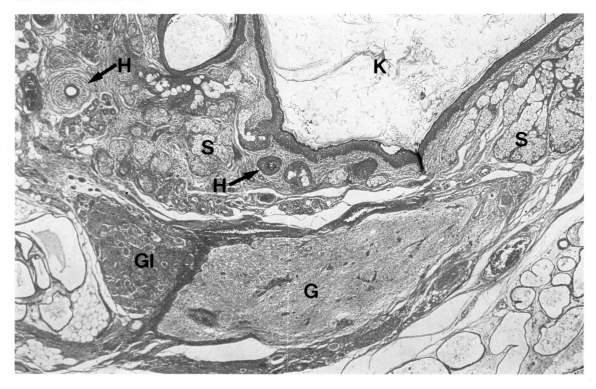

Fig. 16.19   Benign cystic teratoma (MP)

This tumour, formerly known as *dermoid cyst of the ovary,* is an example of a benign, well-differentiated teratoma in which ectodermal elements usually predominate. The lesion takes the form of a unilocular, thin-walled cyst filled with a thick, yellowish, pasty material composed of masses of degenerating keratin **K**, often containing hair. This is produced by the lining epithelium of the cyst which is keratinising stratified squamous epithelium resembling skin. At one end of the cyst wall can usually be found a raised area within which are other teratomatous components including hair follicles **H**, sebaceous glands **S** and occasionally teeth. Although ectodermal derivatives predominate, particularly skin and skin appendage components,

mesodermal (e.g. cartilage and smooth muscle) and endodermal (e.g. respiratory and gut epithelium) elements occur in some tumours. Neuroectodermal tissues may also be found and in the example illustrated, note the area of glial tissue **G** and a ganglion **Gl** alongside.

Cystic teratomas are most common in young women, and are almost always benign. Rarely, malignant change may occur in the squamous epithelial component and this is seen in elderly patients who have harboured a cystic teratoma for many years.

In addition to benign cystic teratomas discussed here, solid malignant ovarian teratomas occur in children and pubertal girls and are prone to widespread metastasis.

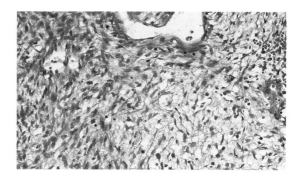

Fig. 16.20   Theca cell tumour (thecoma) (MP)

This is but one example of a number of ovarian tumours which may secrete hormones. Theca cell tumours are spherical, solid tumours with a yellowish cut surface appearance. The tumour is composed of plump spindle cells containing fine lipid droplets which have dissolved out of this preparation leaving vacuoles. This tumour secretes excessive amounts of oestrogens and may be associated with endometrial hyperplasia (see Fig. 16.9) or even endometrial carcinoma.

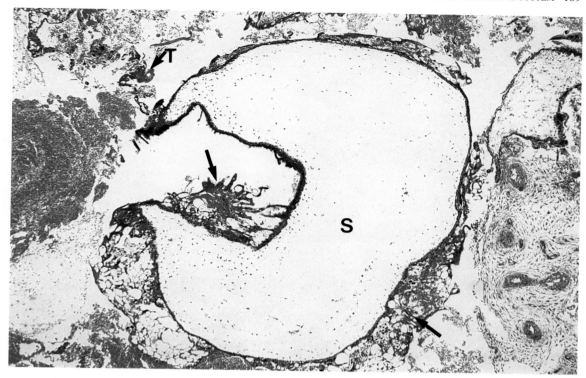

Fig. 16.21 Hydatidiform mole (MP)

The condition known as *hydatidiform mole* arises in a small proportion of non-productive pregnancies. The fetus fails to develop but the membranes remain viable; the chorionic villi become markedly swollen and expanded as a result of hydropic swelling of the villous stromal core **S** which contains none of the vessels usually present in functional villi. These cyst-like translucent swellings are invested by a layer of cytotrophoblast and syncytiotrophoblast, which in normal chorionic villi are a single layer thick. In

hydatidiform mole, the layers of the trophoblast become thickened (arrowed) and there may be disconnected masses of trophoblast cells **T** lying apparently free of the main tumour mass and showing features of cellular pleomorphism.

Hydatidiform moles exhibit a wide spectrum of behaviour; some are eradicated by simple curettage, others persist despite repeated curettage, and a small number develop into undoubtedly malignant choriocarcinoma (see Fig. 16.22).

Fig. 16.22 Choriocarcinoma (HP)

Choriocarcinoma is a malignant tumour derived from trophoblast cells usually from abnormal gestations. They are composed of pleomorphic masses of cytotrophoblast cells **C** and syncytiotrophoblast cells **S** showing no evidence of chorionic villus formation. This tumour is remarkably invasive, metastasising widely via lymphatics and the blood stream particularly to the lungs. Haemorrhage and necrosis in the tumour are common.

Choriocarcinoma may also develop as a component of a teratoma, for example in malignant teratoma of the testis (Fig. 18.3), where it puts the tumour into a poor prognostic group.

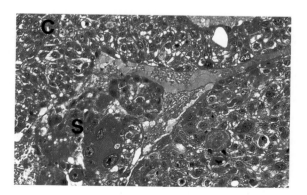

17. Breast

Introduction

The female breast, being dependent on a variety of hormones for its normal activity, exhibits considerable structural and functional variation through life. Apart from the overt changes occurring at puberty, pregnancy, lactation and menopause, more subtle changes also occur within the normal menstrual cycle; as a corollary, hormonal disturbances probably underlie various disorders of the breast, notably *fibroadenosis,* but probably also play some part in the pathogenesis of more serious conditions such as breast tumours. Likewise, the male breast normally remains rudimentary unless breast enlargement, *gynaecomastia* (see Fig. 17.8), is induced by exogenous or endogenous hormone imbalance; it may also result from the use of certain drugs, e.g. spironolactone.

Most clinically significant breast disorders present as a lump and the major imperative is to identify those which are malignant tumours so that the patient may be treated promptly. Several national screening programmes now use radiological techniques *(mammography)* to identify early suspicious breast lesions which are then subject to excision biopsy in the hope that removal of early-stage malignancy will prevent metastasis.

Inflammatory disorders of the breast

Infections of the breast are uncommon and mainly occur during lactation, the organisms (usually *Staphylococcus aureus*) gaining access through cracks and fissures in the nipple and areola; without early antibiotic therapy the resulting *bacterial mastitis* is often followed by the development of a *breast abscess* which may require surgical drainage. More commonly, localised areas of inflammation of the breast follow trauma, which may be of sufficient severity to produce a condition known as *fat necrosis* (see Fig. 17.1).

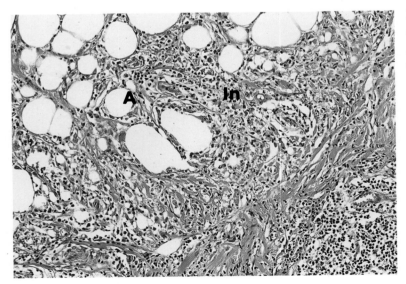

Fig. 17.1 Fat necrosis (MP)

Trauma to the breast, sometimes apparently quite trivial, may result in necrosis of mammary adipose tissue. Following a typical initial acute inflammatory response, the continuing presence of necrotic adipose tissue **A** excites a chronic inflammatory cell infiltrate **In**, in which lipophages (macrophages containing lipid) and plasma cells may be present in large numbers. Fibrous proliferation at the margins of the damaged area produces a hard, often irregular, breast lump which may resemble a breast carcinoma on palpation.

Fibroadenosis

The most frequent disorder of the female breast is *fibroadenosis*. This condition is common in the breasts of mature women, increasing in frequency and severity towards the menopause. Also known by a variety of other terms including *fibrocystic disease*, *cystic mammary dysplasia* and *cystic hyperplasia,* the condition is characterised by proliferative changes affecting components of the mammary unit (lobule, ducts and supporting stroma) probably in response to subtle disturbances of hormone levels, particularly oestrogen. Unequal growth of epithelial and stromal elements gives rise to a variety of solid and cystic nodules within the breast which are clinically important as they must be distinguished from malignancy. The basic lesion is illustrated in Figure 17.2, and common variants shown in Figure 17.3.

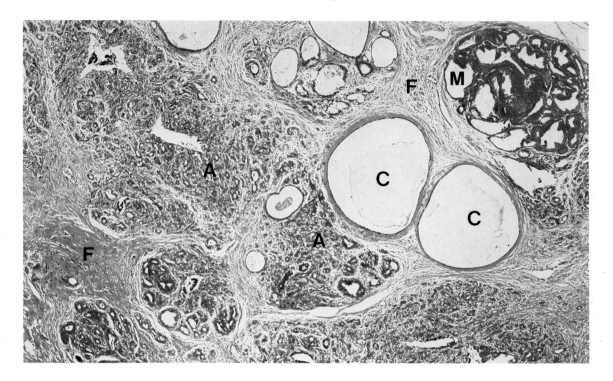

Fig. 17.2   Fibroadenosis - typical lesion (MP)

In essence, the changes of fibroadenosis are the result of various different patterns of distortion and overgrowth of the functional breast unit, including ducts, lobules and supporting fibrous stroma. The epithelial components show hyperplastic overgrowth *(adenosis)* and the fibrous tissue increases *(fibrosis).*

This micrograph shows the histological appearances of a typical lesion of fibroadenosis. There is hyperplasia of breast acinar tissue in the lobules *(adenosis)* to produce islands of dark-staining epithelium **A**; a prominent feature is fibrosis **F** surrounding the areas of adenosis. A frequent feature is marked dilatation of the ducts, to produce cystic lesions **C** lined by flattened ductular epithelium. The epithelium in areas of adenosis often develops strongly eosinophilic cytoplasm and comes to resemble the epithelium in apocrine sweat glands; this is termed *apocrine metaplasia* and is shown in the top right of the micrograph **M**

Several variants of fibroadenosis are commonly encountered which produce histological patterns which can be confused with carcinoma; these variants are illustrated in Figure 17.3.

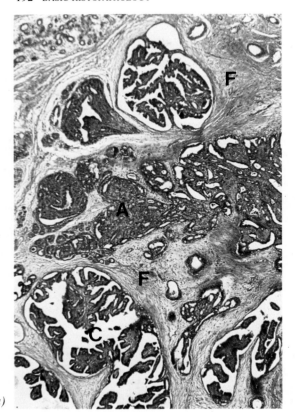

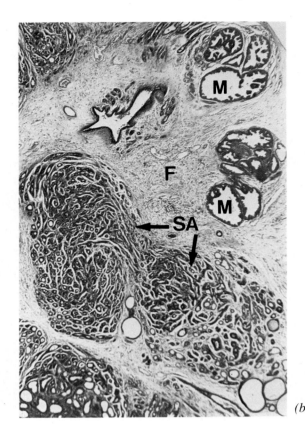

(a)   *(b)*

Fig. 17.3   Fibroadenosis variants
(a) adenosis and duct papillomatosis (MP)   **(b) sclerosing adenosis** (MP)

The hyperplastic overgrowth of epithelium and stroma in fibroadenosis may preferentially affect one tissue component giving rise to patterns which can superficially resemble carcinoma. Two of the more common variants of fibroadenosis are illustrated in these micrographs.

Sometimes marked epithelial overgrowth results in the cystically dilated ducts **C** being filled by papillary ingrowths from the wall, a condition known as *duct papillomatosis*; this is shown in micrograph (a). Solitary duct papillomas of similar appearance may occlude the larger mammary and nipple ducts (see Fig. 17.5). Note the areas of adenosis **A** and fibrosis **F** which constitute more usual components of fibroadenosis.

The changes which may occur in the mammary lobules in fibroadenosis are essentially those of hyperplastic proliferation of lobular acini *(adenosis)* and of the terminal part of the mammary duct within the lobule *(terminal duct hyperplasia)*. In some variants, there is proliferation of the specialised hormone-responsive lobular stromal element, splitting the acini apart and compressing them into elongated strips. This change, known as *sclerosing adenosis* **SA**, is seen in micrograph (b). The importance of this condition is that it may be difficult to distinguish histologically from some invasive patterns of carcinoma, particularly in frozen sections of breast biopsies. This micrograph also illustrates apocrine metaplasia, **M**.

Some areas of fibroadenosis occasionally contain ill-defined nodules which are histologically identical to benign fibroadenoma (see Fig. 17.4).

At one extreme, fibroadenosis may show only replacement of mammary adipose tissue by dense fibrous tissue, with the only epithelial component being dilated mammary ducts; this is particularly seen in women after the menopause, and is described as *mammary fibrosis with duct ectasia*.

Neoplasms of the breast

The most common benign neoplasm of the breast is the *fibroadenoma* (see Fig. 17.4), a localised proliferation of breast ducts and stroma. Such lesions occur most frequently in isolated form in women aged 25-35 ('breast mice'), but nodules of histologically identical tissue may also be a component of fibroadenosis; fibroadenoma may therefore be a form of hormone-dependent nodular hyperplasia rather than a true benign tumour. The only other benign tumour of much clinical significance is the benign *intraduct papilloma* (see Fig. 17.5), usually occurring as a solitary lesion in one of the larger mammary ducts. Histologically similar papillary lesions may also be multifocal, occupying some of the ectatic (dilated) ducts as a component of some patterns of fibroadenosis (see Fig. 17.3); here the lesion is known as *duct papillomatosis* and probably represents hormone-induced hyperplasia rather than a true neoplasm.

Malignant tumours of the female breast are extremely common, with a peak incidence in the decade before the menopause. Most are adenocarcinomas arising from the epithelium of either the mammary lobules *(lobular carcinoma)* or the mammary ducts *(ductal carcinoma)*; the range of histological appearances is illustrated in Figure 17.6 and Figures 6.4 (c) and (d). In some cases the development of invasive breast cancer may be preceded by carcinoma in situ in which the malignant cells proliferate within the mammary ducts or lobules but do not breach the basement membrane *(intraduct or intralobular carcinoma)*. In addition to the main groups of lobular and ductal carcinoma there is a small group of special breast carcinomas which are associated with distinct clinical and pathological features, often with a good prognosis; examples are *tubular carcinoma of the breast* and *medullary carcinoma of the breast*. Carcinoma of the breast does occur in males but is extremely uncommon.

In some cases of breast carcinoma, both in situ and invasive, malignant cells may spread within mammary and lactiferous ducts onto the surface of the nipple resulting in *Paget's disease of the nipple* (see Fig. 17.7).

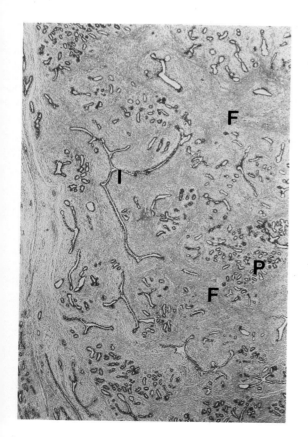

Fig. 17.4   Fibroadenoma (MP)

This condition commonly arises in the breasts of young women (25-35) as a solitary lesion but may occur as a component of fibroadenosis (see Fig. 17.2) particularly in older women approaching the menopause. It is usually considered to be a benign tumour but may well represent a nodular form of benign mammary hyperplasia (fibroadenosis). The mass is well circumscribed by a condensation of connective tissue and is composed of both epithelial and fibrous stromal components. The epithelial components form glandular structures lined by mammary duct-type epithelium, whilst the stromal component is a loose, cellular form of fibrous tissue **F**. In very large masses, the stroma may be myxomatous.

Two patterns of growth are seen, often in the same lesion. In the *pericanalicular pattern* **P**, the epithelial component takes the form of rounded ducts which remain small and undistorted, with the stroma arranged round them in a roughly symmetrical and regular manner. By contrast, in the *intracanalicular pattern* **I**, the ducts appear elongated but actually represent sections cut through flattened spaces compressed by the stromal component which appears to proliferate in an irregular nodular manner; in general, this latter pattern is more prominent in the larger fibroadenomata. In both patterns of fibroadenoma, hormonal changes such as occur in pregnancy and lactation may induce marked proliferation of the epithelial component.

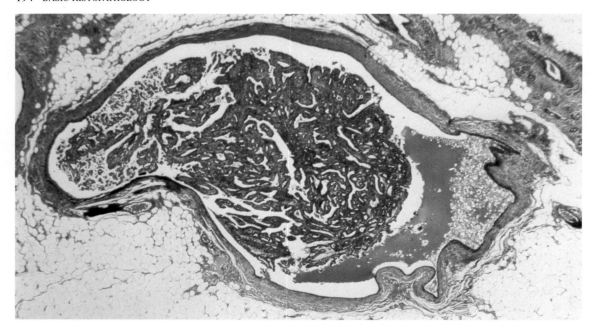

Fig. 17.5 Intraduct papilloma (LP)

Papillomas of mammary duct epithelium may arise as solitary or multiple lesions; solitary lesions as shown here are usually located in the larger lactiferous ducts near the nipple and present with blood-stained discharge from the nipple. The lesions are usually small, consisting of a delicate pink-staining supporting stroma covered by a single or double layer of cuboidal or low columnar epithelial cells resembling those lining the mammary duct from which the papilloma has arisen; with larger lesions, the duct is often dilated. Multiple duct papillomata (florid duct papillomatosis) occur as a component of fibroadenosis (see Fig. 17.2). Malignant change is rare.

Fig. 17.6 Carcinoma of the breast *(illustrations opposite)*
(a) intraduct carcinoma (HP)   **(b) lobular carcinoma in-situ** (HP)
(c) invasive ductal carcinoma (HP)   **(d) invasive lobular carcinoma** (HP)

Carcinoma of the breast may originate in the epithelium of the mammary ducts or the breast lobular glands (*ductal* and *lobular carcinoma* respectively); the vast majority are of ductal origin. Both ductal and lobular carcinomas may have an in situ stage exhibiting the cytological characteristics of malignancy yet showing no evidence of invasive behaviour, being still confined by the epithelial basement membrane of the duct or lobule.

In non-invasive *intraduct carcinoma,* tumour cells fill and distend the ducts. In micrograph (a), note a small duct filled with tumour **T** surrounded by normal acini **A**. The tumour cells are large and pale staining with large nuclei; there may be evidence of increased mitotic activity. Sometimes, duct distension is marked and the tumour cells at the centre undergo necrosis *(comedo pattern)*. Note that there is no infiltration into surrounding stroma **S** and that the epithelial basement membrane is not breached. Infiltration eventually supervenes with development of an *invasive ductal carcinoma;* as shown in micrograph (c), cords of tumour cells **T** then spread out from their ductal origin into the surrounding fibrous stroma **S**.

In non-invasive *lobular carcinoma in situ* as shown in micrograph (b), the normal lobular mammary architecture is maintained but the mammary lobules are increased in size as a result of proliferation of lobular epithelial cells with the cytological characteristics of malignancy. The cells fill and expand the acini of the mammary lobule, but the basement membrane remains intact and the general architecture of the lobule thus remains undisturbed.

In *invasive lobular carcinoma* as shown in micrograph (d) , the tumour cells **T** broach the basement membranes of the acini and spill out into the surrounding stroma **S**, whence they infiltrate into the fibroadipose breast tissue, often in narrow cords and rows of cells described as 'Indian file' pattern of invasion.

Lobular carcinoma has a high risk of bilateral breast involvement.

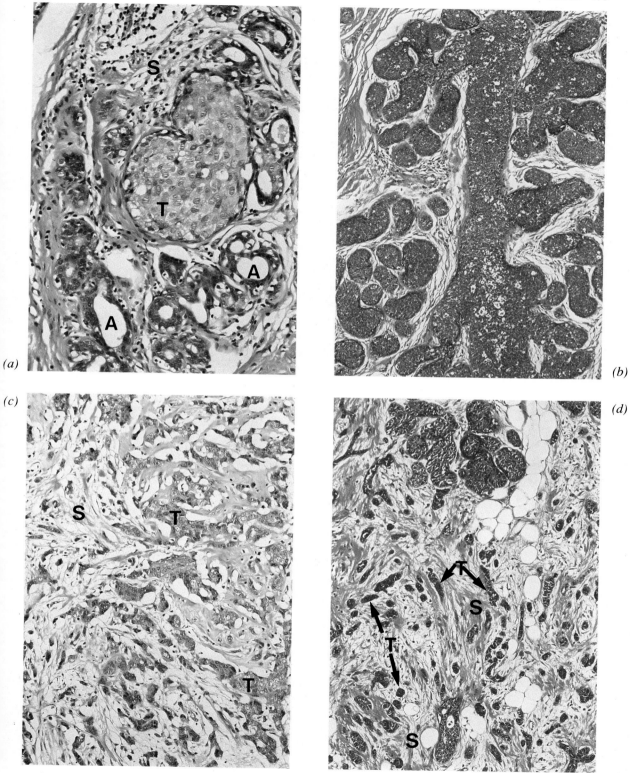

(a)

(b)

(c)

(d)

Fig. 17.6 Carcinoma of the breast *(caption opposite)*

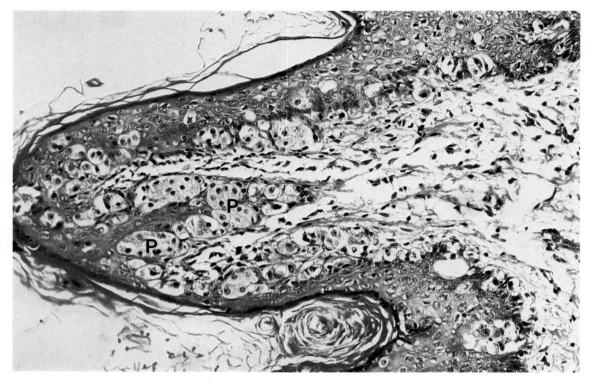

Fig. 17.7 Paget's disease of the nipple (HP)

Some patients with carcinoma of the breast (usually of ductal origin) develop reddening and thickening of the skin of the nipple and areola, occasionally followed by ulceration. The epidermis of the nipple and areola becomes infiltrated by large pleomorphic epithelial cells with hyperchromatic nuclei and pale cytoplasm. These cells, known as *Paget's cells* **P**, are breast carcinoma cells which are presumed to have spread along the epithelium of the mammary and nipple ducts to the surface from an intraduct or infiltrating ductular carcinoma, which is invariably present in the underlying breast tissue.

This phenomenon is known as *intraepithelial spread* of malignant cells.

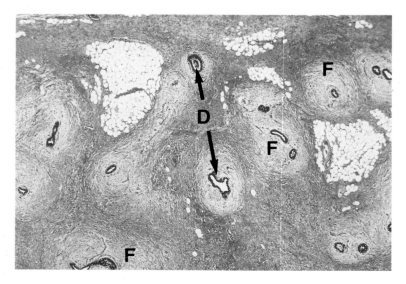

Fig. 17.8 Gynaecomastia of male breast (MP)

The male breast is normally rudimentary and inactive, consisting of fibroadipose tissue containing atrophic mammary ducts.

Oestrogen excess, either endogenous (e.g. puberty) or exogenous (e.g. stilboestrol therapy for carcinoma of prostate), causes breast hyperplasia *(gynaecomastia)*. The simple mammary ducts **D** become enlarged, often with thickening of the epithelial layer and an increase in periductal fibrous tissue **F** which may be markedly collagenous.

18. Male reproductive system

Testis and epididymis

Inflammation of the testis *(orchitis)* may result from virus infections, e.g. mumps, and the testis may also be the site of a gumma in the tertiary stage of syphilis (see Fig. 3.20). Bacterial infections usually arise as a complication of infection of the lower urinary tract or following surgical instrumentation. A non-infective cause of testicular inflammation is *granulomatous orchitis* (see Fig. 18.1) which may follow an episode of trauma to the testis, or sperm retention, e.g. after vasectomy. The most important pathological lesions of the testis are the tumours *seminoma* and *teratoma* illustrated in Figures 18.2 and 18.3. Venous infarction of the testis due to *torsion* is an important cause of testicular pain in childhood and young adulthood and is illustrated in Figure 18.6.

Like the testis, the epididymis may become infected by pyogenic bacteria associated with lower urinary tract infection and surgical instrumentation; when infection occurs, both the testis and epididymis are commonly involved together, a condition known as *acute epididymo-orchitis.* The epididymis is occasionally the site of metastatic tuberculous infection, *tuberculous epididymitis,* (see Fig. 3.17), usually secondary to active pulmonary or renal tuberculosis.

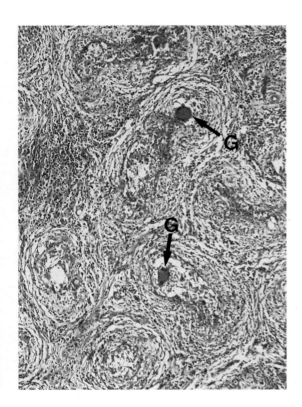

Fig. 18.1 Granulomatous orchitis (MP)

This form of inflammatory disease of the testis most commonly follows trauma to the testis or surgery to the spermatic cord. The testis becomes uniformly firm and enlarged and has a homogeneous pallid cut surface appearance. Histologically, there is diffuse chronic inflammatory cell infiltration, mainly lymphocytes and plasma cells, with numerous granulomata containing giant cells **G**. These inflammatory changes are associated with destruction and atrophy of the seminiferous tubules which in this specimen have been almost entirely destroyed. The cause of this inflammation is not known but it may represent an abnormal response to extruded spermatozoa.

Tumours of the testis

The most important tumours of the testis are the *germ-cell tumours* which are derived from multipotential spermatocytic cells of the seminiferous tubules; they are subdivided into two major types :

- **Seminomas** - cells in this type of tumour resemble the normal cells lining the seminiferous tubules.

- **Teratomas** - this group of tumours is composed of cells which exhibit patterns of differentiation into endodermal, mesodermal and ectodermal elements. If a strict definition of the term teratoma is applied, then a tumour should possess all three lines of differentiation, however the term has come to be used in a more general sense to include many of the non-seminomatous germ-cell tumours with the assumption that differentiation in the tumour has become restricted to only one element. Variation in the latitude with which different workers have included tumours under the umbrella term teratoma is reflected in several classification systems; the most important differences are between those used in Britain and those used in America, from which the classification of the World Health Organization (WHO) is derived. The most noticeable difference in nomenclature is for tumours composed of sheets of undifferentiated cells, termed *malignant teratoma undifferentiated* in the British classification but *embryonal carcinoma* in the WHO classification.

A small proportion of testicular tumours arise from the non-seminiferous cells in the testis, e.g. Leydig cells and Sertoli cells; the majority are benign and may secrete inappropriate sex hormones.

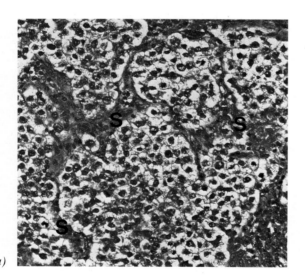

(a)

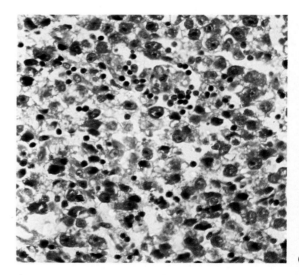

(b)

Fig. 18.2 Seminoma
(a) well differentiated (HP) **(b) poorly differentiated** (HP)

Seminoma is the most common tumour of the testis, with a peak incidence between 30 and 45 years. On cut surface, the tumour is pale, creamy-white and homogeneous with a faint lobular pattern; necrosis and haemorrhage are rare unless the tumour is very large. Histologically, most seminomas show the classical appearance illustrated in micrograph (a). The tumour consists of sheets of uniform, tightly packed, polygonal cells with clear cytoplasm and a round central nucleus; the cells are divided into clumps by fine fibrous septa **S** in which there is a variable accumulation of small lymphocytes. Less differentiated histological variants occur, as shown in micrograph (b); the tumour cells are more variable in size and shape with pleomorphic nuclei and showing greater mitotic activity. Seminoma is a malignant tumour and tends to spread via lymphatics, initially to iliac and para-aortic lymph nodes.

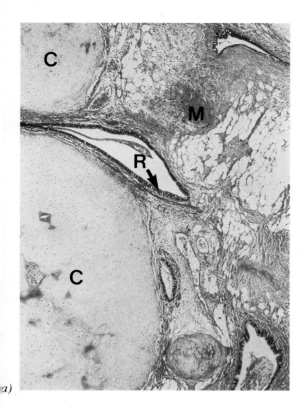

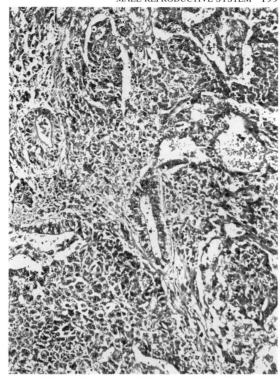

(a) *(b)*

Fig. 18.3 Teratoma of testis
(a) differentiated teratoma (MP)   (b) malignant teratoma undifferentiated (HP)

Testicular teratomas are slightly less common than seminomas with a younger peak incidence at between 20 and 35 years. Teratomas are thought to be derived from multipotent cells capable of differentiating into derivatives of all three germ layers, mesoderm, ectoderm and endoderm; this feature is seen in well-differentiated teratomas as illustrated in micrograph (a). In general, teratomas have a partly cystic cut surface appearance, and necrosis and haemorrhage are extensive, even in quite small tumours; this offers a most useful distinguishing feature from the homogeneous seminoma. Teratomas of the testis are malignant and spread early via the blood stream, often to the lung. Among the teratomas, however, there is a wide range of malignant behaviour: the aggressiveness of the tumour, tendency to metastasise and prognosis vary according to the histological form of the tumour.

Micrograph (a) shows the least aggressive pattern of teratoma, associated with the best prognosis. It contains any of a wide variety of differentiated tissues closely

resembling those of the mature adult; derivatives of mesoderm (e.g. cartilage **C**, smooth muscle **M**), ectoderm (e.g. squamous epithelium) and endoderm (e.g. respiratory epithelium **R**) may all be present. This form closely resembles the benign cystic teratoma of the ovary (see Fig. 16.17) and is most common in children. This type of lesion is termed *differentiated teratoma (TD)* (British) or *mature teratoma* (WHO).

In the histological variant shown in micrograph (b), no differentiated elements are seen and poorly differentiated tumour cells are arranged in carcinoma-like patterns, often part glandular or tubular, with frequent solid patternless tumour masses. No differentiated organoid elements such as cartilage are present. This type is known as *malignant teratoma undifferentiated (MTU)* (British) or *embryonal carcinoma* (WHO). This type of teratoma behaves aggressively with propensity for wide metastatic spread. Modern chemotherapy, particularly with agents containing platinum, has revolutionised treatment and greatly improved prognosis in this type of tumour.

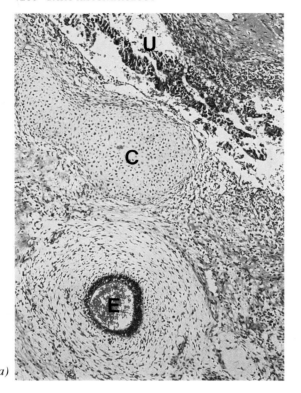

(a)

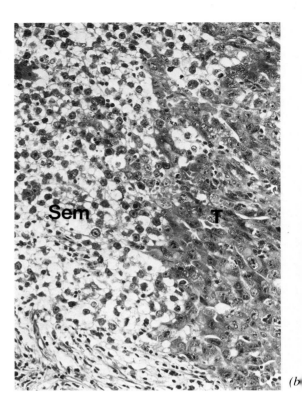

(b)

Fig. 18.4 Teratoma of testis
(a) malignant teratoma intermediate (MP) (b) mixed germ-cell tumour (HP)

Micrograph (a) shows a germ-cell tumour in which both differentiated and undifferentiated elements are present. It is termed *malignant teratoma intermediate (MTI)* (British) or *teratoma with embryonal carcinoma* (WHO). Part of the tumour **U** is of the undifferentiated (embryonal carcinoma) type, whilst other areas show some tendency to differentiation into organoid structures, though rarely as well differentiated as in a differentiated teratoma; in this example there is some immature cartilage **C** and formed epithelium **E**.

Certain germ-cell tumours are composed of a mixture of elements. One such lesion is illustrated in micrograph (b) where seminomatous areas co-exist with teratomatous areas. In this micrograph, note the pale-staining cells of the seminoma component **Sem** contrasting with the darker-staining undifferentiated cells of teratoma **T**. This is termed *malignant teratoma undifferentiated plus seminoma (MTU+S)* (British) or *embryonal carcinoma with seminoma* (WHO).

Germ cell tumours may also contain foci of *trophoblastic differentiation (choriocarcinoma or MTT)* or *yolk sac differentiation* as part of a mixed germ cell tumour. Alpha-fetoprotein is produced by yolk sac tumours and β-HCG is produced by trophoblastic elements; these can be used as biochemical markers for the presence of these elements as well as being used to detect tumour recurrence at an early stage.

Fig. 18.5 Classification of testicular teratomas

British classification	WHO classification
Teratoma differentiated (TD) (Fig. 18.3a)	Mature teratoma (Fig. 18.3a)
Malignant teratoma intermediate (MTI) (Fig 18.4a)	Embryonal carcinoma and teratoma (Fig 18.4a)
Malignant teratoma undifferentiated (MTU) (Fig.18.3b)	Embryonal carcinoma (Fig.18.3b)
Malignant teratoma trophoblastic (MTT)	Choriocarcinoma
Yolk sac tumour	Yolk sac tumour

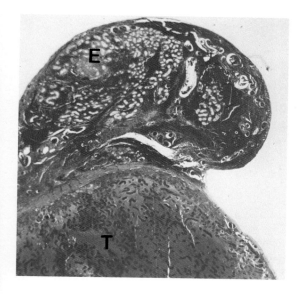

Fig. 18.6 Torsion of the testis (LP)

The arterial supply and venous drainage of the testis pass in the long course of the spermatic cord to and from the major vessels in the abdomen and pelvis. The spermatic cord is liable to twist, leading to compression of the thin-walled veins and obstruction of venous drainage from the testis. If this state persists for several hours or more without correction, the testis **T** and epididymis **E** may become deeply congested and subsequently undergo *venous infarction,* in which necrosis is associated with severe congestion and extravasation of blood. The histological changes are similar to those seen in venous infarction of the bowel following volvulus or strangulation, and described in Figure 9.5.

Prostate gland

The prostate gland frequently undergoes *benign nodular hyperplasia (hypertrophy)* in elderly men, probably due to an alteration in hormone balance. This important lesion, shown in Figure 18.7, produces obstruction to bladder outflow as a result of pressure on the prostatic urethra; in turn, the obstruction may produce pressure effects on the proximal conducting system of the urinary tract, leading to *hydroureter* and *hydronephrosis* with pressure atrophy of the renal parenchyma. As with other abnormalities of the tract, prostatic hyperplasia also predisposes to infection and stone formation.

Invasive *carcinoma of the prostate* is a common and important malignant tumour in men, and is illustrated in Figure 18.8. Small foci of tumour with the histological characteristics of prostatic adenocarcinoma but exhibiting little tendency to enlarge, invade or spread, are commonly seen as an incidental finding at autopsy or in prostates removed for benign hyperplasia in the very elderly; such lesions are called *latent carcinomas*.

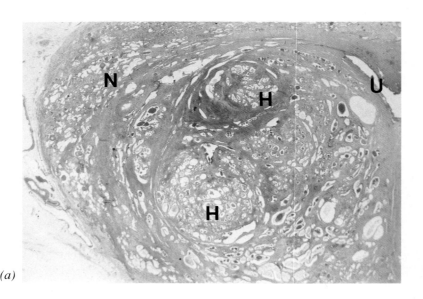

(a)

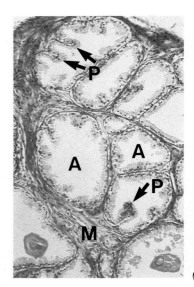

(b)

Fig. 18.7 Benign prostatic hyperplasia
(a) (LP) **(b)** (HP)

Benign prostatic hyperplasia is a common condition affecting elderly men in which the inner para-urethral components of the prostate gland undergo nodular glandular hyperplasia accompanied by hyperplasia of the intervening fibromuscular stroma of the gland. The peripheral glandular components of the prostate (making up the prostatic gland proper) are not involved in the hyperplastic process and become compressed and atrophic at the outer margin. At low magnification in micrograph (a), note the rounded nodules of hyperplastic prostatic tissue **H** in the inner (para-urethral) part of the gland, and the compressed non-hyperplastic zone **N** at the periphery. Since the para-urethral component of the prostate gland is involved, compression of the urethral lumen **U** is a

frequent occurrence, being responsible for typical clinical features such as hesitancy, poor urinary stream and urinary retention. On cut surface, the typical hyperplastic prostate has a nodular microcystic appearance, the tiny cysts representing enormously dilated hyperplastic prostatic glandular acini.

At high magnification as in micrograph (b), the acini **A** are lined by tall prostatic epithelial cells with small basal nuclei; the cells have a regular arrangement but are sometimes thrown up into papillary folds **P**. Adjacent acini are separated by a variable amount of fibromuscular connective tissue **M** in which the muscular component may be hypertrophied; muscular hypertrophy is particularly prominent in the region of the bladder neck.

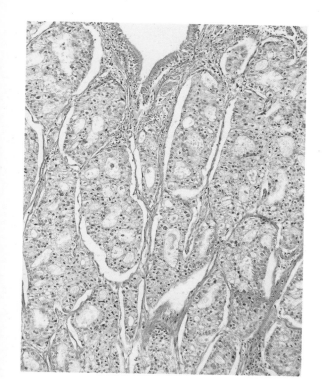

Fig. 18.8 Carcinoma of the prostate (HP)

This common tumour usually arises in the peripheral component of the prostate gland, as opposed to benign prostatic hyperplasia, which characteristically develops in the para-urethral glandular component (see Fig. 18.7). This tumour, being derived from glandular cells of the prostatic acini, takes the form of an adenocarcinoma. In this well-differentiated example, there is a well-defined acinar pattern of tumour replacing normal gland. These neoplastic acini are very irregular in shape when compared to those seen in normal tissue. Carcinoma of the prostate has a propensity for metastatic spread to bone (see Fig. 15.10) where it may cause an osteosclerotic reaction. Poorly differentiated tumours also spread to pelvic and para-aortic lymph nodes.

Penis

The most important pathological lesion of the penis is *squamous carcinoma* (see Fig. 18.9) which is usually located on the glans or prepuce; the glans penis is also the site of a form of non-invasive carcinoma in situ known as *erythroplasia of Queyrat,* histologically similar to intra-epidermal carcinoma (see Fig. 20.17). It probably represents a form of dysplasia falling just short of frank carcinoma.

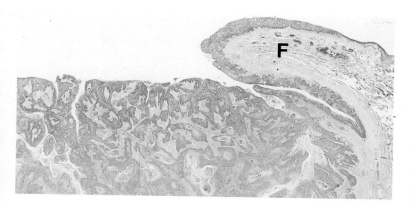

Fig. 18.9 Squamous carcinoma of penis (LP)

This micrograph illustrates, at low magnification, a well-differentiated keratinising squamous carcinoma of the glans penis; part of the uninvolved foreskin **F** is included. In this example, islands of purple-staining tumour extend deeply into the glans towards the urethra (not shown). Carcinoma of the penis is rare in circumcised men and chronic irritation and poor hygiene may be predisposing factors; metastatic spread is by lymphatics to superficial inguinal nodes.

19. Endocrine system

Pituitary gland

Structural defects of the pituitary gland are few, although functional abnormalities are potentially numerous, leading to under- or over-production of one or more of the many hormones produced by the pituitary and its target endocrine glands.

The most important histopathological lesions of the pituitary gland are benign *adenomas* derived from the adenohypophysis. These are commonly endocrinologically active and result in the development of endocrine syndromes. Adenomas may be derived from any of the normal anterior pituitary cell types:

- **prolactinomas** – lead to infertility, and occasionally inappropriate breast milk production
- **corticotroph adenomas** – secrete ACTH and result in Cushing's syndrome (see Fig. 19.1)
- **somatotroph adenomas** – secrete excess growth hormone and lead to gigantism or acromegaly
- **thyrotrophs and gonadotroph adenomas**– both types are rare
- **non-secretory adenomas -** a large number of pituitary adenomas have no demonstrable hormone secretion; such tumours thus only become manifest by impinging on vital local structures such as the optic chiasma causing visual disturbance, or by expanding to a size large enough to destroy the surrounding normal functioning tissue resulting in clinical hypopituitarism.

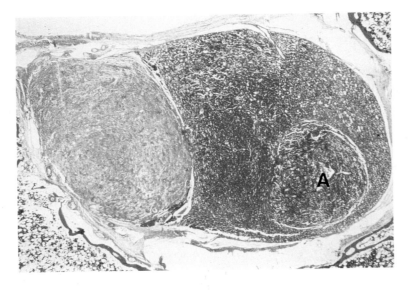

Fig. 19.1 Pituitary adenoma (LP)

The micrograph shows a pituitary gland *in situ* in the pituitary fossa and cut in sagittal section. Within the substance of the anterior pituitary lies a small benign *pituitary adenoma* **A** composed of cells of a uniform type. The tumour is benign as evidenced by its well-circumscribed, non-invasive, spherical appearance, and small enough to have caused no distortion of the pituitary outline or undue compression of adjacent normal pituitary cells. In this particular case, the tumour cells secreted ACTH in gross excess and the patient died as a result of the metabolic and cardiac complications of *Cushing's disease;* in all his illness lasted no more than 7 or 8 weeks despite its 'benign' pathogenesis.

Thyroid and parathyroid glands

The thyroid gland is the seat of many pathological processes which may lead to either diminished or excessive output of thyroxine. Hypothyroidism *(myxoedema)* may result from a variety of causes, some of which have an autoimmune basis, e.g. *Hashimoto's disease* (see Fig. 19.2). By the time the thyroid is examined histologically in cases of long-standing hypothyroidism, the thyroid often shows only shrinkage, fibrosis and destruction of most of the thyroid acini, with a sparse residual infiltrate of chronic inflammatory cells. This change, known as *primary atrophic thyroiditis,* is analogous to the 'end-stage' of long-standing kidney damage (see Fig. 14.2) and provides little evidence of the nature of the original thyroid abnormality.

Hyperthyroidism is usually the result of diffuse hyperplasia of the thyroid acinar cells, most commonly in the condition known as Graves' disease (see Fig. 19.3); sometimes the hyperplasia is confined to a single *benign thyroid adenoma,* or to one or two nodules in an otherwise inactive multinodular goitre ('goitre' is the term now applied indiscriminately to almost any thyroid swelling). Nevertheless, the vast majority of thyroid adenomas and multinodular goitres are non-functional and do not lead to disturbances of thyroid hormone output. Examples are shown in Figure 19.4.

Three main forms of *thyroid carcinoma* occur; these are also non-functioning and are illustrated in Figure 19.5. *Medullary carcinoma of the thyroid* is an uncommon malignant tumour of calcitonin-producing cells and is particularly notable for its production of amyloid (see Fig. 4.7).

The parathyroid glands show only two important pathological abnormalities, hyperplasia and benign adenoma (see Fig. 19.6); in both cases there are associated primary or secondary abnormalities of parathormone and calcium metabolism.

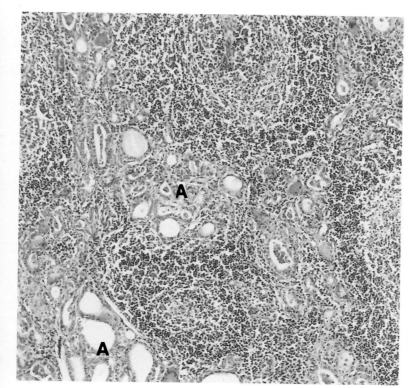

Fig. 19.2 Hashimoto's thyroiditis (MP)

This disease is an autoimmune thyroiditis in which thyroid acini **A** are progressively destroyed by immunological processes and the gland becomes diffusely infiltrated by lymphocytes. In some areas, these small darkly staining cells tend to aggregate and often form typical lymphoid follicles with germinal centres. In the early stages of the disease, the extensive lymphoid infiltrate produces a diffusely enlarged firm thyroid gland with a pale cut surface appearance. As thyroid follicles are progressively destroyed over the years, the patient, who at the outset is euthyroid, or even mildly hyperthyroid, becomes increasingly hypothyroid (myxoedematous). When almost all thyroid acini are destroyed, the lymphoid infiltrate becomes less obvious and fibrosis supervenes, with progressive reduction in size of the gland.

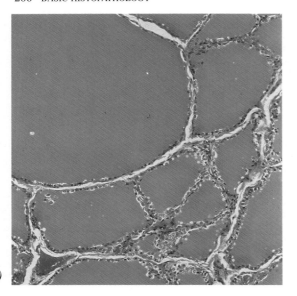

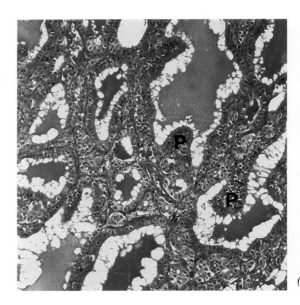

(a)

(b)

Fig. 19.3 Thyrotoxic hyperplasia
(a) normal thyroid (HP) **(b) hyperplastic thyroid** (HP)

Thyroid function is normally under the control of the hypothalamic-pituitary system via the release of TSH which stimulates thyroid acinar cells to liberate thyroxine. The resulting level of circulating thyroxine then regulates TSH production by a negative feedback mechanism.

Certain circumstances disrupt this balance resulting in prolonged excess production of TSH or a functionally similar substance which then promotes hyperplasia and hypertrophy of thyroid acinar cells; this gives rise to the histological appearance known as *thyroid hyperplasia*. Depending on the underlying cause, the patient may be clinically euthyroid or thyrotoxic.

Graves' disease is by far the most common cause of pathological thyroid hyperplasia. In this autoimmune disease, a circulating immunoglobulin known as *long*

acting thyroid stimulator (LATS) is produced which binds to thyroid acinar cells, mimicking the effects of TSH and resulting in excess secretion of thyroxine. The resulting glandular appearance is described as *thyrotoxic hyperplasia* and is illustrated in micrograph (b).

Compared to the normal thyroid shown in micrograph (a), the hyperplastic acinar cells are tall and have large nuclei reflecting a greater degree of metabolic activity. The acini themselves are smaller than normal because of the reduced amount of colloid resulting from increased thyroxine secretion. The hyperplastic acinar cells may crowd up on one side of the acini so as to project into the lumen as papillary structures **P**. In Graves' disease, the thyroid may sometimes contain prominent lymphocytic aggregates (not shown in this specimen).

Fig. 19.4 Thyroid adenoma and nodular goitre *(illustrations opposite)*
(a) colloid adenoma (LP) **(b) microfollicular adenoma** (LP) **(c) multinodular goitre** (LP)

Thyroid adenomatous nodules are a common clinical finding and are often so numerous as to occupy the entire gland which may become considerably enlarged. Although described as 'adenomas' there is disagreement whether these should be regarded as true benign tumours, or as foci of hyperplasia, since identical lesions can arise in the thyroid as a result of dietary lack of iodine, congenital lack of enzymes or the activity of goitrogens. Whatever the pathogenesis, the nodules are usually spherical and of highly variable size; their internal structure may be of many different types, two of the more common being illustrated here.

Micrograph (a) shows the *colloid nodule* variety, in which the acini are markedly distended by normal-looking colloid and the lining epithelium is much flattened; there is minimal interacinar stroma.

Micrograph (b) shows a *microfollicular adenoma*, composed of small tightly packed acini virtually devoid of luminal colloid, giving the adenoma a more solid and compact appearance.

Micrograph (c) shows a *multinodular goitre* which consists of numerous adenomatous nodules of varying size and histological type; the largest nodules **C** are usually of the colloid type.

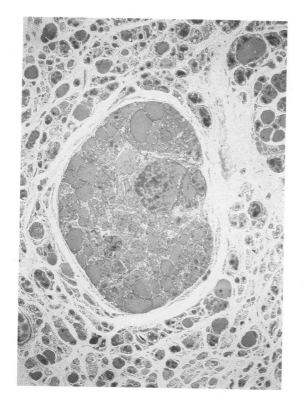

(a)

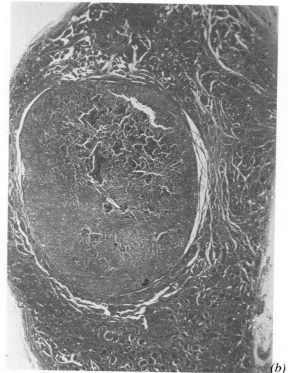

(b)

(c)

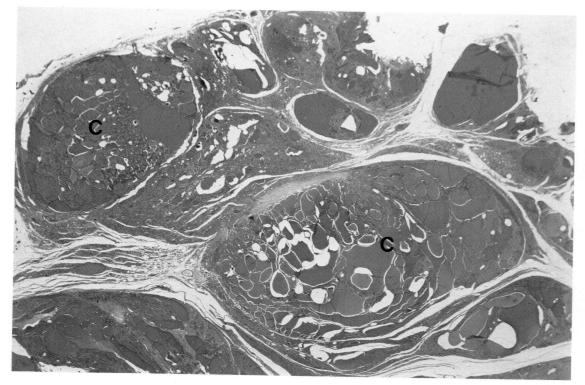

Fig. 19.4 Thyroid adenoma and nodular goitre *(caption opposite)*

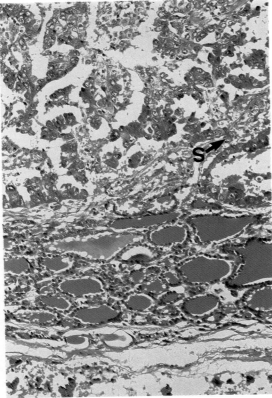

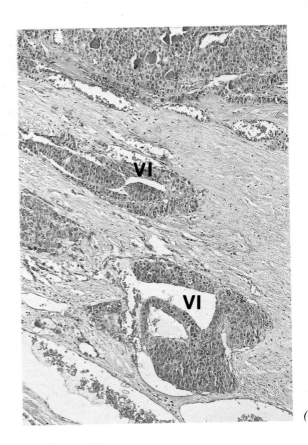

(a)

(b)

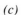

(c)

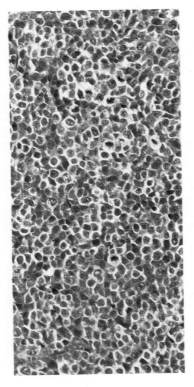

Fig. 19.5 Carcinoma of thyroid
(a) papillary (HP)   **(b) follicular** (MP)   **(c) anaplastic** (HP)

Carcinoma of the thyroid takes three common histological forms.

Papillary adenocarcinoma, shown in micrograph (a), is the most common type, found particularly in young women under 40. The tumour is in the form of complex papillary structures, each composed of a narrow stromal core **S** covered with a layer of glandular epithelium. The stromal cores sometimes contain small calcified laminated bodies known as *psammoma bodies* (not shown here). Note the normal thyroid tissue at the bottom of this field. The tumour tends to spread via lymphatics to regional nodes, and has the best prognosis of all thyroid cancers.

Follicular carcinoma illustrated in micrograph (b) has, as its name implies, a well-structured follicular pattern and may be difficult to distinguish from a benign follicular adenoma (see Fig. 19.4); evidence of vessel invasion **VI** at the tumour edge provides clear evidence of malignancy. Bloodstream spread is the major method of metastasis, and lung and bone are common sites of secondary tumour deposits.

Anaplastic carcinoma, as shown in micrograph (c), usually occurs in the very elderly and is composed of sheets of small, very poorly differentiated cells, with little cytoplasm; such tumours may be confused with large cell malignant lymphomas (see Fig. 15.4d). These tumours grow very rapidly and extensively invade local tissues, often presenting as a bulky mass in the neck associated with symptoms of tracheal compression.

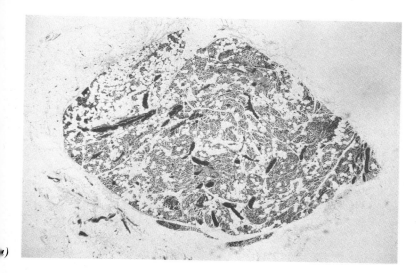

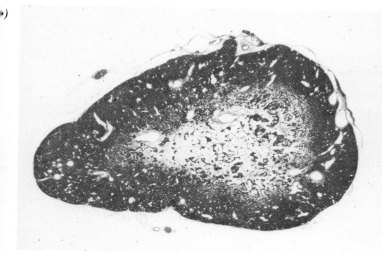

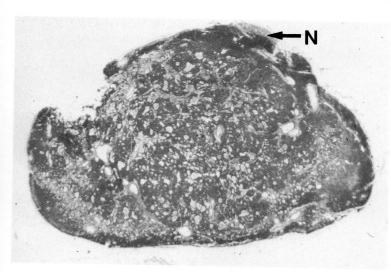

Fig. 19.6 Parathyroid hyperplasia and adenoma
(a) normal gland (LP)
(b) hyperplastic gland (LP)
(c) parathyroid adenoma (LP)

The normal adult parathyroid gland contains small endocrine cells arranged in clumps or cords within highly vascular adipose tissue; with increasing age, more of the gland becomes replaced by adipose tissue. Should the need arise for a greater output of parathormone, for example in cases of excessive urinary calcium loss in chronic renal failure, the endocrine cells undergo hyperplasia with loss of the adipose tissue.

Compare the hyperplastic gland in micrograph (b) with the normal parathyroid in micrograph (a); the hyperplastic gland is only marginally larger than the normal gland, yet the hormonally-active endocrine component has increased two or threefold by replacing the adipose tissue component. If demand for excess parathormone persists, the gland may become markedly enlarged; these hyperplastic changes affect all four parathyroid glands uniformly.

In contrast, autonomous benign tumours of the parathyroid gland, *parathyroid adenomas,* usually only affect one of the four parathyroid glands, although occasionally they may be multiple. In micrograph (c), a parathyroid adenoma replaces the whole gland, with just a fragment of normal parathyroid tissue **N** remaining at the periphery. The cellular arrangement in parathyroid adenoma is variable, with the cells arranged in sheets or in a microacinar pattern. The finding of a peripheral rim of compressed normal gland is a useful clue in distinguishing an adenoma from hyperplasia.

In cases of parathyroid adenoma, the non-involved glands may show the *suppressed parathyroid pattern,* in which the endocrine component atrophies, being replaced by adipose tissue; the gland as a whole therefore remains a normal size.

Adrenal gland

The adrenal gland has two distinct morphological and functional components:

- the cortex – this secretes three groups of steroid hormones, namely glucocorticoids (e.g. cortisol), mineralocorticoids (e.g. aldosterone), and small quantities of sex hormones

- the medulla – this forms part of the neuroendocrine system and is responsible for the production of the catecholamines, adrenalin and noradrenalin.

Disorders affecting the adrenal cortex

In response to stress, the normally lipid-rich cells of the adrenal cortex metabolise lipid in the production of steroid hormones and become *lipid depleted*; this is commonly seen in adrenal gland at post-mortem, particularly when a patient has died with features of shock. It is manifest by loss of the normal lipid vacuolation in adrenal cortical cells.

Atrophy of the adrenal cortex (see Fig. 19.7b) may result from primary autoimmune disease, but is now more commonly iatrogenic, the result of steroid therapy. Hyposecretion of adenocortical steroids, known clinically as *Addison's disease,* may also result from destruction of the gland by tuberculosis (see Fig. 3.12).

Hyperplasia of the adrenal cortex (see Figs. 19.7c and d), usually the result of prolonged stimulation of the adrenal cortex by pituitary ACTH or tumour-derived ACTH-like substance, results in *Cushing's syndrome* (excess cortisol production).

The adrenal cortex may be the site of benign *adrenal cortical adenomas* (see Fig. 19.8) or rarely malignant *adrenal cortical carcinomas*. These tumours of the adrenal cortex may be functional and result in the following endocrine syndromes:

- *Cushing's syndrome* – caused by tumours which secrete cortisol

- *Conn's syndrome* – results from tumours that secrete aldosterone

- *adrenogenital syndrome* – due to excess production of androgens.

Often, cortical hyperplasia is nodular rather than diffuse and it may be difficult to distinguish between a benign cortical adenoma and a large nodule arising as part of nodular cortical hyperplasia.

Disorders affecting the adrenal medulla

The most important lesions of the adrenal medulla are tumours. *Phaeochromocytoma* (see Fig. 19.9) produces excessive adrenalin and noradrenalin and is usually benign; the neuroblastoma (see Fig. 10.10) is a highly malignant embryonal tumour of neuroblasts seen in childhood. Both these tumours may also arise elsewhere in the abdomen in sites corresponding to components of the paraganglia system such as the organ of Zukercandl.

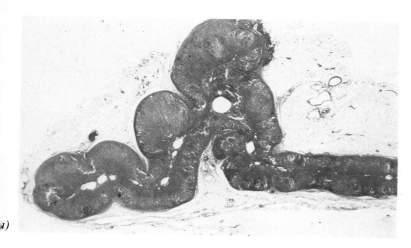

(a)

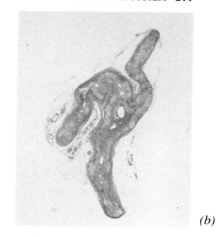

(b)

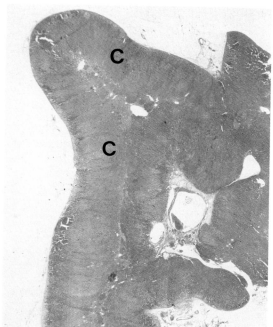

(d)

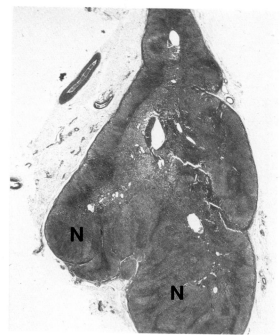

Fig. 19.7 Adrenal cortical atrophy and hyperplasia
(a) normal gland (LP) **(b) atrophic gland** (LP)
(c) diffuse hyperplasia (LP) **(d) nodular hyperplasia** (LP)

These micrographs, taken at the same magnification, compare adrenal atrophy and hyperplasia with the normal.

In *adrenal atrophy* as shown in micrograph (b), marked reduction in gland size is due to cortical atrophy. In this example, the atrophy was caused by long-term administration of corticosteroids which suppresses pituitary ACTH output.

Adrenal cortical hyperplasia occurs in either *diffuse* or *nodular* forms as illustrated in micrographs (c) and (d) respectively. In the diffuse form, the cortex **C** is uniformly and regularly thickened, often by cells of one type. In the much more common nodular form, the cortex contains adenoma-like nodules **N** of hyperplastic cortical cells, usually of zona fasciculata type. Diffuse adrenal cortical hyperplasia is usually caused by excess stimulation by ACTH from the pituitary (*Cushing's syndrome*) or by an ACTH-like substance, e.g. from an oat cell carcinoma; rarely, it results from a congenital enzyme deficiency. Nodular hyperplasia is commonly idiopathic and non-functional.

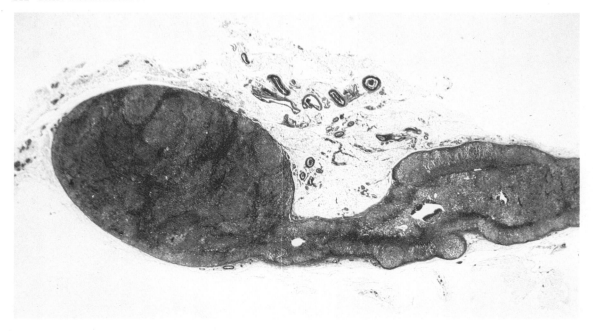

Fig. 19.8 Adrenal cortical adenoma (LP)

Hyperadrenal syndromes may result from excessive secretion of hormones by a solitary benign *adrenal cortical adenoma,* the activity of which is independent of regulation by pituitary ACTH. These tumours form a circumscribed, spherical mass within the cortex and may be composed of a single cell type, e.g. zona glomerulosa cells in Conn's syndrome, but more often contain a mixture of cortical cell types. Note how similar the adenoma is to the nodules in nodular cortical hyperplasia seen in Figure 19.7 (d). Cortical adenomas are a fairly frequent incidental finding at necropsy, a fact which leads to the belief that most are non-functioning and asymptomatic. Almost all cortical adenomas have a yellow cut surface, thereby distinguishing them from phaeochromocytomas which appear brown.

Fig. 19.9 Phaeochromocytoma (HP)

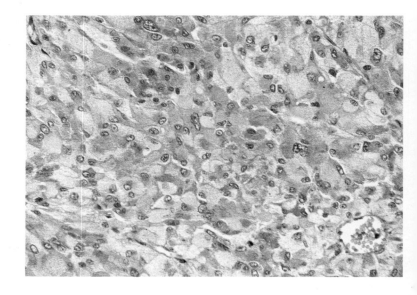

Phaeochromocytoma is a tumour arising from the adrenal medulla which secretes adrenalin and noradrenalin. Most tumours are benign in their growth characteristics but excess catecholamine secretion may cause potentially lethal hypertension. Macroscopically, the cut surface of the tumour is pale brown in colour. Histologically, the tumour is composed of nests of plump irregular cells, often with pink granular cytoplasm reflecting a high content of endocrine granules.

True malignant variants do occur, but diagnosis must be based on evidence of invasion and spread since purely cytological criteria are unreliable.

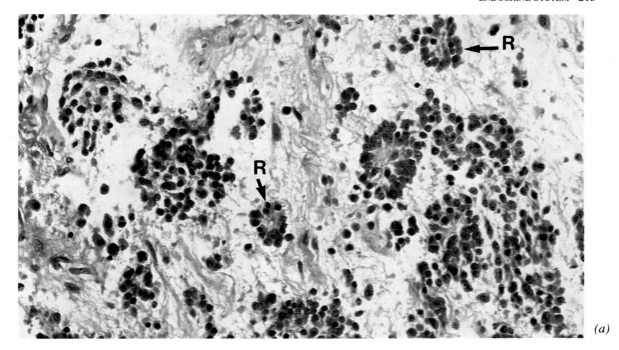

(a)

Fig. 19.10   Adrenal embryonal tumours
(a) neuroblastoma (HP)
(b) ganglioneuroblastoma (HP)

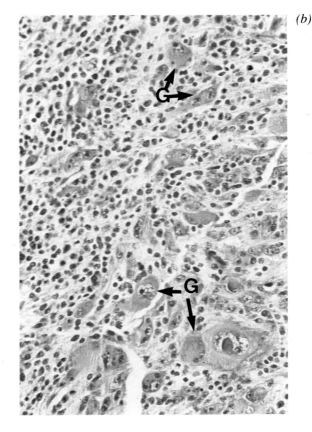

(b)

Neuroblastoma is an example of an embryonal tumour
(see Ch. 6) and is believed to be derived from primitive
neuroblastic cells in the adrenal medulla. It occurs in
children and is highly malignant, spreading mainly via
the blood stream to internal organs, especially the liver,
and to the bones, particularly those of the face and skull.

The typical appearance of the neuroblastoma is shown
in micrograph (a); there is usually extensive haemorrhage
and necrosis, but the viable areas (as here) are composed
of small undifferentiated tumour cells in a pink-staining
fibrillar stroma. Cells have a densely stained nucleus
with scanty cytoplasm. A characteristic feature is
occasional clumps of cells arranged in the form of a
rosette **R** surrounding a central zone of neurofibrils.

A somewhat less aggressive form of this tumour is the
ganglioneuroblastoma and is illustrated in micrograph
(b). These tumours exhibit some degree of
differentiation, and ganglion cells **G** of varying degrees
of maturity are found mixed with the small dark-staining
undifferentiated neuroblasts. Such tumours have a rather
better prognosis than those composed entirely of the
undifferentiated neuroblasts.

These tumours commonly secrete catecholamines and
a diagnostic marker is to measure *vanillyl mandelic acid*
(VMA), a metabolite, in the urine.

20. Skin

Introduction

Many systemic diseases have manifestations, both clinical and pathological, in the skin. For example, skin rashes are a feature of many generalised viral infections such as measles, chicken pox and herpes. Systemic immunological diseases such as scleroderma, systemic lupus erythematosus and dermatomyositis, and some vasculitic disorders such as Henoch-Schönlein purpura, have major manifestations in the skin. In addition, the skin is the subject of many specific primary disorders, mainly inflammatory or neoplastic in nature.

While there are many different causes of tissue damage in the skin, it has only a limited repertoire of reactions to the damage; the most important of these patterns of reaction are illustrated in Figures 20.1 to 20.4. Various skin disorders show these basic changes in different combinations and with varying degrees of severity. Few skin conditions have any absolutely pathognomonic histological features, and in most cases a precise diagnosis can only be made when the clinical history, macroscopic features, distribution and duration of the lesions are considered in conjunction with the histological appearances.

Dermatitis is a commonly used clinical term and is used to describe a wide variety of inflammatory skin conditions with many different causes. Histologically, non-specific features of acute or chronic inflammation are seen (Figs. 20.5 and 20.6), but in some cases there are other histological changes which give a clue to the precise diagnosis or most likely cause. Two specific and relatively common types of dermatitis with characteristic histological features, are *lichen planus* (Fig. 20.7) and *psoriasis* (Fig. 20.8).

Viruses are responsible for many common skin lesions; some, like *viral warts* (Fig. 20.9), *keratoacanthoma* (Fig. 20.10) and *molluscum contagiosum* (Fig. 20.11), are probably primary skin lesions. Others, such as the vesicular lesions of herpes simplex, chicken pox and herpes zoster, are merely the cutaneous manifestations of a more generalised viral illness, the last two being different manifestations of infection by the same virus. *Pyogenic granuloma* (Fig. 20.12) is a common, localised, nodular inflammatory lesion which frequently follows trauma.

Numerically, the commonest skin lesions of all are the ubiquitous pigmented lesions known colloquially as 'moles'. This non-specific term encompasses a range of lesions called *naevi* characterised by the presence of aggregates of pigmented (melanin-producing) cells in various sites in the skin. Three important histological types, *junctional, intradermal* and *compound naevi,* are compared in Figure 20.13. Clinically, the most important pigmented lesion is the *malignant melanoma* (Fig. 20.14), potentially a highly malignant tumour of epidermal melanocytes.

Epithelial tumours derived from the epidermis and its appendages are also common, the most frequent being the *basal cell carcinoma,* an invasive tumour of low grade malignancy derived from the basal cells. Basal cell carcinoma (Fig. 20.15) has characteristic histological features which enable it to be easily distinguished from *squamous cell carcinoma* (Fig. 20.16), a rather more aggressive malignant tumour derived from the prickle cell layer of the epidermis. The latter may be preceded by a type of carcinoma in situ in which the epidermal cells exhibit the cytological criteria of malignancy but show no evidence of invasive behaviour by breaching the epidermal basement membrane. Examples of this type of epidermal dysplasia include *solar ('senile') keratosis* and *Bowen's disease* (Fig. 20.17), analogous to the so-called erythroplasia of Queyrat of the penis and carcinoma in situ of the cervix (see Fig. 16.6). Malignant lymphomas may involve the skin secondarily, however occasionally the skin is the site of the first manifestation of malignant lymphoma, including a variant known as *mycosis fungoides* (Fig. 20.20).

Two common skin lesions which are difficult to classify are *epidermal cysts* (Fig. 20.18) and the so-called *seborrhoeic keratosis* of the elderly (Fig. 20.19). The former, known to generations of clinicians by the inaccurate name *sebaceous cyst,* is probably an epidermal inclusion cyst, and the latter (also known as *seborrhoeic wart*) has formerly been widely regarded as a benign tumour of the basal cells of the epidermis, a belief perpetuated in the little-used synonym, *basal cell papilloma.*

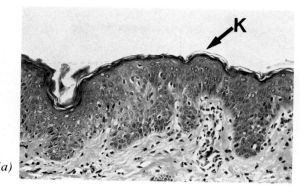

(a)

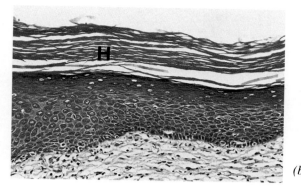

(b)

(c)

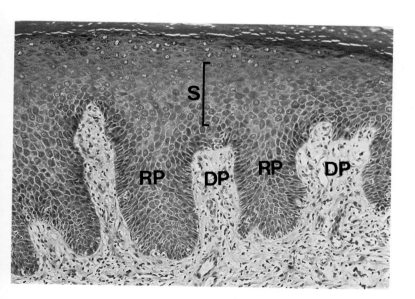

Fig. 20.1   Abnormalities of surface keratin
(a) normal keratin (HP)
(b) hyperkeratosis (HP)
(c) parakeratosis (HP)

This series of micrographs compares the normal keratin **K** of thin skin with two common abnormalities of keratin, *hyperkeratosis* and *parakeratosis*. In hyperkeratosis **H**, the keratin layer is thickened but otherwise normal *(orthokeratosis)*. In parakeratosis **P** the keratin is also thickened, but shows the persistence of purple-staining nuclear remnants; the granular layer is absent.

Fig. 20.2   Abnormal epidermal thickening - acanthosis (HP)

Acanthosis is the term given to thickening of the epidermis, usually due to an increase in the thickness of stratum spinosum **S** (prickle cell layer) and is a common feature of many skin conditions, particularly chronic inflammatory conditions (see Fig. 20.6). The thickening of the epidermal layer is particularly marked in the rete pegs **RP** which are expanded and elongated with prominent interdigitating dermal papillae **DP**.

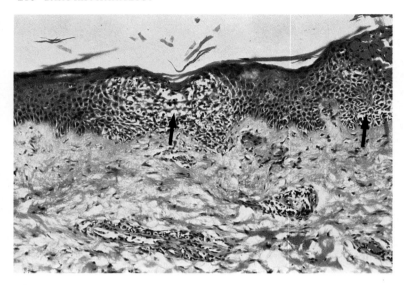

Fig. 20.3 Intraepidermal oedema - spongiosis (HP)

Oedema of the epidermis causes separation of epithelial cells, particularly in the prickle cell layer, a condition known as *spongiosis*. Accumulation of fluid between epidermal cells causes gaps to appear (arrow), which may coalesce with increased severity to form fluid-filled intraepidermal vesicles. Spongiosis with vesicle formation is a feature of acute dermatitis (see Fig. 20.5).

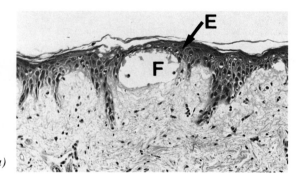

(a)

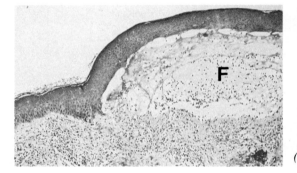

(b)

(c)

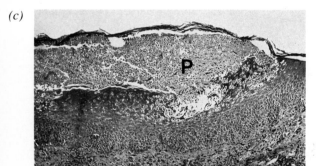

Fig. 20.4 Other epidermal inflammatory reactions
(a) vesicle (HP)   (b) bulla (MP)   (c) pustule (HP)

Accumulations of fluid beneath or within the epidermis may cause small raised blebs on the skin; most are due to inflammation in the epidermis. When small, such lesions are termed *vesicles;* in micrograph (a), note the area of fluid accumulation **F** elevating and thinning the epidermis **E**. Larger collections of fluid are termed *bullae*. A bulla is shown in micrograph (b) at lower magnification than in (a); the collection of serous fluid **F** is larger and may include small numbers of inflammatory cells. The term *pustule is* used to describe a collection consisting mostly of neutrophils with some serous fluid within or beneath the epidermis. Micrograph (c) shows a pustule **P** beneath the corneal layer of the epidermis.

Vesicles, bullae and pustules are further categorised as to location either *subepidermal, intra-epidermal* or *subcorneal*.

Fig. 20.5 Acute dermatitis
(HP)

In early *acute dermatitis* the major changes are epidermal, with fluid accumulating between the prickle cells causing spongiosis **Sp**. As the lesion progresses, the spongiotic areas may become converted into fluid-filled vesicles containing a few inflammatory cells, mainly lymphocytes and neutrophils, and there is variable infiltration of the epidermis by these cells. If the vesicles rupture onto the surface, crusts or scabs composed of fibrin and polymorph nuclei form. In the earlier stages, the upper dermis shows only oedema, but later there may be a mixed acute and chronic inflammatory cell infiltrate, particularly around upper dermal blood vessels **V**.

In *subacute dermatitis,* the changes are less severe, with less obvious oedema and vesicle formation, and an inflammatory infiltrate which is proportionately more lymphocytic.

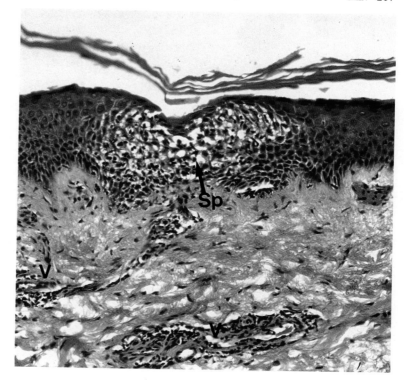

Fig. 20.6 Chronic dermatitis
(MP)

The histological features of *chronic dermatitis* are seen in many skin rashes with a variety of causes. The characteristic feature is epidermal thickening due to acanthosis **A** and a variable degree of hyperkeratosis **H**. There is no infiltration of the epidermis by inflammatory cells, but the upper and mid-dermis shows a moderate to heavy infiltrate of chronic inflammatory cells **C**, mainly lymphocytes and plasma cells, particularly around blood vessels. The acanthosis and hyperkeratosis may produce the clinical appearance of *lichenification,* a feature recognised in the term *lichen simplex chronicus* applied to one of the variants of this chronic non-specific dermatitic picture.

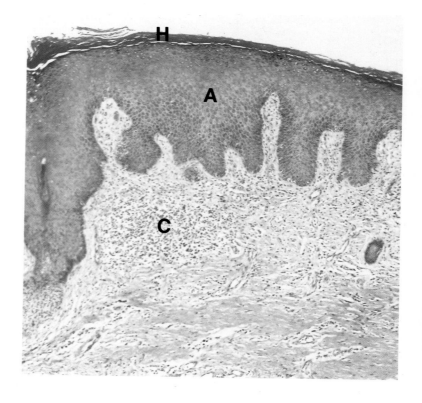

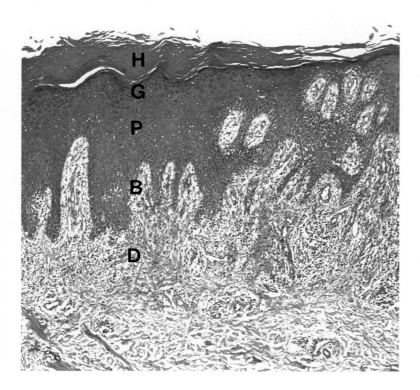

Fig. 20.7 Lichen planus (MP)

Lichen planus is a clinically and histologically distinct type of dermatitis. In the epidermis there is hyperkeratosis **H**, and thickening of the granular layer **G**, whilst in the prickle cell layer **P**, acanthosis is seen. A characteristic feature is the disruption of the normally regular basal layer **B** by hydropic degeneration and destruction of basal cells, leaving a ragged and irregular dermo-epidermal junction. The dermis **D** shows a dense chronic inflammatory cell infiltrate mainly confined to the upper third. The combination of the heavy dermal infiltrate and the destruction of the basal layer may produce a jagged saw-tooth appearance of the rete pegs.

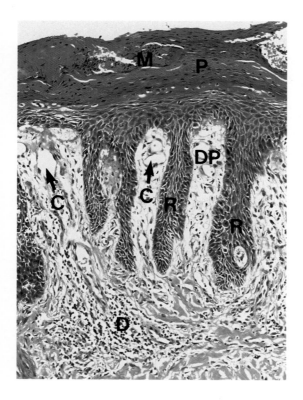

Fig. 20.8 Psoriasis (HP)

Psoriasis is a chronic skin disease characterised by well-demarcated, erythematous scaly lesions. Histologically, the major feature is acanthosis with greatly elongated narrow rete pegs **R**. Between the rete pegs, the epidermis is thinned over oedematous and prominent dermal papillae **DP** in which dilated capillaries **C** are prominent. The alternately thick and thin epidermis is covered by a parakeratotic layer **P** and may contain small aggregations of neutrophils forming microabscesses **M**.

There is a variable chronic inflammatory infiltrate in the upper dermis **D** and swollen dermal papillae.

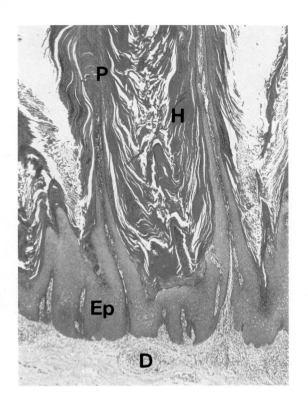

Fig. 20.9 Viral wart (verruca vulgaris) (MP)

Viral warts on non-traumatised skin have an exophytic papillary form. Histologically, the epidermis **Ep** is irregularly thickened and covered by a thick layer of hyperkeratosis **H** in which there are parakeratotic spires **P** over the tips of the more prominent papillary epidermal outgrowths. The epidermal cells in an active viral wart usually show focal prominence of the granular layer, with occasional areas of large, pale, vacuolated cells in the upper stratum spinosum (not seen at this magnification). The dermis **D** shows a chronic inflammatory cell infiltrate. In skin areas prone to trauma warts have a much less papillary form and may be dome-shaped (e.g. in juvenile warts of hands) or involuted (e.g. plantar warts of soles of the foot).

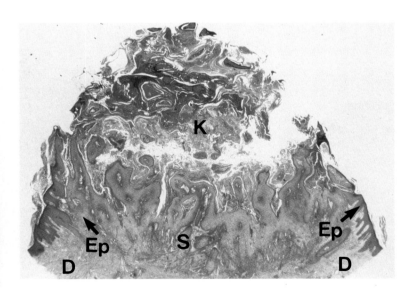

Fig. 20.10 Keratoacanthoma (LP)

This lesion is of unknown aetiology but has many of the features of a viral condition. A localised proliferation of squamous cells **S** produces a nodule in the skin with a central crater containing large masses of keratin **K**.

At its periphery, the nodule has a collar of thin but normal epidermis **Ep** and the junction between normal and proliferating epidermis is abrupt. The proliferating squamous cells may exhibit marked atypia, with large swollen cells showing abnormal nuclei and increased mitotic activity, a feature which often leads to confusion with squamous carcinoma in biopsy specimens. The surrounding dermis **D** shows a heavy chronic inflammatory infiltrate with some inflammatory cells extending into the base of the lesion.

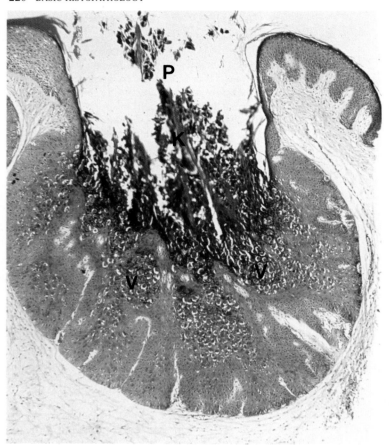

Fig. 20.11 Molluscum contagiosum (MP)

Molluscum contagiosum, like keratoacanthoma, is a localised nodular thickening of epidermis; in this condition, however, the viral aetiology is unquestioned since viral inclusion bodies **V** are easily visible, both in the proliferating epidermis, where they stain reddish, and in the overlying keratin plug **K**, where they stain blue-black. The keratinous plug extrudes through a central pit **P** at the apex of the dome-shaped nodule which is surrounded by normal epidermis.

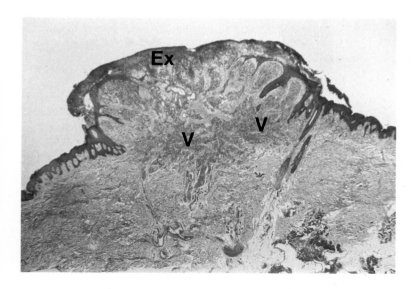

Fig. 20.12 Pyogenic granuloma (LP)

The *pyogenic granuloma* is a common inflammatory lesion which may follow a minor penetrating injury, e.g. rose thorn. It consists of a raised nodule of highly vascular tissue somewhat resembling a capillary angioma and may represent an abnormal overgrowth of the vascular element of normal granulation tissue. At this magnification, the vascular tissue **V** appears as irregular, blue-stained areas. The surface of the lesion is frequently ulcerated; in this example the surface is covered by an inflammatory exudate **Ex**. A characteristic histological feature is a collar of proliferating epithelium at the margin of the lesion.

Melanocytic lesions

In normal skin, melanocytes are scattered in the basal layers of the epidermis, their fine cytoplasmic processes ramifying between the keratinocytes towards the skin surface. Melanocytes are responsible for the synthesis of melanin which is then transferred to adjacent keratinocytes. Exposure to sunlight enhances the process.

The common pigmented moles (naevi) are benign hamartomatous accumulations of melanocytes in the epidermis and/or dermis; three different patterns are recognised according to the location of melanocytes and these are illustrated in Figure 20.13.

Malignant melanoma is a highly malignant tumour derived from melanocytes, the incidence of which is rising dramatically in white-skinned people around the world; excessive sun exposure, and in particular sun burning, is the principal cause. A proportion of melanomas arise in pre-existing pigmented naevi, the clinical signs of malignant transformation being rapid change in size, development of an irregular outline or surface contour, or change in pigmentation. Excision biopsy of any suspicious lesion should be performed without delay as the most important prognostic factor influencing metastasis is thickness of the lesion.

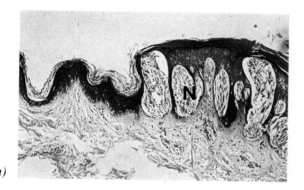

(a)

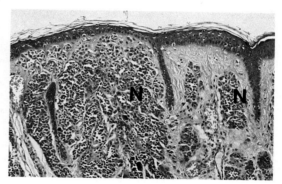

(b)

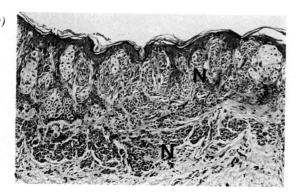

(c)

Fig. 20.13 Benign naevi (HP)
(a) junctional   (b) intradermal   (c) compound

In the *junctional naevus* (a), large melanocytes aggregate in the basal layers of the epidermis (i.e. junction of dermis and epidermis); the aggregations may be so large that the overlying epidermis may be thinned. The *naevus cells* N have pale-staining cytoplasm and may contain melanin. Junctional naevi occur most commonly before puberty.

In adults, *intradermal naevi* (b) are most common and in this type the naevus cells N form clumps in the upper dermis and are not present in the epidermis; these naevus cells are more compact and may also contain melanin pigment.

Compound naevi (c) are considered to represent a transition from junctional to intradermal forms and have naevus cells N both in the basal epidermis and in the upper dermis; with the passage of time the junctional component becomes less prominent and less active.

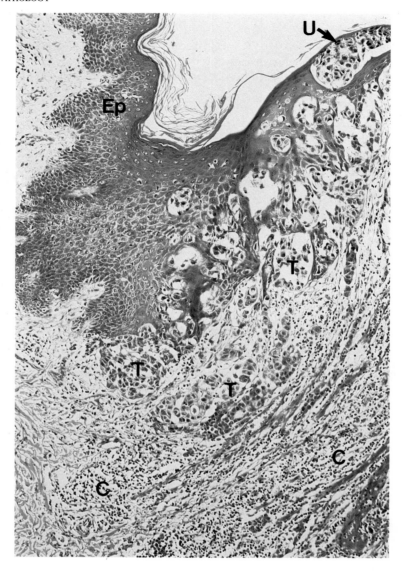

Fig. 20.14   Malignant melanoma (HP)

This highly malignant tumour of melanocytes occurs most commonly in the
skin, although it may rarely occur in the eye and other sites. In the skin, the
tumour appears as a pigmented nodular lesion which may become ulcerated.
The tumour is presumed to originate in naevus cells in the region of the
dermo-epidermal junction and quickly invades downward into the dermis. In
this specimen, note the incipient surface ulceration **U** and adjacent normal
epithelium **Ep**. The tumour cells **T** exhibit marked nuclear and cytoplasmic
pleomorphism and frequent mitoses; many cells contain melanin pigment,
although *malignant melanomas* may sometimes be *amelanotic*. There is
frequently a chronic inflammatory cell infiltrate **C** around the margins of the
tumour. The tumour spreads via dermal lymphatics to the surrounding skin
forming *satellite lesions,* and metastasises early to regional lymph nodes and
thence via the bloodstream to many organs.

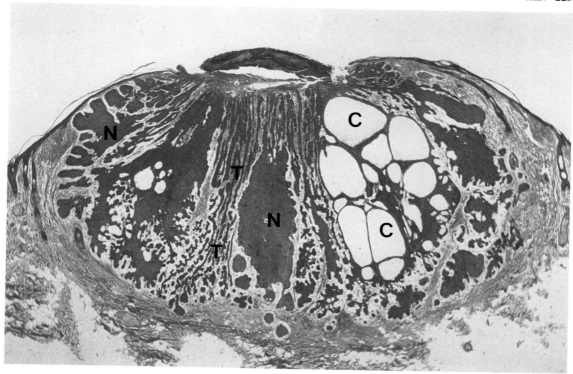

(a)

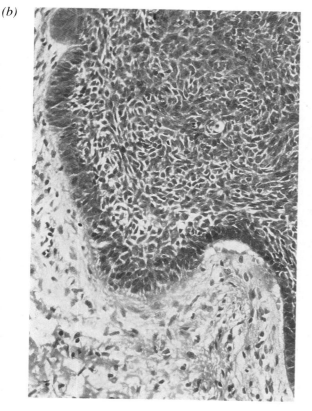

(b)

Fig. 20.15 Basal cell carcinoma
(a) (LP)   **(b)** (HP)

Basal cell carcinoma is a common tumour composed of cells with deep blue-staining nuclei centrally located in sparse, poorly defined cytoplasm. As seen in micrograph (b), the cells at the periphery of the tumour clumps are characteristically arranged in a *palisade pattern*, whereas the central cells are more haphazardly arranged. Micrograph (a) shows the typical growth pattern of the tumour; a nodular pattern **N** is most common but trabecular **T** and cystic **C** patterns are also seen often in the same lesion, as in this example.

Basal cell carcinoma arises from the basal cells of the epidermis or epidermal appendages; it behaves as a malignant tumour in that it invades dermis and any deeper underlying structures, but almost never metastasises. Basal cell carcinomas occur most frequently on the light-exposed areas of skin, particularly the face, and present as nodular lesions which may undergo ragged ulceration giving rise to the colloquial term *rodent ulcer.*

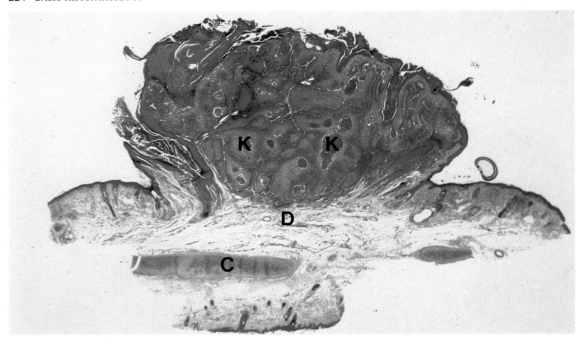

Fig. 20.16 Squamous cell carcinoma (LP)

Squamous cell carcinomas of the skin histologically resemble squamous cell carcinomas in many other sites (see Fig. 6.11), but the skin tumours are usually very well differentiated and highly keratinising, containing numerous keratin pearls **K**. The tumour may invade the dermis **D** and underlying structures, and may spread via the lymphatics to regional lymph nodes. Invasive squamous cell carcinomas of the skin may develop from intraepidermal carcinoma, the skin equivalent of carcinoma in situ, (see Fig. 20.17). In this micrograph the tumour has arisen on the pinna of the ear, but has not yet invaded the underlying cartilage **C**.

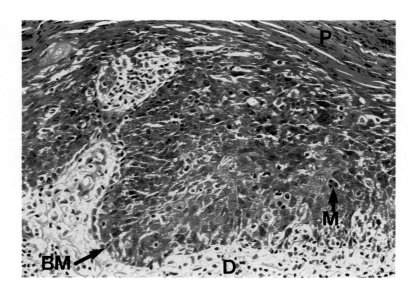

Fig. 20.17 Intraepidermal carcinoma (HP)

Invasive squamous carcinoma may be preceded by epidermal dysplasia. When the dysplasia is severe and involves the full thickness of the epidermis, it is termed *intraepidermal carcinoma*. In this micrograph, note the severe dysplasia extending through the whole epidermis with the loss of normal organisation and stratification; the surface layer exhibits parakeratosis **P.** Note a tripolar mitotic figure **M**. The basement membrane **BM** is intact with no invasion of the dermis **D**.

When the degree of epidermal dysplasia is restricted to lower levels of the epidermis, the condition is known as *actinic (solar) keratosis* (see Fig. 5.6 d).

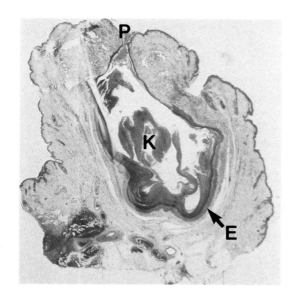

Fig. 20.18 Epidermal cyst (LP)

These common lesions were formerly known as *sebaceous cysts* although they contain no sebaceous material. They occur in the dermis and hypodermis and may open to the exterior through a punctum **P**. The cyst contains masses of degenerating keratin **K**, and is lined by flattened, stratified squamous epithelium **E**. Trauma to the cyst may lead to escape of keratin into surrounding tissues exciting a giant cell inflammatory reaction with swelling, tenderness and redness around the cyst. Clinically this change is inaccurately referred to as infected sebaceous cyst.

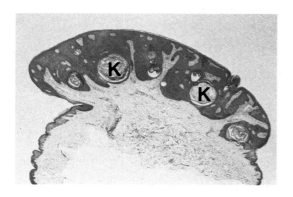

Fig. 20.19 Seborrhoeic keratosis (LP)

Seborrhoeic keratosis is a common lesion of the elderly, composed of a localised proliferation of basal cells forming a raised warty lesion. Such outgrowths are vulnerable to chronic trauma leading to overlying hyperkeratosis and formation of keratin nests **K** in the lesion. The aetiology of seborrhoeic keratosis is unknown, although in the past it has been regarded as a benign skin tumour *(basal cell papilloma)*.

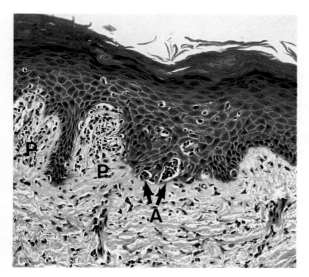

Fig. 20.20 Cutaneous lymphoma (HP)

Lymphoma may occur in the skin as part of spread of systemic lymphoma but also as as primary skin tumours. B-cell lymphomas are usually part of systemic disease. T-cell lymphomas of the skin represent a distinct restricted form of lymphoma encompassing two conditions called *mycosis fungoides* and *Sézary syndrome*. In these conditions neoplastic T-cells first involve the skin but with progression later involve lymph nodes and, in Sézary syndrome, circulate in the blood.

The typical skin lesion of cutaneous T-cell lymphoma shows acanthosis of the epidermis which contains scattered abnormal lymphoid cells, some forming small aggregates known as *Pautrier abscesses* **A**. There is also a heavy infiltrate of dark-staining lymphoma cells in the upper dermis, most obvious in the dermal papillae **P**. These can be shown to be T-cell in type using immunohistochemical techniques.

21. Skeletal system

Bone

Bone is a highly specialised type of connective tissue formed by the deposition of calcium salts within a dense matrix comprising collagen fibres and ground substance; the unmineralised matrix is known as *osteoid*. Osteocytes maintain the integrity of bone structure and participate in calcium homeostasis by mediating the continuous turnover of matrix and mineral constituents. On a wider scale, bone is being constantly remodelled by the resorptive activity of osteoclasts and redeposition by osteoblasts so as to reinforce bone architecture in response to changing functional demands. In normal bone, dynamic balance thus maintains total bone mass at a relatively constant level whilst providing a potentially large calcium pool which can be drawn upon to maintain serum calcium homeostasis.

Bone fracture

Bone fracture is a common and important result of trauma, although where there is some underlying bone abnormality (e.g. osteoporosis, osteomalacia, Paget's disease, metastatic tumour), the trauma or extra stress required to produce bone fracture may be minimal; this is termed *pathological fracture*. The healing of a bone fracture is briefly outlined in Figure 2.12 as an example of a specialised form of tissue repair. Torn ligaments and tendons and sprained joints are even more commonplace sequelae of accidents and sporting injuries; repair of such tissues occurs by the usual method of scar formation (see Figs. 2.10 and 2.11).

Bone infections

Infections of the bone are now comparatively uncommon, though bacterial osteomyelitis, both pyogenic and tuberculous, were formerly important crippling diseases. *Acute osteomyelitis* caused by pyogenic bacteria (usually *Staphylococcus aureus)* usually occurs in infants and young children, the bacteria gaining access to the marrow cavity via the bloodstream; it may also follow penetrating trauma in people of any age, e.g. compound fracture. Pathologically, acute osteomyelitis represents abscess formation in the medullary space of the bone, but the course of the disease in bone is complicated by two factors. Firstly, increased pressure in the confined space causes infarction of further large areas of bone; secondly, masses of dead bone *(sequestra)* behave as foreign bodies inhibiting normal repair processes and providing a haven for bacteria inaccessible to body defence mechanisms. *Chronic osteomyelitis* may follow if treatment is delayed or inadequate. *Tuberculous osteomyelitis* is illustrated in Figure 3.15.

Metabolic bone diseases

Osteoporosis (osteopaenia) is a condition in which total bone mass is decreased by reduction of bone trabeculae in number or size (usually both) and thinning of cortical bone; nevertheless the bone otherwise appears structurally normal. In contrast, *osteomalacia* is a disease in which osteoid fails to undergo normal mineralisation, usually due to deficiency of vitamin D, although other causes of total body calcium depletion may also be responsible; *rickets* is the childhood equivalent of osteomalacia. The appearance of normal bone, osteoporosis and osteomalacia are compared in Figure 21.l.

Paget's disease of bone (Fig. 21.2) is a condition of unknown aetiology occurring in the elderly; it is characterised by haphazard inappropriate osteoclastic erosion of formed bone and concurrent osteoblastic deposition of new bone. *Hyperparathyroidism* may cause somewhat similar haphazard osteoclastic erosion of bone; this condition is rare and therefore not illustrated in this chapter.

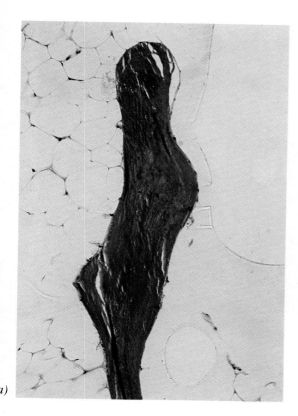

(a)

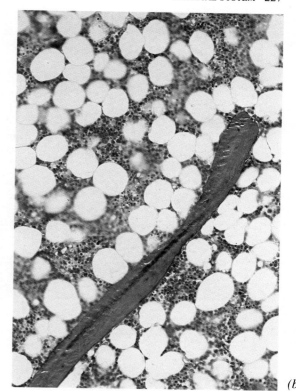

(b)

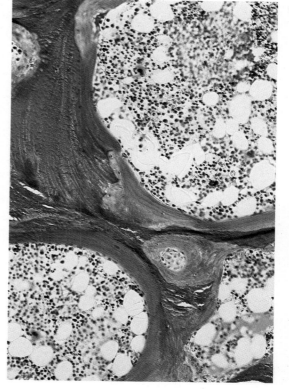

(c)

Fig. 21.1   Osteoporosis and osteomalacia
(undecalcified resin sections, Goldner's trichrome; MP)
(a) normal bone
(b) osteoporotic bone
(c) osteomalacia

In *normal trabecular bone* (a), the entire trabeculum is fully calcified (stained green by the Goldner trichrome method).

In *osteoporosis,* the bone appears qualitatively normal but its mass is diminished with the trabeculae being reduced in both number and size. Osteoporosis is extremely common in the elderly, especially in post-menopausal women, and is exacerbated by immobility. It may also occur in an isolated limb if immobilised for any reason and probably represents disuse atrophy. Osteoporosis is also caused by some endocrine disorders and is particularly seen with corticosteroid excess.

In contrast, in *osteomalacia,* the trabeculae are of normal or increased thickness, but there is deficient mineralisation so that each trabeculum has a central core of calcified bone (stained green) coated by an outer shell of unmineralised osteoid (stained orange-red). Osteomalacia is usually the result of vitamin D deficiency. Vitamin D deficiency in the growing child *(rickets)* is identical to osteomalacia pathologically; it results in gross skeletal deformity by disruption of bone mineralisation at growth plates.

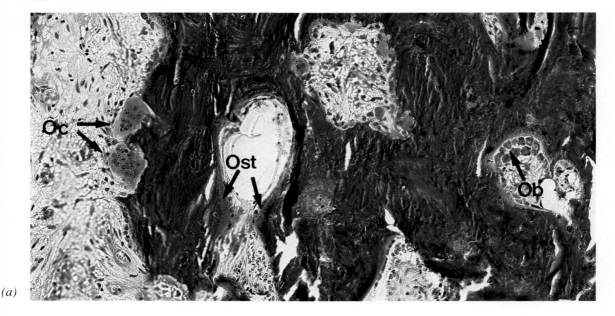

(a)

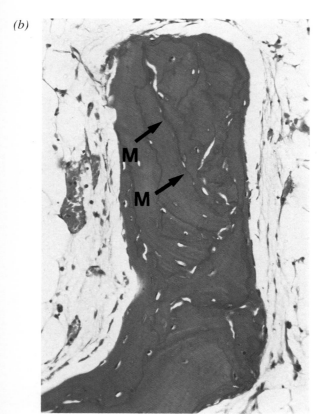

(b)

Fig. 21.2   Paget's disease of bone

(a) active osteolytic lesion (undecalcified resin section, Goldner's trichrome; HP)
(b) inactive sclerotic lesion (decalcified paraffin section, H&E; HP)

In Paget's disease of bone there is indiscriminate and uncontrolled osteoclastic erosion of bone followed by excessive osteoblastic activity producing excess osteoid which subsequently becomes mineralised, leading to irregular trabecular thickening. Micrograph (a) shows typical large multinucleate osteoclasts **Oc** lying in lacunae formed by active erosion of bone. The trabecular surface shows a layer of newly deposited red-staining osteoid **Ost** underlying rows of large active cuboidal osteoblasts **Ob**. This progressive haphazard remodelling results in gross distortion of bone often with marked thickening; the condition tends to be confined to a relatively small number of long bones, vertebrae or cranial bones which may become inadequate to withstand functional stresses leading to severe skeletal deformity, e.g. bowing of long bones, or even pathological fracture.

With time, the bone cell activity slowly diminishes, the initially highly cellular bone becoming progressively sclerotic; usually the bone is left thicker than before but paradoxically weaker, as much of the former strong lamellar bone is replaced by weaker woven bone. The disruption of the optimum lamellar pattern can be readily viewed by polarising microscopy, and in old lesions as in micrograph (b), the limits of separate episodes of previous bone destruction and irregular new bone formation marked by thin dark mosaic lines **M**.

Bone tumours

Primary tumours of bone may arise from all the cell types found in bone and the essential features of the more important of these tumours are tabulated in Figure 21.5. In addition, there is a miscellaneous group of tumour-like lesions also found in bone, the main features of which are presented in Figure 21.4. *Osteosarcoma* is of great clinical importance and is shown in Figure 21.3. Malignant tumours may also arise from lymphoid cells of the bone marrow, e.g. myeloma, lymphoma, leukaemia etc. (see Ch. 15). Bone is a frequent and important site of haematogenous metastatic spread of malignant epithelial tumours, particularly carcinomas of bronchus, breast, kidney, thyroid and prostate. Metastatic tumour deposits usually destroy bone trabeculae, although carcinoma of the prostate sometimes stimulates excessive new bone formation resulting in *osteosclerotic* rather than the more usual *osteolytic* deposits.

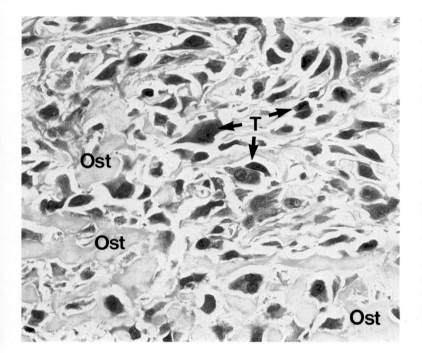

Fig. 21.3 Osteosarcoma (HP)

This tumour, although relatively uncommon, is nevertheless the most frequently occurring primary malignant tumour of bone. Most cases occur in children and adolescents (usually around the knee), but it may occasionally occur in elderly patients with long-standing Paget's disease. Histologically, the tumour has a very variable appearance, but islands of delicately pink-stained osteoid **Ost** are usually present, although some parts may be irregularly mineralised. The tumour cells **T**, which are derived from osteoblasts, are usually poorly differentiated and pleomorphic with much mitotic activity. These tumours are generally highly vascular and early bloodstream metastasis to the lungs is common.

Fig. 21.4 Tumour-like lesions in bone

Name	Age and sex incidence	Common sites	Behaviour
Cartilage-capped exostosis	Child/Adol M>F	Upper tibia, lower fibula	Benign (?hamartomatous) cartilage and bone outgrowth from bone surface, rare potential for malignant transformation
Aneurysmal bone cyst	Adol/Young adult M>F	Shaft of long bones, spine	Osteolytic, predispose to fracture
Fibrous dysplasia	Child/Adol M>F	Femur, tibia, ribs, facial bones	Osteolytic, predispose to fracture
'Brown tumour' of hyperparathyroidism	Adults M>F	Anywhere	Osteolytic lesions, often multiple

Fig. 21.5 Important primary tumours of bone

Name	Presumed cell of origin	Age and sex incidence	Common sites	Behaviour
Osteoid osteoma	Osteoblast	Adolescents M>F	Lower limb	Benign, osteosclerotic; painful
Non-ossifying fibroma	Uncertain	Child/Adol M>F	Long bones of lower limb	Benign, osteolytic; occasionally multiple
Chondromyxoid fibroma	Uncertain	Adol/Young adult M>F	Long bones, esp. tibia	Benign osteolytic
Enchondroma	Chondrocyte	Young adults M>F	Bones of hands	Usually benign and expansile
Giant cell tumour	Osteoclast	20-40 yrs M>F	Around knee	Mostly benign, may recur; rarely malignant
Chordoma	Notochord tissue	40+ yrs M>F	Sacrum	Local bone destruction and invasion
Osteosarcoma	Primitive osteoblast	(i) 10-25 yrs (ii) over 65 yrs M>F	(i) Around knee (ii) At site of Paget's disease	Highly malignant; early metastasis to lungs
Chondrosarcoma	Chondrocyte	30-60 yrs M>F	Spine and pelvis	Malignant; local spread and distant metastasis
Ewing's tumour	Uncertain	Child/Adol M>F	Midshaft of long bones	Malignant; early and extensive metastasis
Myeloma	Marrow plasma cells	50+ M>F	Any	Monostotic, multifocal or diffuse marrow involvement

Joint disease

The two most important disorders of joints are *rheumatoid arthritis* and *osteoarthritis*. Osteoarthritis (Fig. 21.6) is the name given to the wear and tear degenerative changes which occur in some joints with increasing age, and appears to be clearly distinct pathologically from rheumatoid arthritis (Fig. 21.7), a chronic inflammatory synovitis and arthritis of probable autoimmune origin.

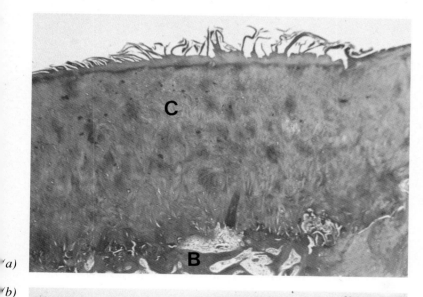

(a)

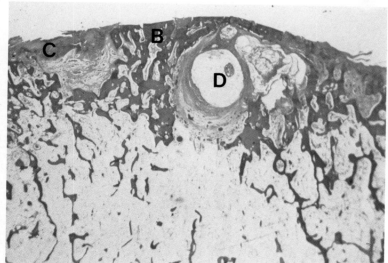

(b)

Fig. 21.6 Osteoarthritis
(a) early changes (LP)
(b) established lesion (LP)

Osteoarthritis is a degenerative disorder of articular cartilage believed to occur as a result of excessive wear and tear although there may be secondary inflammatory changes in the soft tissue components of the joint. In the earliest stages, the articular cartilage **C** loses its smooth appearance and develops surface fibrillations and flaking as shown in micrograph (a). The damaged cartilage is progressively eroded until the underlying cortical bone **B** is exposed. After prolonged articulation of naked bone with the opposing surface, the bone becomes slightly thickened, hard, dense and highly polished, a process known as *eburnation*. At the same time, there is irregular outgrowth of new bone *(osteophytes)* at the articular margins. In the established case shown in micrograph (b), only a small amount of cartilage **C** remains and the exposed bone **B** has undergone eburnation. The bone underlying the traumatised eburnated surface may undergo cystic degeneration **D**.

All of these changes lead to joint pain and progressive limitation of movement at the joint. The hips and knees are most commonly and severely affected.

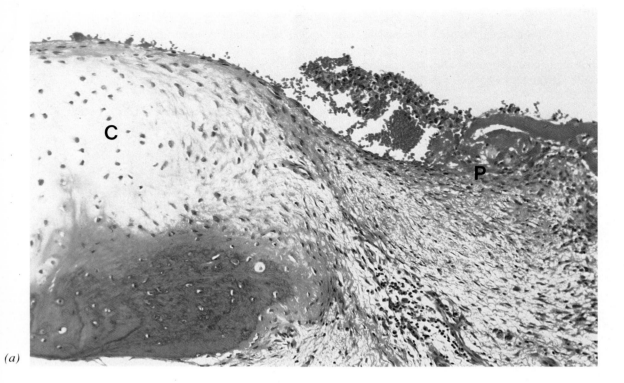

(a)

(b)

Fig. 21.7 Rheumatoid arthritis
(a) articular cartilage changes (HP)
(b) synovial changes (HP)

Rheumatoid arthritis is a systemic disorder, the predominant feature of which is chronic relapsing inflammation of articular joints, particularly in the hands and knees. The disease affects both the synovium lining the joint capsule and the cartilage on the articular surfaces. The earliest changes occur in the synovium which becomes thickened, excessively vascular and thrown up into papillary folds as a result of oedema and heavy lympho-plasmacytic infiltration; this is seen in micrograph (b). This is accompanied by exudation of excess fluid into the joint space with precipitation of fibrin **F** on the synovial surface.

   The articular cartilage changes shown in micrograph (a) follow later and involve localised destruction of cartilage **C** and its replacement by fibrovascular granulation tissue known as *pannus* **P** from the inflamed synovium. Initially, joint mobility is limited by pain and swelling, then later by gross cartilage and bone destruction and fibrous ankylosis across the joint space due to fusion of transjacent granulation tissue pannus.

22. Nervous system

Introduction

There is nothing special about the nervous system and its diseases. It is prone to infection, trauma and the processes of infarction, inflammation, and neoplasia in the same way as other tissues. The main problem with understanding the pathology of the nervous system is the terminology which is often eponymous or derived from outdated concepts of disease.

Diseases affecting the nervous system may be divided into two types:

- **general pathological phenomena** which affect all cellular constituents - for example, processes such as cerebral infarction and acute inflammation affect neurones, specialised support cells (glia), blood vessels and associated connective tissues including the meninges

- **specific disease processes** affecting particular cell types - for example in *Alzheimer's disease* (a form of dementia) neurones alone are affected causing generalised brain atrophy; in *Parkinson's disease* there is focal loss of neurones from the substantia nigra; in *multiple sclerosis*, damage is specific to myelin sheaths and in this case lesions are distributed in a patchy manner throughout the CNS.

Tissues of the CNS

- Neurones are the functional units of the nervous system. A typical neurone is composed of a cell body rich in rough endoplasmic reticulum *(Nissl substance)*, short afferent cell processes termed dendrites, and a main efferent cell process termed the axon. Except in development, neurones are not capable of replication and hence, once a neuronal cell body dies, regeneration is not possible. Damage to the axon with preservation of the nerve cell body can, however, be repaired by regeneration of the axon. The nervous system is particularly vulnerable to relatively transient metabolic insults such as hypoxia or hypoglycaemia, with death of the neurones and their axons; other tissue elements are less immediately affected.

- Specialised support cells (glial cells) are of four types: astrocytes, oligodendrocytes, microglia, and ependymal cells. *Astrocytes*, with their delicate cytoplasmic processes, form a 'fibrillary' supporting framework for the neurones and other cells of the CNS; in this respect, their function is somewhat analogous to the reticulin supporting framework in organs such as the liver and lymph nodes. *Oligodendrocytes* are responsible for myelin formation around axons in the central nervous system; their counterparts in the peripheral nervous system are the Schwann cells. *Microglia* are cells with small processes and are the central nervous system equivalent of quiescent macrophages elsewhere; they appear to perform functions of specialised immune surveillance, antigen presentation and phagocytosis of tissue debris. *Ependymal cells* provide a lining to the ventricles and central canal of the spinal cord.

- Blood vessels in the brain have a specialised structure for maintenance of the blood-brain barrier; this limits transport and diffusion from the vascular compartment into the CNS. Connective tissues in the CNS are limited to the meninges, choroid plexuses, and around blood vessels. The relative paucity of fibroblastic cells means that healing in the CNS is generally not marked by fibrous scarring. In the peripheral nervous system, connective tissue and associated blood vessels are found in association with individual axons (endoneurium), bundles of axons (perineurium) and peripheral nerves (epineurium).

Response of CNS tissues to injury

Neurones have a limited ability to survive significant changes in their metabolic or physical environment and are said to be *selectively vulnerable* when compared to the more robust astrocytes or microglial cells. Neurones may undergo reversible cell damage which is recognisable histologically by swelling of the cell body associated with loss of Nissl substance, a process termed *chromatolysis*. This process is particularly seen in the cell body of a neurone after damage to the axonal process. As discussed in Chapter 1, necrosis of brain tissue usually results in liquefaction, leaving a fluid-filled space.

Following injury or necrosis, healing through granulation tissue and fibrous scarring does not generally occur due to a relative lack of fibroblasts in the CNS. Initially, there is an exudative response with activation of local microglia and recruitment of phagocytic monocytes to phagocytose dead tissue. This is followed by proliferation of astrocytes to form an astrocytic scar. This process is generally termed *gliosis* and is a common end product of damage to the specialised structures of the CNS. If there is extensive tissue necrosis, e.g. following infarction, the gliotic response is insufficient to repair the whole defect and a fluid-filled space lined by glial scar remains.

Healing through granulation tissue and collagenous fibrosis occurs in relation to healing of bacterial inflammatory processes such as around a cerebral abscess; it also occurs in diseases involving the meninges, such as acute meningitis (Fig. 2.6) and tuberculous meningitis (Fig. 3.16).

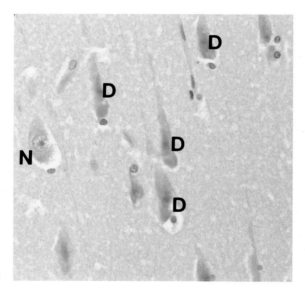

(a)

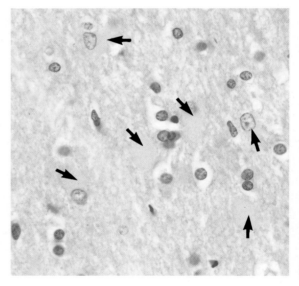

(b)

Fig. 22.1 Neuronal death and astrocytic response (a) early response (HP)   (b) later response (HP)

Neurones are especially vulnerable to hypoxia such as may occur following cardiac or respiratory arrest. At an early stage, dead neurones become shrunken and eosinophilic with pyknosis of the nuclei. This change particularly affects large pyramidal neurones and is shown in micrograph (a) where recently dead neurones **D** in the hippocampus contrast with normal surviving cells **N**. Note that surrounding cells such as oligodendrocytes and astrocytes are unaffected.

Following damage such as this, these dead neurones will be removed by phagocytic cells, and there is associated proliferation of astrocytic cells in the damaged area. This is seen in micrograph (b), which is a similar area of the hippocampus after an episode of hypoxia several weeks before. No neurones are seen and the area is replaced by large pink-stained astrocytic cells (arrows). This process, termed gliosis, is a common end result of damage to neurones in the central nervous system.

Inflammatory and related conditions of the CNS

Inflammatory processes involving the CNS are divided into those involving the meninges (termed *meningitis*) or the CNS proper (*encephalitis* in the brain, *myelitis* in the cord). *Encephalomyelitis* and *meningo-encephalitis* describe conditions where a mixed pattern of involvement occurs. Inflammatory diseases are due to bacterial, viral or immunological causes.

Viral meningitis is commonly due to an enterovirus, rarely fatal, and results in a transient lymphocytic response in the meninges. In contrast, bacterial meningitis is a severe life-threatening disease commonly due to infection by *meningococcus (Neisseria meningitidis), Streptococcus pneumoniae* or *Haemophilus influenzae.* Histologically, there is an acute purulent neutrophilic response in the meninges with secondary thrombosis of many of the blood vessels supplying the CNS. Treatment with antibiotics may allow recovery, however healing may be complicated by fibrosis in the meninges. Tuberculosis may also cause meningitis, which is characterised by a lymphocytic response in the CSF and the formation of caseating granulomata in the meninges (see Fig. 3.16). Fungal meningitis may be caused by *Cryptococcus,* being increasingly seen in immunosuppressed patients. Tertiary syphilis may cause chronic meningitis, meningeal fibrosis resulting in cranial nerve entrapment.

Encephalitis and myelitis are usually caused by viral infections, some having a particular propensity to affect specific types of neurones. In viral encephalitis or myelitis there are three main histological features:

- focal neuronal loss and phagocytosis (direct result of viral infection)
- lymphocytic 'cuffing' of vessels with increase in microglial cells (local immune response)
- astrocyte reaction with increase in number and size (response to cell loss).

Herpes virus causes a severe form of encephalitis with extensive necrosis of brain tissue (Fig. 22.2).

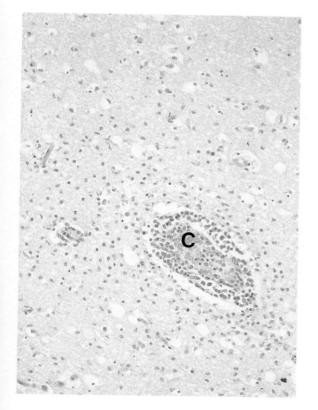

Fig. 22.2 Herpes simplex encephalitis (HP)

Viral encephalitis may be caused by Herpes simplex type 1 (the same virus which causes 'cold sores'). The virus spreads to involve the frontal lobes, limbic system, and temporal lobes of the brain. The typical histological features of an encephalitis are seen, namely neuronal death, lymphocytic cuffing of vessels, and astrocyte proliferation. There is, however, severe necrosis of the affected areas of brain, which become semi-liquid as macrophages phagocytose dead tissue.

This micrograph shows an area of cortex replaced by a mixture of macrophages and astrocytes (the cytological detail is not discernible at this magnification), with a small vessel cuffed by lymphoid cells **C.** Careful examination of tissue may reveal eosinophilic viral inclusion bodies in nuclei of remaining neurones. Immunofluorescence tests can detect Herpes viral antigen and are used diagnostically. Electron microscopy is another method to detect the virus. Prompt treatment with the drug Acyclovir may halt progression of the disease, however late presentation commonly results in death or severe neurological deficit.

The *polio virus* tends to attack motor cells of the anterior horn of the spinal cord causing *poliomyelitis* and for this reason is termed a *neurotropic virus* (see Fig. 22.3). *Rabies virus* is also neurotropic and results in a meningo-encephalitis with virus inclusions visible in neuronal cells. *Papova virus* infection of the CNS occurs in immunosuppressed patients and particularly affects oligodendroglial cells resulting in loss of myelin in white matter; the disease is termed *progressive multifocal leucoencephalopathy*. The *human immunodeficiency virus* (HIV1) which causes AIDS also affects the central nervous system and results in an 'AIDS' encephalopathy causing dementia. Persistent viral infection of the brain occurs in some cases with *measles virus* and results in a chronic degeneration of nerve cells in a disease termed *subacute sclerosing panencephalitis*.

Cerebral abscesses may develop as a part of a meningitis or may be the result of direct spread of infection from the middle ear (into the temporal lobe) or by blood-borne spread from an infection elsewhere in the body such as the lung. In cerebral abscesses there is commonly a mixed infection including anaerobic organisms. Histologically there is a pus-filled cavity walled off by fibrosis generated through granulation tissue derived from local blood vessels. Around this fibrous cavity wall there is a reactive astrocytic response.

Fungal infections of the CNS proper are mainly confined to immunosuppressed patients and are most commonly due to *Aspergillus*, *Zygomycoses* and *Cryptococcus* species; lesions usually take the form of a brain abscess. The CNS is also affected by parasitic infection, particularly *Toxoplasmosis*, a disease which affects neonates and increasingly those who are immunosuppressed.

The most common pattern of *immunologically mediated* damage to the CNS is lymphocytic infiltration around blood vessels and immune-mediated destruction and phagocytosis of myelin. One type of disease in which this process is seen is *post-infectious encephalomyelitis*, where the trigger to such an immune reaction is a recent viral infection or vaccination. *Multiple sclerosis* is a much more common disease which is also thought to be mediated by an abnormal immune response causing myelin destruction (see Fig. 22.4), although the triggering factor in this disease is as yet unknown.

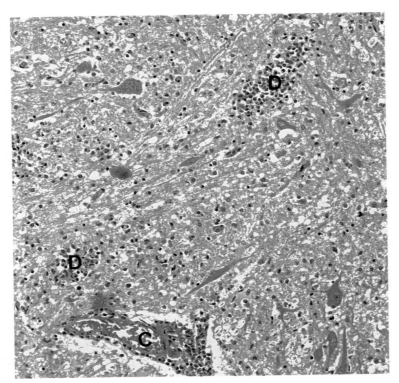

Fig. 22.3 Poliomyelitis (HP)

Although it may cause a diffuse encephalomyelitis, the polio virus most commonly attacks the anterior horn cells of the spinal cord (lower motor neurones), resulting in paralysis of associated skeletal muscle. It may also affect cranial nerve motor nuclei and result in a bulbar paralysis. Nerve cells are invaded by viral particles and die. The dead cells excite a phagocytic response and are marked by clusters of microglial cells engulfing cellular debris **D**. As with other viral infections of the nervous system, the histological hallmark of vascular cuffing by lymphoid cells **C** is prominent. The spaces occupied by the destroyed cells are replaced by gliosis.

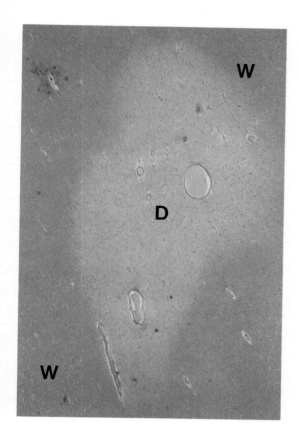

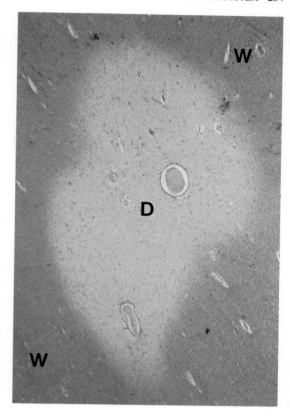

(a) *(b)*

Fig. 22.4 Multiple (disseminated) sclerosis
(a) H&E stain (LP)   (b) Loyez staining method (LP)

Multiple sclerosis is a disease caused by the selective destruction of myelin in the central nervous system; hence it is termed a demyelinating disease. It is postulated that there is an abnormal immunological reaction in the central nervous system, possibly triggered by a viral infection, resulting in focal myelin destruction. There are three histological stages in the demyelinating process. First, during an acute episode, myelin breakdown occurs associated with lymphocyte and macrophage infiltration of the affected area (termed a plaque); at this stage there is clinical evidence of focal neurological dysfunction. Although this process is directed against myelin, secondary damage to axons also occurs. In the second phase of the process, astrocytes proliferate and gradually infiltrate the demyelinated area which exhibits continued evidence of lymphocytic infiltration. In the final phase of evolution of the plaque, cellularity is reduced, astrocytes shrink in size, and the process becomes 'burnt out'.

Macroscopically, areas of old demyelination appear as pale-grey, rubbery, sharply defined areas in the white matter.

Micrograph (a) shows the typical H&E appearance of an established focus of demyelination. The pale-staining demyelinated area **D** is easily distinguished from the normal-staining white matter **W**. Micrograph (b) illustrates the same lesion stained by a method to demonstrate myelin; the demyelinated area is unstained.

Multiple sclerosis runs a variable but usually prolonged course characterised by periods of focal demyelination which are disseminated both in location within the CNS and time of occurrence. During episodes of active demyelination, focal neurological signs often appear, but at times of remission there may be partial or even complete resolution of the neurological deficit, possibly as a result of resolution of inflammatory oedema surrounding the active lesions.

Vascular disorders of the CNS

Cerebral arteries are prone to all of the diseases affecting vessels described in Chapter 10, particularly atheroma, arteriosclerosis, thrombosis, aneurysm formation and vasculitis.

The main consequence of disease of cerebral blood vessels is *stroke*, a term used to describe the sudden onset of a persistent focal neurological deficit such as paralysis, disturbance of speech, co-ordination, or sensation. The majority of strokes are due to *cerebral infarction* as a result of atheroma, thrombosis or embolism. *Cerebral haemorrhage* is also a major cause of stroke and is the consequence of rupture of small intracerebral vessels. A generalised term used clinically to describe these sudden vascular events is *cerebro-vascular accident* (commonly abbreviated to CVA).

Cerebral infarction may be due to thrombosis of a cerebral artery, commonly superimposed on atheroma of cerebral vessels. This is commonly seen in the vertebro-basilar territory resulting in brain stem infarction. Cerebral infarction may also be due to occlusion of a vessel by embolus. Emboli most commonly arise from the left side of the heart, frequently from mural thrombus after myocardial infarction, from atrial thrombosis in atrial fibrillation, or from thrombotic vegetations on the aortic or mitral valves. A more insidious disease process results from progressive arteriosclerosis in the brain causing degeneration of white matter with small areas of micro-infarction in the cerebral cortex. This is a common cause of dementia (progressive intellectual deterioration) in the elderly and is termed *multi-infarct dementia.*

Intracerebral haemorrhage is usually a complication of hypertension. The muscular walls of small vessels in the brain are replaced by collagenous tissue and the vessels are then prone to rupture. The three most common sites for intracerebral haemorrhage are in the basal ganglia, the pons and the cerebellum.

Intracranial haemorrhage may also occur from vessels outside the brain. *Subarachnoid haemorrhage* is due to rupture of vessels in the subarachnoid space; the most common reason is rupture of a small aneurysm arising on the main cerebral arteries descriptively termed a *berry aneurysm* (see Fig. 10.9). Intracerebral or subarachnoid haemorrhage may also be due to congenital abnormalities of cerebral vessels forming *arterio-venous malformations. Subdural haemorrhage* results from bleeding from fragile veins which traverse the subdural space. This most commonly occurs in the elderly as a result of trauma which may be relatively trivial. Extradural haemorrhage is a result of bleeding from arterial vessels outside the dura. This is a common complication of trauma to the head, especially with skull fracture; the middle meningeal artery is most vulnerable.

(a)

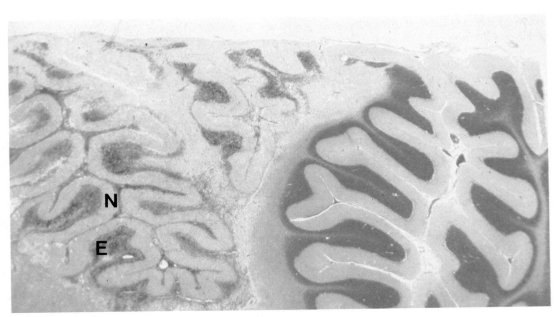

Fig. 22.5 (a) Cerebral infarction *(caption opposite)*

Fig. 22.5 Infarction of the brain
(a) early infarct (LP) *(illustration opposite)*
(b) later infarct (MP)
(c) old (cystic) infarct (LP)

These three micrographs illustrate important histological features of cerebral infarction.

The earliest histological manifestations are seen in neurones which become shrunken, eosinophilic and exhibit nuclear pyknosis. These changes are seen between 6 and 12 hours after infarction and are accompanied by microscopic disruption of small capillary vessels with extravasation of red cells. Unlike other tissues, in cerebral infarction a neutrophilic response is only transient and macrophage infiltration dominates the cellular reaction in necrotic tissue from about 2 days post-infarction. This is accompanied by proliferation of small vessels at the margin of the infarcted territory. Macroscopically, cerebral infarcts can be either haemorrhagic or 'anaemic' (pale). The haemorrhagic pattern is thought to be caused by blood flowing back into capillaries damaged by the initial ischaemic episode. Micrograph (a) illustrates an area of infarction in the cerebellum of a patient dying 2 days after infarction. The infarcted area on the left exhibits loss of basophilia due to necrosis **N** of the small neurones of the granular layer and extravasation of erythrocytes **E**.

Following the infarct, organisation and repair take place. The dead tissue becomes infiltrated by macrophages recruited from blood monocytes which phagocytose lipid-rich myelin and take on a foamy appearance. By about 7 to10 days post-infarction, the infarct has become liquefied and partly cystic. Micrograph (b) shows this phase in a cortical cerebral infarct; the infarcted area **I** consists of a homogeneous mass of necrotic tissue with remnants of karyorrhectic nuclei. Surrounding this area is a zone of lipid-containing macrophagic cells **C** and beyond this a peripheral zone of proliferating astrocytic glial cells and blood vessels **G**. Glial proliferation *(gliosis)* is the equivalent of granulation tissue in infarcts elsewhere in the body and is intended to fill the infarcted territory. The resulting *glial scar* is formed not of fibrous tissue but of the cell bodies and processes of astrocytes. This phase lasts up to 2 months post-infarction.

When an infarct is large, the process of gliosis does not completely fill the defect and a cyst-like cavity remains lined by dense astrocytic tissue. Micrograph (c) shows an old cystic infarct in the internal capsule with the central cavity **C** surrounded by glial tissue **G**. There is no neuronal regeneration following a cerebral infarct. Some of the early clinical manifestations of cerebral infarction may be due to oedema occurring in the relatively undamaged tissue at the margins of the infarcted territory. This oedema resolves and explains some of the clinical improvement which a patient may experience with time.

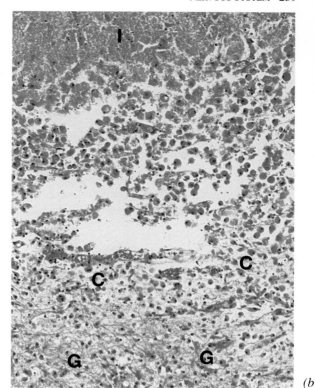

(b)

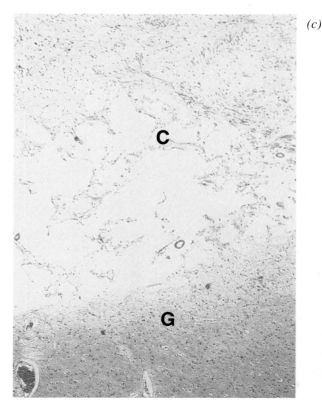

(c)

Degenerative diseases of the CNS

Certain diseases of the CNS are characterised by progressive degeneration of neurones, and/or white matter.

- **Alzheimer's disease** causes dementia mainly in the elderly. The disease is of unknown aetiology but there are distinct histological abnormalities (Fig. 22.6) which distinguish the condition from multi-infarct dementia and cortical Lewy body disease.

- **Parkinson's disease** (Fig. 22.7) causes clinical features of tremor, slow movement, and rigidity and is a result of degeneration of nerve cells in the substantia nigra. The cause is unknown.

- **Cortical Lewy body disease** is similar to Alzheimer's disease and causes dementia. It has brain-stem pathology identical to that seen in Parkinson's disease but, in addition, the same type of neuronal pathology destroys cortical neurones and causes dementia.

- **Motor neurone disease** is the result of specific degeneration of motor neurones in the cerebral cortex, brain stem, and spinal cord. Cells degenerate over a period of a few years and this results in progressive denervation of muscle with insidious paralysis and death. The cause of this disease is unknown.

- **Creutzfeldt–Jakob disease** is a cause of rapid dementia resulting from extensive death of neurones in cerebral cortex. The disease is unique amongst degenerative diseases in that a transmissible cause has been demonstrated although poorly characterised. The infective agent is closely related to that which causes scrapie in sheep and bovine spongiform encephalopathy in cattle, termed 'slow virus' diseases.

- **Leukodystrophies** are a group of degenerative diseases of white matter usually resulting from an inborn error of metabolism; they usually cause progressive neurological impairment in childhood.

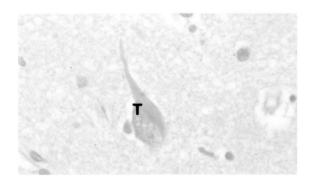

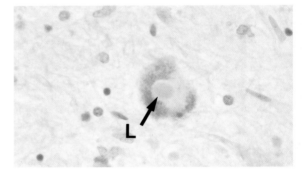

Fig. 22.6   Alzheimer's disease (HP)

Alzheimer's disease is a cause of dementia usually occurring after the age of 70 years but in some cases at an earlier age. The cause of the disease is unknown, however there are distinctive changes in the brain which allow the diagnosis to be made histologically. Macroscopically there is thinning of gyri (cerebral atrophy), particularly of the frontal and temporal lobes.

Neurones accumulate abnormal filaments forming flame-shaped skeins termed *neurofibrillary tangles* **T**. In addition there is extracellular deposition of an amyloid (see Fig. 4.2) in association with distorted dendrites which form structures termed *senile plaques*.

Fig. 22.7   Parkinson's disease (HP)

Parkinson's disease is caused by idiopathic destruction of neurones in the *substantia nigra* resulting in loss of the transmitter *dopamine*. Histologically distinctive inclusions are seen in the remaining neurones. This specimen, from the substantia nigra of a patient with Parkinson's disease, shows a typical melanin-containing neurone containing a rounded pink-staining inclusion known as a *Lewy body* **L**. These bodies are composed of aggregates of neurofilaments and non-filament proteins. Similar inclusions occur in neurones of the cerebral cortex in *cortical Lewy body disease*, which is recently recognised as a common cause of dementia.

Tumours of the CNS

Primary tumours of the CNS arise from four main cell types: neurones and their precursors, glial cells, meningeal arachnoidal cells and lymphoreticular cells. Primary tumours of the nervous system vary greatly in behaviour from slow-growing *(low grade)* to rapidly-growing *(high grade)*. They exert harmful effects by growing into vital structures or by causing swelling of the brain around the tumour resulting in secondary compression of vital structures. The different types of primary brain tumour have preferred sites of origin and patterns of age incidence, summarised in Figure 22.8.

Fig. 22.8 Primary tumours of the CNS

Tumour	Cell of origin	Site	Age	Behaviour
Astrocytoma	Astrocyte	Hemisphere Cerebellum	Adult Childhood	Low to high grade Low grade
Oligodendroglioma	Oligodendrocyte	Hemisphere	Adult	Low to high grade
Glioblastoma	Primitive glial cell	Hemisphere	Adult	High grade
Ependymoma	Ependyma	IV ventricle Cord	Childhood Adult	High grade Low grade
Lymphoma	Lymphocyte	Hemisphere	Adult	High grade
Meningioma	Arachnoidal	Meninges	Adult	Low grade
Medulloblastoma	Neurectoderm	Cerebellum	Childhood	High grade
Haemangioblastoma	Unknown	Cerebellum	All ages	Low grade

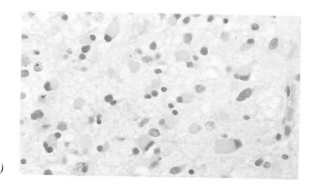

(a)

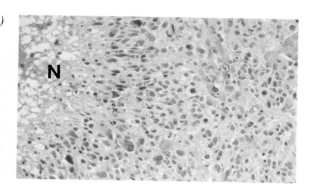

(b)

Fig. 22.9 Tumours of astroglial origin
(a) astrocytoma (HP)
(b) glioblastoma (HP)

There is a spectrum of differentiation in tumours of glial origin from low grade (benign) to high grade (malignant).

A *low grade astrocytoma* in the cerebral hemispheres is illustrated in micrograph (a). Tumour cells have pink cytoplasm and cellular processes characteristic of astrocytic cells. Low grade astrocytomas do not exhibit great cellularity, and show no necrosis or endothelial proliferation in blood vessels.

Glioblastoma (b) is a tumour composed of a mixed population of cells, varying from small cells which exhibit little tendency to differentiation, to cells exhibiting astrocytic morphology as seen in (a), through to large bizarre giant tumour cells. Necrosis **N** is a typical feature of this type of tumour, together with a high cellularity and proliferation of endothelial cells in blood vessels. These tumours have a very poor prognosis even when treated by surgery and radiotherapy.

In between these two extremes are astrocytomas which exhibit high cellularity and endothelial proliferation in blood vessels. These are termed *anaplastic astrocytomas* and have an intermediate pace of growth and recurrence.

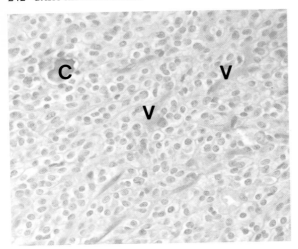

Fig. 22.10 Oligodendroglioma (HP)

These tumours are most commonly seen in the cerebral hemispheres and are believed to derive from oligodendrocytes on the basis of cytological similarity rather than any proven biological marker. The tumour is composed of homogeneous sheets of cells with rounded uniform nuclei, a vacuolated cytoplasm forming a 'halo' around each cell and a network of finely branching small blood vessels **V**. Microscopic foci of calcification **C** are frequently seen in this type of tumour.

While many oligodendrogliomas behave in a relatively low grade manner, the presence of nuclear pleomorphism, necrosis, a high mitotic count and endothelial proliferation in blood vessels is associated with rapid growth and recurrence. Tumours exhibiting such features are termed *anaplastic oligodendrogliomas.*

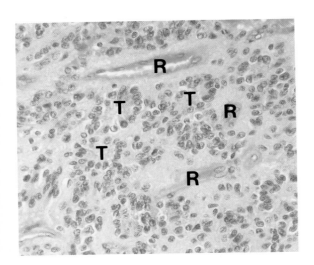

Fig. 22.11 Ependymoma (HP)

These tumours are derived from the ependymal cells which normally line the ventricular system. Histologically, tumour cells are uniform and arranged in a rosette pattern **R** around blood vessels to leave a perivascular 'nuclear free zone'. In addition, small areas of tumour form epithelial tubules **T** which recapitulate the structure of the central canal of the spinal cord.

Ependymomas are most commonly seen in the region of the fourth ventricle and are also the commonest intrinsic tumour of the spinal cord in childhood. A peculiar variant of this tumour is the *myxopapillary ependymoma* of the filum terminale where the tumour produces large vacuolated cells with a mucinous intercellular matrix.

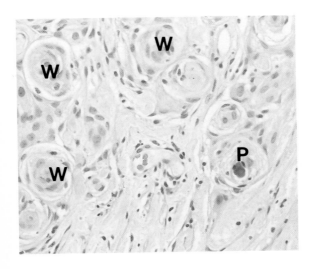

Fig. 22.12 Meningioma (HP)

Meningiomas are thought to arise from arachnoidal epithelial cells of the meninges and are common tumours in adults. The tumours are nearly always benign and produce symptoms by slow compression of underlying brain or spinal cord. There are several histological patterns of meningioma varying from epithelial-type lesions to spindle-cell lesions.

This micrograph illustrates a meningioma composed of a mixture of spindle cells and epithelial cells arranged in characteristic whorls **W**. At the centre of the whorls may be areas of calcification termed *psammoma bodies* **P**. Mitotic figures are not common in meningiomas, however their presence is associated with increased chance of recurrence following excision.

Disorders of peripheral nerves

Diseases of the peripheral nerves, *peripheral neuropathies*, result in abnormal motor or sensory function in the territory of the nerve affected. Generalised peripheral neuropathies may be found in association with a variety of diseases such as diabetes mellitus, lead poisoning, alcoholism, uraemia and some malignancies. Several specific peripheral neuropathy syndromes are associated with segmental loss of myelin; these include *post-infectious polyneuropathy (Guillain-Barré syndrome)*, and a large group of *hereditary sensory-motor neuropathies*. Axonal degeneration underlies other causes of peripheral neuropathy such as trauma or ischaemia. As a world problem, an important cause of peripheral nerve disease is *leprosy* in which nerve trunks are infiltrated by large numbers of macrophages filled with *Mycobacterium leprae* with resulting loss of nerve fibres.

Tumours of peripheral nerve are common and are derived from Schwann cells (the cells forming peripheral myelin sheaths) and perineurial cells; examples are shown in Figures 22.13 and 22.14.

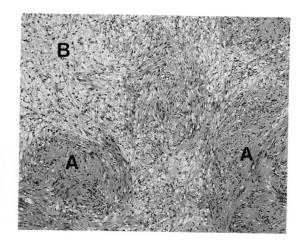

Fig. 22.13 Schwannoma (MP)

These tumours, derived from Schwann cells, typically arise in peripheral nerves; they are commonly seen arising from the eighth cranial nerve when they are termed *acoustic neuromas*.

There are two patterns of growth seen histologically. Compact areas of spindle cells with pink cytoplasm forming palisades and whorls are termed *Antoni-A tissue* **A**, while degeneration in the tumour results in loosely arranged vacuolated tumour areas termed *Antoni-B tissue* **B**.

Schwannomas are usually solitary, rounded tumours found in relation to nerve trunks. They are benign and usually slow growing. Rare malignant forms of also exist.

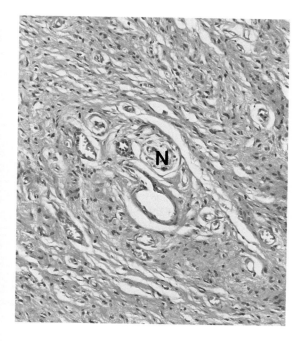

Fig. 22.14 Neurofibroma (HP)

The neurofibroma is a tumour of peripheral nerves derived from perineurial cells. Tumours may be solitary but are frequently multiple, especially in the genetically determined disease *neurofibromatosis*. Lesions on peripheral nerves are visible as subcutaneous nodules; lesions on spinal nerve roots within the spinal canal may cause spinal cord compression.

Histologically, the tumour is composed of loosely arranged spindle cells with varying amounts of intervening collagen. A frequent feature is accumulation of connective tissue mucopolysaccharides resulting in a gelatinous or myxoid tumour. In contrast to the Schwannoma, these tumours expand the nerve trunks in a diffuse manner and, as in this micrograph, it is possible to identify axons and nerve fibres of the underlying nerve **N**. Neurofibromas are benign tumours, however malignant tumours may also arise from perineurial cells when they are termed *neurofibrosarcomas*.

Disorders of skeletal muscle

Diseases of skeletal muscle present clinically with weakness, wasting of muscle, or pain on exercise. These symptoms and signs can be either due to primary disease of muscle *(myopathy)* or may be secondary to degeneration in the innervation of the muscle *(denervation)*; for this latter reason muscle diseases are commonly considered together with diseases of the nervous system. Histology often provides the only satisfactory method for distinguishing between myopathies and certain neuropathies. Myopathies can be classified according to aetiology into three main groups: genetically determined disorders collectively known as *muscular dystrophies*, inflammatory diseases termed *myositis*, and *myopathies* secondary to systemic diseases.

The muscular dystrophies are genetically determined disorders characterised by degeneration of muscle fibres resulting in muscle wasting and weakness. There are several syndromes differing in age and sex incidence, time of onset, and clinical course. Histologically there are abnormalities of size and internal structure of muscle fibres, often associated with fibrous replacement of damaged muscle.

Myositis is most commonly due to immunologically-mediated muscle damage in a disease termed *polymyositis*. Cushing's disease, thyrotoxicosis and carcinomatosis may be associated with muscle weakness and wasting secondary to the systemic disease process.

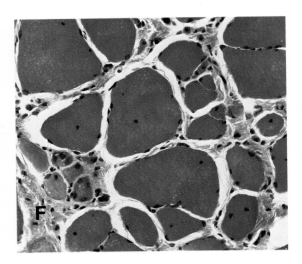

Fig. 22.15 Duchenne muscular dystrophy (HP)

This form of dystrophy is transmitted as an X-linked recessive trait and is therefore almost exclusively manifest in boys. Symptoms of proximal muscular weakness develop early in childhood causing difficulty in standing up.

Histologically, there is destruction of muscle fibres with replacement of the muscle by fibrous tissue **F**. Residual muscle fibres exhibit a markedly abnormal variation in fibre size due to atrophy of some and hypertrophy of others. As the disease progresses the muscle becomes virtually replaced by fibrosis and later adipose tissue. This gives rise to apparent swelling of the affected muscles and accounts for the pseudohypertrophy of the calf muscles seen in affected children.

Duchenne dystrophy has a relentless course and results in death in early adult life. Other forms of muscular dystrophy may have a more benign clinical course.

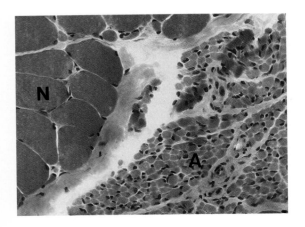

Fig. 22.16 Neurogenic muscular atrophy (HP)

Weakness and wasting of skeletal muscle may occur as a result of lower motor neurone damage rather than primary muscle disease. Histologically, neurogenic muscle atrophy affects groups of muscle fibres supplied by single motor units in contrast to the haphazard pattern of atrophy seen in the muscular dystrophies.

In this micrograph, normal-sized fibres **N** contrast sharply with a large group of atrophic fibres **A** from a denervated motor unit. This is an example of *spinal muscular atrophy* in which there is failure of development of certain anterior horn cells. Similar changes are seen in a variety of peripheral nerve diseases.

Index